# The
# Canary
## and
# Chronic Fatigue

# Majid Ali, M.D.

Associate Professor of Pathology (Adj)
College of Physicians and Surgeons
of Columbia University, New York
Director, Department of Pathology, Immunology and Laboratories
Holy Name Hospital, Teaneck, New Jersey
Consulting Physician
Institute of Preventive Medicine, Denville, New Jersey
Fellow, Royal College of Surgeons of England
Diplomate, American Board of Environmental Medicine
Diplomate, American Board of Chelation Therapy

Library of Congress Catalog Card Number
93-79990
ISBN 1-879131-04-8

Ali, Majid
The Canary and Chronic Fatigue  Majid Ali.--1st ed.

Includes bibliographical references and index

1. Chronic Fatigue: Oxidative Molecular Injury
2. Human Canaries and Injured Enzymes
3. Up-Regulation of Energy Enzymes
4. Oral Nutrient Protocols for Chronic Fatigue
5. Intravenous Nutrient Protocols
6. Limbic Exercise for Chronic Fatigue

10 9 8 7 6 5 4 3 2 1

Published in the USA by

**LIFE SPAN PRESS**
95 East Main Street, Denville, New Jersey 07834
(201) 586-9191

# *Human Canaries*

Chronic fatigue sufferers are human canaries — unique people who tolerate poorly the biologic stressors of the late 20th century. They are genetically predisposed to injury to their energy and detoxification enzymes by agents in their internal and external environments. Their molecular defenses are damaged by undiagnosed and unmanaged allergies, chemical sensitivities, environmental pollutants, microbes, sugar-insulin-adrenaline roller coasters, stress and hostility of speeded-up lives. Under their skin, they carry oxidative storms — the Fourth-of-July chemistry.

This book offers information and guidance about nondrug therapies that *do* work for the fatigue sufferer as well as the professional.

The case histories included in this volume are true to life. Names, genders and some minor details have been changed to protect the identity of the subjects.

**I do not recommend that chronic fatigue sufferers consider the therapies I describe in this volume as recipes for treating chronic fatigue on a self-help basis. Such an approach would be fraught with many dangers. I strongly urge the readers who suffer from persistent fatigue to seek out physicians knowledgeable and experienced in the use of nondrug therapies.**

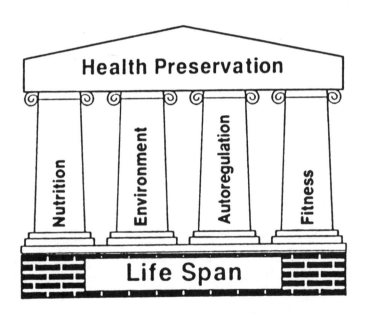

## Dedication

*I dedicate this book to chronic fatigue sufferers who continue their search for the true answers to their suffering in spite of a multitude of diagnostic labels and symptom-suppressing drugs given by drug doctors,*

*and*

*to physicians who, at great peril to their integrity and their licenses, courageously defy the dogma of drug medicine, continue to search for the true causes of chronic fatigue states, and try innovative, nondrug therapies to restore the damaged energy enzymes of their human canaries.*

## Acknowledgments

I am grateful to my human canaries who persist with me against all odds, sometimes for months, as I struggle to explain what I believed is the true nature of their suffering. I am grateful to them for agreeing to try my nondrug nutritional, environmental and self-regulatory approaches to restore their energy enzymes.

Because no one can attempt to solve any significant problem of his time in a vacuum. I am deeply indebted to my colleagues in nutritional and environmental medicine, too numerous to name here, who listened and critiqued my essential theory about the true nature of chronic fatigue state. They generously shared their clinical experiences with me, and offered guidance and encouragement.

I thank Jerrold Finnie, M.D., Dolores Finnie, R.N., Maria Sumberac and Lisa Rosen for their editorial work; Ronald Rizzio and his staff at the library of Holy Name Hospital, Teaneck, for complying with endless requests for literature searches; and the staff at Life Span Press for their unfailing support.

I am especially grateful to Sister Patricia Lynch, President, Holy Name Hospital for her support of my work with preventive medicine.

Talat, my wife, is my best resource. There is much of her reflected in the pages of this book.

# Table of Contents

## *Preface*

In this book, my patients define with their true-to-life stories what chronic fatigue is and what it isn't. For my part, I define the scientific basis of this malady as accelerated oxidative molecular injury. Clinical outcome data obtained with nondrug therapies that I present in this book — I believe — validate my patients' definition of chronic fatigue as well as my essential viewpoint about its cause and effective management.

The core messages of this book are the following:

Chronic fatigue will be the dominant chronic health disorder of the 21st century.

Chronic fatigue sufferers are human canaries — they are unique in that they poorly tolerate biologic stressors imposed on their internal and external environments.

Chronic fatigue is preventable and reversible.

Chronic fatigue is caused by accelerated oxidative molecular injury, and such injury cannot be reversed with drugs.

Chronic fatigue states require holistic, integrated,

*nondrug* nutritional and environmental therapies. Training in effective methods of self-regulation and slow, sustained exercise for restoring normal energy patterns is also necessary.

Although predictions in medicine are risky, I make four predictions in this book.

First, chronic fatigue states — more than other chronic disorders — will budge mainstream medicine from the dogma of drugs and scalpels toward energetic-molecular medicine — a medicine that focuses on energetic-molecular events that occur *before* tissues are damaged and not on structural damage as seen with microscopes *after* the tissues have been ravaged with disease.

Second, chronic fatigue states — more than any other disease — will force drug doctors to learn the use of nontoxic, nondrug therapies of nutritional and environmental medicines as well as effective methods of self-regulation and physical fitness.

Third, chronic fatigue states — more than any other factor — will usher in participatory medicine: a medicine in which the patient actively guides the physician in molecular restorative work, rather than merely accepting a prescription for temporary symptom suppression.

Fourth, hope and spirituality will become integral parts of medical literature. Physicians will no longer scoff at the essential healing qualities of hope and spirituality.

These predictions do not spring forth from the delusional plausibility of an idealogue. Rather, these conclusions seem inescapable to me as I look at how the lives of so many are devastated by incapacitating chronic fatigue, how drugs used to "cure" their fatigue inevitably deepen their suffering, and how they recapture their normal energy patterns with the steady, sustained — and often painfully slow — use of nondrug therapies put forth by the new energetic-molecular medicine.

Two questions have preoccupied me in my clinical work with chronic fatigue during the last several years:

*How are energy enzymes down-regulated?*
*How can down-regulated energy enzymes be up-regulated?*

In the chapters What Is Chronic Fatigue? and How Does It All Begin?, I present evidence for my viewpoint that chronic fatigue states are states of accelerated oxidative molecular injury. In the last six chapters, I outline the nondrug therapies I recommend to manage chronic fatigue states, and present clinical outcome data obtained with such therapies. For the professional readers, I published my theory in the *Journal of Advancement in Medicine* (6:83-96;1993). That article is reproduced with the kind permission of Human Health Sciences Press in the Appendix of this book.

---

## McPATIENTS, McDOCS, McCLINICS
## AND CLINTON'S McHEALTH PLAN

There is a somber — and a growing — sense among Americans that health care is a steam engine, speeding down a track on a steep hill with failed brakes, gathering momentum at a frightening rate. They know a devastating explosion is imminent. Yet, they stand, frozen in time, paralyzed with fear.

Some political pundits are incubating grand schemes in their clever minds to solve, in one large swoop, all the health care problems of their countrymen. They think they can resolve all problems by prescribing the great McDonalds recipe for Americans. If McDonalds can serve up its large cheeseburgers and french fries sizzling hot and fast, why can't the American people benefit from similar marketing and organizational genius? They dream of the day when patients will become McPatients; physicians, the McDocs; and physician offices, McClinics. And all this shall be achieved with one brilliant legislative stroke — Clinton's McHealth Plan.

The problem with such political pundits is this: They cannot see the difference between *front-end* medicine and *tail-end* medicine. Drug medicine in the United States is utterly committed to keeping the ill incarcerated in the illness mold. Physicians do not believe in preventive medicine because they know what is being pushed as preventive medicine simply does not work. Even when we celebrate our success in the early diagnosis of cancers of the breast and cervix, we know it is *not* preventive medicine. As desirable as it is, early diagnosis is not prevention. Disease prevention requires focus on nutrition and our internal and external environments. That, of course, as everyone knows, is quackery.

The political pundits know American medicine is superb medicine. What they do not know is that it is superb medicine only for those who are near death. Compared with nondrug therapies, it has little to offer those who are not yet near death yet. How can it? It considers nutritional medicine a fraud; environmental medicine, the treatment of diseases that do not exist; and hope and spirituality, subjects for the feeble-minded.

All our McHealth plans will — and can — do is divert funds from physicians to entrepreneurs who will own McClinics and hire McDocs to treat McPatients. These McEntrepreneurs know well that money is in CAT and MRI scans and in procedures and not in listening to the sick. Listening in medicine is not — as our attorneys say — billable. There is no CPT code for reimbursing listening. The McClinic McEntrepreneurs know all this. They are investing for high returns from procedures, not from listening to the sick to find out what ails them.

*"Medical-Industrial Complex: Who Wins Among the winners under Mr. Clinton's proposal would be doctors who join a health plan...medical specialists would lose...Lawyers may also be winners. New limits on the historically independent*

*practice of medicine could produce many a
legal battle... Consulting firms may win.*"

*The New York Times*
November 14, 1993

Now the *Times* cannot be wrong. Or can it be? Does the *Times* really think that our grand edifices of Star Wars medicine are simply going to shrivel down just because Mr. Clinton believes — rightly, for valid reasons — that America needs more preventive medicine? The requirements of momentum for the furnaces of the nation's surgical suites are enormous, and they have insatiable appetites for human flesh — no laws can save people from their jaws. No grand plans for managed care can keep people away from operating and endoscopy tables. No quality assurance activity in the hospitals can reduce the number of unnecessary diagnostic procedures.

The dominant problems of our time are problems of nutrition, environment, stress and fitness. Neither our scalpels nor any miracles of synthetic chemistry can solve any of these problems. Mr. Clinton will find this out with time.

*The significant problems we face cannot be
solved with the same level of thinking we
were at when we created them.*

Albert Einstein

I do not believe true solutions to our health problems will come from our lawmakers nor from mainstream medicine. Both groups are trying to solve the 21st century problems of nutrition and environment with 19th century medical thinking about diseases and drugs. I believe the inevitable changes will come from those who understand the real issues by their true-to-life suffering. The suppressed truth of our time is that nutritional and environmental therapies work. Chronic fatigue sufferers speaking out in this book give eloquent testimony to this fact. Where drug therapies fail for chronic degenerative and immune disorders, nondrug therapies succeed. People are discovering this truth in ever increasing numbers. These are the people who will bring forth the medicine of the future. These are the people who will demand *real* preventive medicine that *does* work — and will forcefully reject the frivolous double-blind cross-over notions of drug doctors. This change is inevitable because our blind devotion to drugs and scalpels of drug medicine is exacting much too high a price from Americans.

I do not underestimate the enormous stakes of the different economic interests in health care. I do not believe they will relinquish their powerful grips on health care largesse simply because the true potential of nutritional and environmental medicines and the medicine of self-regulation become widely recognized. I am fully aware of how clinical research and the wisdom of experienced holistic physicians is laughed at by drug doctors who serve on the editorial boards of our medical journals. I am sadly aware of the unbearable punishment meted out to holistic doctors by the practitioners of disease medicine who sit on state licensing boards.

## PRUNING POWER OF PROBLEMS

Dead and dying ideas in medicine, like radioactive isotopes, have long lives. The annals of medicine are replete with accounts of drug therapies that endured long after they were proven ineffective or perilous or both.

The case this time around is different. Drugs are *interruptive* in their modes of action, and so cannot serve as *enabling* agents for healing. Drugs are chemicals, and so cannot solve problems caused by chemicals. Drugs drain energy, and so cannot promote physical fitness. Drugs deplete energy enzymes, and so cannot revive injured energy enzymes in fatigue states. Chronic fatigue *is* a difficult problem for disease doctors of drug medicine. This problem has an enormous pruning power. Unresolved problems eventually do strip the tree of medicine of its dead branches, though this process is maddeningly slow for the sick. The physicians of the future will go nondrug or they will have no patients with chronic immune and degenerative disorders.

*A new scientific truth does not triumph by convincing its opponents and making them see the light, but, rather, because its opponents die and a new generation grows up that is familiar with it.*

Max Planck

New ideas, as Max Planck saw so clearly, do not get accepted because of their intrinsic truth. They get accepted when the opposition dies out. This — it seems to me — is far more pertinent to medicine than it could be to physics. We physicians fiercely fought sanitation. How can engineers, who know nothing of *our* diseases, cure them by diverting human refuse? We physicians fought Pasteur. How can a chemist, who knows nothing of *our* maladies, prevent them by his serum? We fought Semmelweis. How can anyone prevent childbirth fever simply by washing his hands? We fought Hahnemann. How can anyone treat real diseases by giving a weak dilution of a substance that is supposed to cause the disease in the first place? (We conveniently forget that Hahnemann based his system of homeopathy on the Law of the Similars propounded by Hippocrates, the father of medicine, among others.) How can oxidative injury to enzymes cause chronic fatigue syndrome? I can hear fatigue experts screaming at me in disgust. How can a simplistic notion like that explain a complex disease like chronic immunodeficiency fatigue syndrome? How can nutrients work where drugs fail? How can quacks with their foolish notions of food and mold allergy, chemical sensitivity, abnormal bowel responses to foods, sugar-insulin-adrenaline roller coasters, impaired immune defenses, and damaged self-esteem succeed with their potions where our professors dismally fail with all their miracles of synthetic chemistry?

This is not merely of philosophic interest to me. I witness a profound change every working day. *Almost every patient I see with chronic fatigue consults me to see if I can help them become drugfree.* I worked as a disease doctor for the first 25 years of my life in medicine. It never once occurred to me during those years that in my life time, I would see a total reversal of objectives of my patients: They do not consult me so that I may begin drug therapies but so I may discontinue drugs they are prescribed by other physicians. We are just beginning to witness the pruning power of the problem of chronic fatigue.

The pandemic of chronic fatigue is real. And so are the problems caused by our polluted environment, contaminated foods, stress and lack of fitness. The pruning power of these problem, with time, will — I am certain — free us from the tyranny of drug medicine.

Majid Ali, M.D.
Teaneck, New Jersey
March 1, 1994.

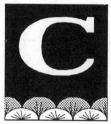

# Chapter 1

# Seven
# Canaries

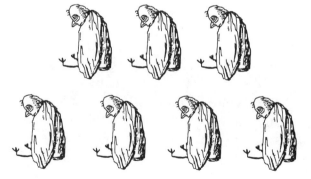

Chronic fatigue — I write in the preface — will be the dominant chronic health disorder of the 21st century. *This is the first core message of this book.*

"Chronic fatiguers" are human canaries. In old mining days, miners carried canaries in cages deep into their mine shafts. The birds were a sort of intelligence system. If there were any poisonous gases in the shafts, the birds would warn the miners. When the birds collapsed or died, the miners knew there were toxic gases in the shaft even though they could not smell them. They left the birds and ran out to escape the poisonous mine gases.

Why did the canaries die when exposed to poisonous mine gases but not the miners? Why did the miners not suffer any ill-effects most of the time even though they were exposed to the same poisons that killed the canaries? The canaries died because of their small size — there was so little of their molecular defenses to be destroyed, so little of their energy and life span enzymes to be poisoned. Yet, the miners didn't die because there was so much of them to be poisoned. The differences between the canaries and miners are entirely *quantitative* — the basic chemical equation of life — the redox reaction — is the same in both. Oxidative molecular defenses in man and canary are identical, and so it is for such diverse living beings as single-celled bacteria, monkeys and monstrous dinosaurs.

*Chronic fatiguers are human canaries.* This is the second core message of this book. It must be understood by those who suffer from chronic fatigue states, and those who care for them, that chronic fatiguers are *different*. Viral infections that common people can clear in days leave chronic fatiguers exhausted for weeks and months. Ordinary people do not even recognize when they are exposed to common environmental pollutants such as formaldehyde, organic solvents such as xylene and toluene, perfumes, paints and car exhaust fumes. Most chronic fatiguers are debilitated by such exposures. Most people breeze through sugar, insulin and adrenaline roller coasters without blinking an eye until degenerative and immune disorders make their appearance years later. Not so with chronic fatiguers. Even an occasional ice-cream cone can put them in bed for hours. Most people are not aware of foods that cause adverse bowel responses and allergic reactions. Not so with chronic fatiguers. Minor indiscretions exact major tolls from them. A large number of common people go about their business with aluminum, mercury or lead overload, never knowing how these toxic metals are poisoning their life span enzymes. Not so with chronic fatiguers. Their immune and molecular dynamics cannot sustain such burdens. We all recognize what stress is and how it injures us — at least theoretically. Stress has altogether different dimensions for chronic fatiguers. Most people intellectualize about anger at dinner tables. Not so with chronic fatiguers. Anger is a constant companion for chronic fatiguers — except for those few who find new spiritual dimensions through windows of suffering opened by chronic fatigue.

*Chronic fatiguers are different.* The critical element for chronic fatiguers is not what microbes and toxins do; rather, *it is how their molecular defenses fail to cope with such injury.* For the human canaries, the soil (energetic-molecular defenses) is more important than the seed (the virulence of microbes and toxicity of chemicals).

*DNA sequences set us up for oxidative injury; environmental triggers set off the oxidative reactions that cause chronic fatigue states.*

Environmental elements, of course, include those that surround us externally and those that exist within our internal ecosystems. Looked at another way, chronic fatiguers are people who have been genetically programmed to respond differently to microbial invasions and environmental toxins. Their vulnerabilities are woven into their genes.

## GENES, ENVIRONMENT, CHRONIC FATIGUE AND CHOICES

Diseases, I wrote in *The Cortical Monkey and Healing,* are burdens on biology. These burdens are imposed upon our genetic makeup by our external and internal environment. The intensity of suffering — diseases as they evolve with time — caused by these burdens is profoundly influenced by a third element: the choices we make in our response to these burdens. I show these relationships schematically in the diagram on the next page.

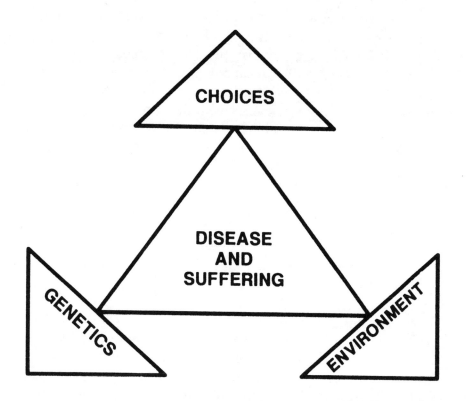

The core problem of medicine today — my friend Choua
often says — is that we have raised generations of physicians
who believe treatment of diseases without drugs or surgical
scalpels is quackery. Choua calls the prevailing drug medicine
in the United States $N^2D^2$ medicine — a medicine that starts with
the name of a disease and ends with the name of a drug. It is
a medicine, Choua says in elaborating his theory, in which all
our deliberations, concerns, thinking and efforts are limited to
finding a disease name for a patient and then finding a drug for
that disease. He expresses it with the following formula:

$$N^2D^2 \text{ medicine } =$$
$$\textbf{Name of Disease } \textbf{ X } \textbf{ Name of Drug}$$

We are paying a prohibitive price for $N^2D^2$ medicine.
There are effective, natural, nondrug and nonsurgical methods
for the reversal of degenerative and immune disorders. Acute
diseases, with rare exceptions, are not sudden departures from
health. These are the protocols of nutritional medicine,
environmental medicine, medicine of self-regulation and
medicine of fitness. This is a different and much less expensive
medicine.

The universe of electrons and cells within our skin is just
as fascinating as the universe of Star Wars technology outside.
The marvels of biology within us are much more relevant to our
health and life span than are the miracles of medical
technology. Patients need us physicians to help them look
inward for disease reversal much more than they need the
output of our prescription pads. This is the central issue facing

medicine today.

Perhaps nowhere are these considerations and the relationships between genes, environment, illness and suffering as relevant as in chronic fatigue states. Chronic fatiguers have to make some choices.

## *First,*

whether to search for one or more of those trendy diagnostic labels in vogue among the practitioners of drug medicine, or dispense with such frivolous notions and to think holistically about the energetic-molecular events that cause chronic fatigue states.

## *Second,*

whether to opt for one of the megabuck, tail-end work-ups that definitely "proves" that we suffer from chronic fatigue syndrome or whether to select tests that reveal burdens on our  biology that impair our energy and detoxification enzyme pathways and lead to chronic fatigue states.

## *Third,*

whether to seek treatment from one or more of the "experts" of drug medicine who prescribe antidepressants, steroids, toxic antiviral agents and a host of other drugs for chronic fatigue, or to consult one of the physicians who integrate in their care protocols of nutritional medicine; environmental medicine; medicine of self-regulation; and slow, sustained exercise for restoring impaired energy enzyme pathways back to their normal states.

The essential issues in chronic fatigue states are mold and pollen allergy, food sensitivities, body burden of environmental pollutants, toxic metal overload, body temperature dysregulation and electrophysiological patterns that set us up for states of absence of health. These conditions lead to accelerated oxidative molecular injury and subsequent chronic fatigue states. Sound, long-term strategies must address these issues in order to restore normal energy pathways. The tools of Star Wars medicine have little to offer chronic fatiguers.

*Important*

Long-term success *depends* upon choices. *Nothing is more important than those choices for chronic fatiguers.*

---

## CHRONIC FATIGUE STATES: A SPREADING EPIDEMIC

---

A state of undue tiredness is not a new discovery. A diminished level of general energy — and the sense of decreased vigor that accompanies it — has been known to health practitioners and lay people throughout history. Modern notions of fatigue are often traced to descriptions of George Beard — a New York City neurologist — who in the 1960s called it neurasthenia. Since then, Beard's neurasthenia has largely been regarded pejoratively — not unexpected in view of the "nervous weakness" implicit in the term. The terms "shirker's syndrome" and "yuppie plague" attempt to cloak this bias in contemporary vernacular. In the decades that followed Beard's description, the search for the cause of chronic fatigue often focused on infection with a host of organisms such as Brucella species, Epstein-Barr virus and, more recently, retroviruses. In 1985, a group of investigators at the Centers for Disease Control (CDC) formulated a set of criteria for the diagnosis of chronic fatigue syndrome. These criteria, as I show later, have done nothing to elucidate the true nature of this problem; rather, they have served as a diagnostic label to test the efficacy of drug therapies for chronic fatigue prescribed by practitioners of $N^2D^2$ medicine.

Chronic fatigue — I repeat for emphasis — will be the dominant chronic health disorder of the next century. How prevalent is it at present? Twenty one percent of 500 patients visiting a primary care clinic in Boston and 24% of 1,159 patients presenting at two adult care clinics in Texas complained of chronic fatigue. As comic relief, I cite a recent CDC estimate of the incidence of the chronic fatigue syndrome (reported by *Science* 254:1726;1991) which puts the number of total cases in the United States at 100,000. The wisdom of government experts often escapes me, and this is a good example. New York City alone has several times that number of people whose lives are severely limited by chronic fatigue states. Almost 90% of patients who consult me these days suffer from chronic fatigue. I wonder what could possibly be the motive behind such a ludicrous estimate by the folks at the CDC.

## WHEN I WENT TO MEDICAL SCHOOL IN THE LATE 1950s, CHRONIC FATIGUE SYNDROME DID NOT EXIST IN MEDICAL TEXTS

When I went to medical school in the late 1950s, chronic fatigue as a disorder didn't exist in medical texts. Indeed, it still does not exist in most medical texts. There were a few reports in the literature of chronic fatigue that followed some viral and bacterial infections such as chronic brucellosis, coxsackie and CMV viral infections and a host of other bacterial infections. It was not a subject worthy of serious study. Now, hardly a day goes by that I do not see patients with disabling chronic fatigue. Where did this epidemic of chronic fatigue come from? What makes previously healthy people severely fatigued? Most important, why are our children suffering from chronic fatigue states in such frightening numbers?

## CHRONIC FATIGUE STATES CANNOT BE UNDERSTOOD THROUGH SIMPLISTIC ONE-DISEASE-ONE-DRUG THINKING

States of chronic fatigue cannot be understood through the prevailing reductionistic medical thinking that regards diseases as drug-deficiency syndromes, to be cured by supplying the missing drugs. Nor can chronic fatigue states be successfully managed with narrow-focused drug "cures." What is required is a "systems study" of man and his environment — a holistic view of the impact upon a person's genes of environmental factors, nutritional status, microbes, stress and lack of physical fitness. Instead, millions of dollars are being spent on fragmentary studies of single issues. Isolated studies of epidemiology, immunology and virology, and clinical response to drugs have not — and I am certain will not — lead to effective therapies for restoring normal energy enzyme pathways in chronic fatigue states. What we need are integrated programs of fundamental research into human enzymatic energy mechanisms that are impaired by incremental molecular oxidant stress. Recognition and elimination of specific causes of increased oxidant stress, whenever possible, remain the true answers. Environmental, nutritional, self-regulatory and fitness approaches to reducing excessive oxidant stress are the keys to solving this global problem.

## HOW DO WE CAPTURE LOST ENERGY?

This question has preoccupied me for some years now. During this time, my theory that accelerated oxidative molecular injury is the true nature of chronic fatigue states gradually took form in my mind. Also during this time, I formulated — and validated with clinical outcome studies — my nondrug strategies for restoring normal energy enzyme pathways. As my clinical and research interests became sharply focused on chronic fatigue states, I started writing this book, and began to search for a suitable term for my work — some word that would fully express my notions of the true nature and optimal management of these states. I considered and rejected several different words for this purpose. Recently, between seeing patients in my office, my eyes fell on a draft of this chapter and I saw the question that appears in the heading of this paragraph. My eyes remained fixed first on the word "capture" and then on "energy." In a flash, I saw how the letters in the two words could express my total conceptual clinical approach.

The three letters in the word "cap" stood out for the three essentials of my core philosophy of caring for chronic fatiguers and the six letters in "energy" for the core elements in my clinical strategy. Thus:

**C**atch in early stages

**A**void drugs

**P**revent relapses.

In the same flash image, the word "energy" stood for:

**E**nvironment

**N**utrition

**E**xercise

**R**estoration   (of energy enzyme pathways)

**G**od

**Y**ou

**C**atching chronic fatigue states early is the first of the three core elements of my philosophy of caring for chronic fatiguers. From extensive clinical experience, I know that chronic fatigue states are easy to reverse if caught early. I also know that chronic fatigue states can be prevented. There are two essential requirements for this.

*First,*

we must dispense with silly notions of searching for the cause of chronic fatigue in frivolous diagnostic labels.

*Second,*

we must diligently address *all* factors that increase oxidant stress on human biology.

Avoiding drugs for chronic fatigue is the second core element. Nearly every working day I see the tragedy wrought by misuse of drugs for chronic fatigue states. Nearly every working day I see patients suffering from unrecognized and unmanaged functional nutritional disorders, sugar-insulin-adrenalin roller coasters, allergy and chemical sensitivity, temperature dysregulation and Fourth of July chemistry under the skin. None of these issues can be truly addressed with drugs, though drugs may be necessary for temporary symptom suppression. I address this subject at length in the chapters Lamppost Labels for Chronic Fatigue, What Is Chronic Fatigue? and Where Does It All Begin?

Preventing recurrence of chronic fatigue after initial success is the third core element. Not uncommonly I see chronic fatiguers who make slow and sustained recovery only to be plunged back into physically and emotionally exhausting states of fatigue by mindless use of drugs for sheer symptom suppression. Chronic fatiguers *need* to understand this. They must find physicians who have a global view of how our environment affects our genes and injure our energy and detoxification enzymes.

## ENERGY: THE ESSENTIAL CLINICAL STRATEGY

Environment sustains life. On page 5, I schematically express the relationship between environment, genes, choices and suffering earlier in this chapter. Chronic fatigue is a state of accelerated oxidative molecular injury. The increasing oxidizing capacity of planet Earth, in my view, is the principal threat to mankind and the other living creatures that share this planet with us. I return to this subject several times because it is the essence of this subject. I suggest that the professional reader consider my article "Hypothesis: Chronic Fatigue is a State of Accelerated Oxidative Molecular Injury" published in the Journal of Advancement in Medicine (6:83-96; 1993) and reproduced with the kind permission of Human Sciences Press, Inc., at the end of this volume. For the general reader, I devote the chapters What Is Chronic Fatigue? and Where Does It All Begin? to this subject. I discuss some other aspects of this subject in the companion volume *RDA: Rats, Drugs and Assumptions*.

Here I briefly state that the environment — as it relates to matters of human health and disease and states of chronic fatigue — includes not only the bedroom environment, the workplace environment, air pollution etc., but also the internal environment of our body organs such as the bowel ecosystem, the lung ecosystem, the cell ecosystem and, indeed, the ecosystem of the microcosms of life that exist within single cells and individual cell organelles such as mitochondria — the tiniest powerhouses where energy enzymes are arranged on submicroscopic shelves.

Specifically, I include in environmental concerns the issues of mold and other types of inhalant allergy, chemical sensitivity and toxicity and toxic metal overload.

Nutrition is what makes up our internal ecosystems. Few things sadden me more than the disdain of my colleagues in drug medicine for the essential role nutrition plays not only in preserving health but in *restoring* health by reversing chronic diseases. There are three essentials in this area: 1) optimal food choices in the kitchen; 2) oral nutrient protocols; and 3) intravenous nutrient protocols. I devote *The Butterfly and Life Span Nutrition* to the first subject and strongly recommend that volume to fatigue sufferers. I address the latter two subjects later in this volume.

Exercise for chronic fatiguers must be slow, sustained and non goal-oriented. This is a point of considerable importance. Several of my patients who suffered from chronic, disabling fatigue are competition athletes, dancers and fitness trainers. Oxidative injury to energy enzymes does not seem to show any respect for people no matter their status in society. Time and again, I see the tragedy of a chronic fatiguer making herculean efforts to pull himself out of chronic fatigue with sheer willpower. It does not work. I have seen people who worked with one of the popular exercise videos only to collapse for days after strenuous activity. Oxidant injury to energy enzymes, I might add, is equally ignorant of the teachings of mind-over-body gurus. This is also an essential subject to which I devote the companion volume *The Ghoraa and Limbic Exercise*.

R.estoration of energy and detoxification enzyme pathways calls for strategies that are based on a deeper understanding of how human biology succumbs to the onslaught of oxidant injury.

Specifically, the fundamental issues in this area are:

1. Restoration to normal states of bowel ecology.
2. Restoration of even, steady-state molecular dynamics of health (eliminating sugar, insulin, adrenaline and neurotransmitter roller coasters).
3. Restoration of normal body temperature (through self-regulation and normalization of thyroid gland function).
4. Restoration of cell membrane structure and function (through food choices in the kitchen, oral and, when necessary, intravenous nutrient protocols).
5. Restoration of normal energy dynamics by reducing, and eventually eliminating, stress-related molecular events.
6. Restoration of energy systems that have been blocked or impaired by toxic metal overload such as aluminum, mercury, lead and others.

I devote the companion volume *Battered Bowel Ecology — Waving Away a Wandering Wolf* to issues of altered bowel ecology states. For the professional reader, I suggest my monographs *Intravenous Nutrient Protocols in Molecular Medicine* and *Allergy: Diagnosis and management.*

G od and Y ou are taboo subjects in medicine. I know these words will invite derision from my colleagues in "scientific" medicine. Practitioners of $N^2D^2$ medicine, I know, have no respect for "religion" in medicine. That's how come they are so fond of dismissing any dimensions of the healing process that are outside the domain of their wonder drugs. I make no apology to them. But I know that those who care for persons paralyzed with persistent, debilitating, chronic fatigue will immediately see why I choose to give so much importance to this subject in this volume. The way out of unrelenting suffering cannot be found without redefining — at least in some measure — the link that binds us to the gentle guiding energy of that *presence* that always surrounds us. On a mundane level, the goal of reducing total oxidant stress on an individual requires making many changes in choices he makes in his everyday life — and mere martyrdom doesn't work. He cannot reach the stage at which he *wants* to do the things that he *needs to do* without some profound visceral-spiritual changes. Indeed, in my view, some spiritual dimensions are essential for coping with all serious types of illness. Persistent, disabling chronic fatigue states certainly qualify as serious illnesses. I make no apologies to the "scientist" in drug medicine for this statement.

I consider training in effective methods for self-regulation essential for all my patients who suffer from chronic fatigue.

Beyond the issue of understanding energy dynamics in health and disease through self-regulation, there is the matter of opportunity for doing some spiritual work — opening some new spiritual dimensions in one's life. Enlightenment, in both physical and spiritual senses, usually comes to the seriously ill in three phases: awareness, higher states of consciousness and spirituality.

When caring for seriously ill patients, physicians, in general, are deeply troubled by subjects of states of consciousness, enlightenment and spirituality. It is ironic because the sick almost always welcome any opportunity for instruction and training in these areas. Suffering brings new insight into matters of the human condition, states of consciousness and domains of spirituality. It is really that simple. We do not need to invoke esoteric brands of mysticism for such work. Gurus are really not necessary. Good teachers will do. I return to this essential subject in the chapter On Hope, Spirituality and Chronic Fatigue.

## SEVEN CANARIES

Following are seven true-to-life case studies, each illustrating one or more essential issues in the diagnosis and management of chronic fatigue states. Six of these are my patients, but names have been changed for obvious reasons. The seventh case history is that of an engineer whose story was published in the *Wall Street Journal*.

These case histories demonstrate that these individuals

were set up for later events — they were carrying biological
burdens in the form of allergies, chemical sensitivities, viral and
bacterial infections, sugar and adrenaline roller coasters,
battered bowel ecology states, and toxic metal overloads. One
other factor distinguishes them from others: *These persons
developed chronic fatigue in circumstances in which others would
not have. They are human canaries.* What turned them into
canaries? I address this issue at length in the chapters:
Pasteur's Sheep and My Canaries, What Is Chronic Fatigue?
and Where Does It All Begin?

## LITTLE JOE: THE FIRST CANARY

Little Joe's mom consulted me because he was "always
tired." Little Joe had been a colicky baby and had "bad diaper
rash all the time." His mother didn't know he was allergic. He
frequently suffered from sore throats and ear infections, and
required antibiotic therapy to control such infections. Little Joe
finally had tubes put into his ears. The tubes reduced the
frequency of ear infections but didn't save him from yet more
courses of antibiotics. When he was just an infant, his mother
had asked his pediatrician if he needed allergy tests. The
pediatrician told her he was too young for allergy tests. When
Choua heard about this, he chuckled, "Too young for allergy
tests but not too young for antibiotics." I asked Little Joe's
mother if she had sometimes noticed mood swings or if he had
ever thrown temper tantrums after eating ice cream and candy.
The answer was a resounding "yes."

## ZENA: THE SECOND CANARY

Zena was, as Victor Hugo would say, in the youth of her old age. Fiftysomething, she lived a quiet and contented life with her husband, except when her daughter visited with her two grandsons, which didn't happen too often. There hadn't been any surprises at the office for years. The people at work, it seemed to her, had changed even less than the red bricks on the front wall of the company building. Democrats hadn't begun to like Clinton yet. Nobody liked Bush. Perot still hadn't pulled out, and Quayle was still into *Murphy Brown*. Then everything changed.

Zena suffered a cold. Her doctor prescribed antibiotics. Days went by but her cold symptoms didn't clear up. Antibiotics followed more and different antibiotics, and CAT scans followed chest X-rays. Her dry hacking cough persisted, and she felt very tired. Then she switched doctors. She had several blood tests done and yet more antibiotics were prescribed. The Lyme disease test was negative but one for Epstein-Barr virus turned out to be weakly positive. She became progressively lethargic and irritable, developed muscle and joint aches, and grew anxious and depressed. Days turned into weeks. She suffered from recurrent episodes of lightheadedness and numbness in her limbs. Her husband noticed she didn't remember things that had happened just hours before. She consulted still more doctors who suspected chronic fatigue syndrome but thought she needed to see a psychiatrist before they could give her gamma globulin shots and Zovirax for the viral infection. It didn't really surprise Zena. She herself had begun to wonder if the whole thing were all in her head. Zena wondered if she would ever get better or if this was to be the story of her golden years.

## FATHER THOMAS: THE THIRD CANARY

Father Thomas looked his part. He was tall, broad-shouldered and soft-spoken. Listening came to him naturally and effortlessly, virtues that resulted from years of long professional training. I got the sense he wanted me to succeed, not because he consulted me for relief of his chronic fatigue, but because he felt I deserved to succeed. His fatigue, he confided, was not really disabling. It was just that he was tired all the time and knew that was not right. Sometimes he wondered if he was harboring a killer cancer somewhere in his body that was silently eating at his innards, causing fatigue.

## LUCIA: THE FOURTH CANARY

During her initial consultation with me, Lucia, a 39-year-old housewife, smiled and said,

"Dr. Ali, I'm afraid my husband might divorce me if I don't get my energy level up and don't lose some weight. God knows I have tried, but I haven't succeeded."

Patients often make such comments with smiles that do little to hide serious inner concerns. I returned her smile.

Lucia looked like a strong woman, and her interest in body sculpting work showed in her bearing. She did not recall any specific illness that was followed by problems of impaired general health. Rather, she had slowly lost her energy level over several months. This change in energy level was associated with a host of other symptoms that seemed to follow one after another, including muscle aches, undue sensitivity to cold, abdominal bloating and cramps, severe PMS, headache, mood swings, short-term memory loss and depression. She knew she was allergic but her allergies had never been diagnosed and never managed.

## BRUCE: THE FIFTH CANARY

Bruce, a young man in his forties, walked in for a consultation carrying a thick bundle of previous medical records. His shirt was obviously too large for him, and it was equally obvious that he had lost a lot of weight. He looked exhausted as many chronic fatiguers do. His skin was dry and his eyelids swollen. He sat down on the chair and looked at me with deeply doubtful eyes as I studied his history questionnaire.

During the visit, he pulled out from his thick pile of papers a typed summary of his symptoms that I reproduce below in full.

* Birth to three years

    Received prolonged antibiotics at age 6 months for pneumonia
    More antibiotics for pneumonia at age 2

* 3-6 years

    Physically very active
    More antibiotics for recurrent tonsillitis followed by tonsillectomy
    Extended antibiotic therapy for rheumatic fever

* 6-12 years

    Physically very active
    More antibiotics during dental work
    Multiple mercury fillings

* 13-21 years

    Still physically active but with diminishing energy
    Weighed 130 pounds at age 21
    More antibiotics for acne and for dental work
    Started some herbs for health

* 22-23 years

    Physically inactive
    Weight 142
    Antibiotics continued for dental work

* 24-29 years

Very busy with work as financial analyst
Physically active, running 20-45 miles per week
Antibiotics continued for dental work

* 30-35 years

Knee surgery at 30 that followed forced running
Nasal polyp surgery at 31
Physically inactive, weight steadily rising to 152 pounds
Began losing weight and energy at 35 years
Developed food intolerance and chemical sensitivities
Started elimination/rotation diet and homeopathic
remedies. Symptoms progressively worsened despite
therapy

* 35-37 years

Took nystatin continuously, "Life became tolerable, by
far the best I felt in years, but four months after stopping
nystatin, chemical sensitivity became so strong I had to
stop working. Was easy to identify problem substances.
Occasional good days, but produced lots of lifestyle
constraints."

* 37-41 years

Physically inactive, progressive weight loss from 152 to
117
Digestive aids helped. Internal cleansing: No matter
what, the same pattern occurred: A brief period of
improvement, a slow, steady increase in symptom severity
that continued until the method was stopped.

* Long-term symptoms

    Occasional   age 14-19
    Frequent     age 20-29
    Constant     age  30 to present

* Digestive problems

    Excessive gas
    Always hungry
    Always underweight
    Bloated
    Food intolerance
    Leaky gut
    Cold hands and feet
    Sensitive to heat/cold/weather
    Hair loss
    Poor posture
    Depression
    Hyperactive
    Apprehensiveness/anxiety/shoulder   pain/chest pain
    Mood swings
    Difficulty staying focused
    Sensory perception problems (primarily vision, smell)
    Physical balance problems
    Time/space perception problems
    Coordination, motor skill problems
    Chemical sensitivity
    Heavy metal toxicity
    Fatigue
    Hypoglycemia
    Pancreas/liver stressed
    Degree of problems varies with the degree of

food/chemical exposure

## I'M AFRAID OF HOPE

*"I'm afraid of hope."* Bruce spoke those words during his initial consultation with me. The words have stuck in my mind ever since. He was very eager for me to study his whole case — as most chronic fatiguers are, months and sometimes after years of hope roller coasters. Hope, I found out early in my work with chronic fatiguers, is easy to create. It requires much patience and long hours of work to sustain. I know of many sad stories of chronic fatiguers — people whose hopes were raised by the promise of seeing some great fatigue researcher at some great out-of-state fatigue center. Those hopes came crashing down when — after spending thousands of dollars on sophisticated tests — they were rewarded with a prescription for some antidepressant.

The subject of hope creates a dilemma for me in my clinical work. Hope is essential for healing. Yet, hope that does not bring relief is devastating. Then there are those frivolous people around who sit in judgment of the work of holistic physicians and who equate hope with deception, duping, and outright fraud. And finally, there are malpractice attorneys who blatantly advise you against holding out hope for anyone. Hope, they counsel you, is the fuel for malpractice actions.

I told Bruce that I couldn't work without hope. Hope is what sustains my patients — sometimes for those interminable months when relief from symptoms escapes them. Hope is what sustains me — sometimes during months of strong doubt and a punishing sense of personal inadequacy. And — I told Bruce not knowing how he would take it — I truly do not know where true hope ends and false hope begins. Indeed, I do not know if hope is ever truly false. Some attorneys know better. Editors of our prestigious medical journals know better. Some folks who sit on state licensing boards know better. But I don't. Next, I told Bruce that if he wanted me to work with him, we were going to begin with hope. And that it was okay with me that he was afraid of hope.

## JOHN: THE SIXTH CANARY

John was a financial analyst before he became a full-time chronic fatiguer. That happened four years before I first saw him in the conference room, slumped in a chair during a workshop. I was speaking about how some liver enzymes detoxify environmental pollutants in the body. "Speak for yourself," he muttered to himself, but loud enough to be heard by others. When I turned my head to see where the words might have come from, John became flustered. John, I learned later, knows more about chronic fatigue than most people, including most physicians I know. He told me to speak for myself because he knew his detoxification enzymes were not working, and that was his main problem.

Unfortunately for John, long before he educated himself intensively about the impact of his environment upon his genetic makeup, he had been prescribes extensive broad-spectrum antibiotics for recurrent infections and other drugs for symptom suppression during his childhood and teen years, and then again during the early years of chronic fatigue. John developed severe, unrelenting fatigue, muscle aches, and a diffuse, dry, red rash all over his body that sometimes cracked and oozed. He rapidly developed multiple food allergies and chemical sensitivities, lost weight and became emaciated. By the time he learned the true nature of his suffering, he was seriously ill most of the time inspite of the care given him by some knowledgeable holistic New York physicians.

## THOMAS LATIMER: THE SEVENTH CANARY

Mr. Latimer is not my patient. I choose his story as told by the *Wall Street Journal* to illustrate some other aspects of the chronic fatigue pandemic.

*"Thomas Latimer used to be a vigorous, athletic man, a successful petroleum engineer with a bright future. Then he mowed his lawn. On a summer Saturday in 1985, Mr. Latimer spent an hour or so cutting the grass, picking up the clippings and edging the walkway around his modest two-bedroom home. Soon, something was*

*terribly wrong. He felt dizzy and nauseated. His nose was running, and his chest was tight. He had a pounding headache. Ten days later, he was still sick."*

*The Wall Street Journal* October 14, 1991.

This is not an unusual beginning of what, sadly and only too frequently, turns out to be a horror story. The essential clues in such stories stare physicians in their faces but are seldom heeded.

The man in the *Wall Street Journal* story was "a vigorous, athletic man" who was in perfect health and then become suddenly ill after mowing his lawn. Dizziness, nausea, headache, tightness in the chest and runny nose are symptoms that cry out for recognition as a severe systemic reaction to an environmental poison. Was it recognized? The *Journal* continues.

*"Now six years and 20 doctors later —after liver biopsies, spinal-fluid taps, CAT scans, radioactive brain flow studies, sleep studies and many other tests — Mr. L, 36, accepts the diagnosis of doctors: that he was poisoned by an organophosphate pesticide used to treat his yard."*

Why did it take 20 doctors six years to diagnose pesticide poisoning? Because this type of illness does not fit into our *blessed* double-blind, cross-over model of disease classification in the prevailing drug medicine. It is far more convenient for us physicians to deny such illness. The *Journal* continues,

> *"A toxicologist, three neurologists and two neuro-ophthalmologists who examined him all concluded independently that the Tagamet suppressed the normal role of his liver in metabolizing the poison and expelling it."*

How did these specialists arrive at that conclusion? I wondered about this question. After all, that is the precise reason why physicians who practice environmental medicine have been crucified for some decades. What has been the sin of practitioners of environmental medicine? They searched for the cause of illness in their patients in environmental pollutants? When a clinical ecologist suspects that formaldehyde exposure causes headache, or trichloroethylene (dry cleaning solution) causes skin bruising, the drug doctors jump at him and threaten his license because he is not "scientific" enough. When three neurologists and two neuro-ophthalmologists conclude that Tagamet suppressed the normal role of his liver, no one asks how did they support their conclusion? Did they study the cytochrome P-450 enzyme levels in the liver cells in Mr. Latimer? They didn't. Even if they had, how could they prove that liver enzymes were injured several years previously on that fateful day when he mowed his lawn? How can anyone conclude something like that after years of exposure.

The real answer is that practitioners of environmental medicine make clinical judgments based on repeated patterns of symptomatology that follows exposure to environmental agents. Then they exclude those pollutants and manage other related burdens on detoxification enzymes and *clinically observe* the outcome. This is as good a science as any other in medicine.

The canary in Mr. Latimer carries some important message:

## *First,*

seemingly innocent drugs such as Tagamet used for stomach ulcers by millions of people can slowly but relentlessly injure energy and detoxification enzymes and lead to serious chemical consequences.

## *Second,*

drug therapies administered to "treat" such illnesses only compound the problem — they turn mostly easily manageable clinical problems into irreversible immune disorders.

## *Third,*

the practitioners of drug medicine can accept the precepts of clinical ecology only after prolonged drug therapies have inflicted substantial additional damage.

## *Fourth,*

in environmental medicine, we see cases such as that of Mr. Latimer almost every week — most of them recover relatively early with nondrug therapies. When the drug doctors are stuck with such cases, they become media events. What surprised me was not that an organophosphate in pesticide had poisoned an engineer, but that the *Wall Street Journal* was so impressed by the case history that it put the story on the front page.

## GENES AND CANARIES

Little Joe, Zena, Father Thomas, Lucia, Bruce, John and Mr. Latimer are human canaries. Their genes set them up for chronic fatigue states — to render them vulnerable to life in highly polluted and toxic environment. They become chemically-sensitive and tolerate our miracle drugs poorly. They benefit little from our Star Wars medicine.

> *"DNA legislates life,*
> *Environment interprets the laws, "*

Choua once told me. "You physicians seem to

understand that in theory," he continued, "but in clinical practice, it is a different matter. You ignore both essentials. Drugs and knives are the tools of your trade, and there are no drugs nor surgical procedures to cope with either. Chronic fatiguers suffer needlessly because environmental and nutritional medicine have been declared quackery by the high priests of Star Wars medicine. The champions of $N^2D^2$ medicine believe such therapies are treating diseases that really do not exist. Their injured enzymes are ignored because Star Wars medicine has no drugs that can 'undamage' the damaged energy enzymes — 'unoxidize' the oxidized and denatured enzymes. Women and men who bow at the altar of the gods of the double-blind, cross-over and *scientific vigor* have pronounced that all methods of treatment except those that use drugs and scalpels are unproven and unconventional. I have no trouble with the unconventional part, but unproven is simply not true. They are proven for those who use them every day and see their clinical benefits, clearly and unequivocally."

"Choua, you have a one track mind. You can't help yourself. Everything has to end with an indictment of the medical profession," I complained.

"In the old days, miners carried canaries deep into their mine shafts," Choua continued darkly, "so the birds could warn them of poisonous gases. The canaries died, but the men lived. Chronic fatiguers are the canaries that tell us something about the shape of things to come. Are the high priests of your Star Wars medicine listening? Do they see the havoc our technology has wrought upon our environment? Do they see the chemical avalanches we have unleashed upon our planet Earth? Do they recognize the impact upon human and animal biology of environmental pollutants? Do they understand what polluted air, contaminated water and toxic foods do to living things? Do they realize how the delicate gut ecology of babies is destroyed with indiscriminate use of antibiotics?"

"Choua, it's changing. Even *The New York Times* knows antioxidants are good for preventive medicine." I tried to ameliorate the situation.

"Yes, the *Times* has finally learned that! But do you think those men of scientific vigor on the editorial boards of medical journals know that?"

Choua now referred to an editorial I had written for the *Life Spanner* in which I commented on two studies published by the *New England Journal of Medicine*. These two large multimillion dollar studies clearly showed the protective value of vitamin E against coronary heart disease. Yet, the *Journal* concluded both articles with the recommendation that the use of vitamin E beyond the RDA value of 30 units should await further studies. This was a stunning conclusion for practitioners of nutritional medicine, who have safely used 400 to 800 units of this vitamin for years. I said so in my editorial.

"All you think of is drugs," Choua resumed. "Drugs for chemical sensitivity, drugs for immune disorders, drugs for degenerative diseases, and, of course, drugs for chronic fatigue."

"It's changing," I said lamely.

"Changing? Changing, my foot! You have some sense of humor. Don't you? They are revoking Levin's license and you think things are changing. What are the awful things Levin did that he deserves to lose his license and livelihood? He prescribed vitamins! That's the punishable offense! Isn't it?"

"Levin hasn't lost his license yet. With luck, the Board of Regents will see the truth and will rule in his favor," I said

hopefully.
  "Luck! Aha! Waiting for luck. Waiting for Godot!"

---

### MOST PEOPLE WHO SUFFER FROM CHRONIC FATIGUE DO GET BETTER

Little Joe was doing well at my last visit with him two years later. Micro-elisa blood allergy tests for mold and pollen allergy and electrodermal conductance tests for food incompatibilities revealed allergy and incompatibility to numerous agents. It usually takes children a while to see the relationship between what they eat and how they feel. Joe was no exception. Initially, he resented changes in his diet and bitterly fought with his parents. In a few months, he gradually relented and accepted new foods. Sugar was finally and completely eliminated. Once, when he felt very well, Halloween's arrival made him very sick. That did it. He began to link the way he ate and the way he felt. He has not required antibiotics in several months now. His parents have been satisfied with the clinical results. This turned out to be a simple case of accelerated oxidative injury caused by sugar roller coasters and food allergy. The case management was simple, outcome satisfactory.

Zena made dramatic initial improvement. Her fatigue cleared up almost completely with intravenous (IV) nutrient therapy, oral vitamin and mineral therapy, allergy immunotherapy injections and stress control. "It's hard to believe this problem could have been solved so quickly and without any drugs," she told me after a few weeks. Relapses of fatigue after initial recovery are not uncommon. Indeed this happened to Zena. She returned for some more IV therapy. Her fatigue cleared again and didn't return. This was a case of accelerated oxidative molecular injury triggered by a viral infection and compounded by multiple courses of antibiotics, stress and fear of an unknown, disabling disease.

Father Thomas proved to be allergic to multiple molds and pollen with the micro-elisa blood test and had multiple food incompatibilities. With allergy treatment, some nutrient therapies, food rotation and some autoregulation, his fatigue cleared up within several weeks. I didn't think he needed IV therapy. I saw him recently about three years after the first visit. Now his energy level is high. He continues his nutrient therapy and now takes an immunotherapy injection once every four weeks. Again, this case turned out to be a simple case of chronic fatigue caused by allergy and functional nutrient inadequacies that was successfully reversed with simple nondrug therapies.

Lucia got her energy back, but with some ups and downs. Initially, she responded only minimally to my initial nutritional, environmental and self-regulatory protocols (immunotherapy for IgE-mediated allergy always takes weeks to months to produce clinical result). My advice not to undertake any strenuous body sculpting work went unheeded. I then decided to administer intravenous nutrient protocols.

She responded rather dramatically to four infusions. Then I didn't see her for about six months. She returned with the following story:

*"I was well for several weeks after I stopped your therapies. Then slowly — just as I had before I saw you — fatigue returned along with all the other symptoms. My husband became very frustrated. He took me to this specialist at a New York university hospital who ordered a bunch of tests for which we paid over $1,300. His professional fee came to $560. Then he told us that I needed to see a psychiatrist. I was so mad at my husband. I wanted to come here because I got better here the first time, but he insisted I must see a New York City specialist."*

I reviewed the records again and decided to follow exactly the same management program that had worked so well the first time. As she was leaving my office, she turned back and spoke,

*"Dr. Ali, if your fatigue book   is not finished yet, please write about me. Maybe it will save other patients a lot of*

*aggravation and a lot of money. When you suffer from chronic fatigue, and many other problems, it really hurts when a doctor tells you to consult a psychiatrist. "*

Bruce's progress notes in his own clinical chart written after I started my environmental, nutritional, self-regulatory and fitness protocols include the following:

Seven weeks later

> Very concerned about continuing weight loss. Mild improvement in food choices based on food sensitivity profile. Fresh vegetable juices okay. Squashes give a clear mind — then it crashes. Soreness in ileocecal region. Primer I, II and III intravenous infusions prescribed. (In the chapter Intravenous Nutrient Therapies for Chronic Fatigue States, I give my reasons why I defer such therapies for some time after the initial consultation.)

14 weeks later

> First IV (Primer I intravenous Protocol) brought relief for two to three days. Primer II and III brought relief for four to seven days. "IVs really good results if there is no exposure". Overall improvement 2+ (scale 0 to 4+); Fatigue 1.5+ (scale 0 to 4+)

19 weeks later

> IV therapy with autoregulation much more helpful than
> without it. Now, with permission of the other patient
> receiving IV therapy in my room, I turn down the lights
> and we do autoreg. My initial reactions to IV have
> almost disappeared. I feel I am stepping into a
> transition. Overall improvement score 2+; fatigue score
> 2+.

27 weeks later

> "Dr. Ali, I can't believe it happened. I drove my car for
> five hours at a stretch. And that's some thing for me. I
> have been so sensitive to car exhaust I couldn't drive for
> more than half an hour at a time." I told him not to test
> his limits that way that soon, but he seemed too elated
> with his achievement to pay attention to what I tried to
> impress on him.

J ohn and I came to know each other well. When I first
met him several years ago, I had no plans for writing this book.
He was among the first people who felt my work had
relevance for a much larger audience than I could possibly
manage myself. "Doc, you are the most underutilized resource
there is in preventive medicine. And I have been around," he
told me once.

John is highly allergic. We achieved only minimal
success with allergy immunotherapy injections. Those were the

days that I was just beginning my research with intravenous nutrient protocols. One day he dragged himself to the office. He looked very pale and sick, and was obviously in a lot of pain. He had been mugged a few days earlier, he told me. Some of the wounds got infected. Then he developed multiple abscesses under the skin of his legs and abdomen. He wanted me to treat those abscesses with IV nutrient therapy. I thought he was frightened, in pain and irrational. It is one thing to try to manage severe viral infection with intravenous nutrient infusions and altogether different to try to cope with multiple bacterial infections with such therapy. Antibiotics, it is well-known, do not work against viruses. Antiviral drugs such as AZT for AIDS are too toxic to be lightly used for nonlethal viral infections. It is different with bacterial infections that can almost always be controlled with appropriate antibiotic therapies. I told John I could not agree with his request.

"Doc, you don't know my body. Antibiotics will kill me. Please do an IV for me, will you?" John pleaded.

I repeated my detailed explanation all over again. Then I said, "John, I do not have as much freedom as you might think I have. There are such things as malpractice insurance carriers and state licensing boards."

"Give me more credit than that, Doc. I will sign a consent form that you are giving me this therapy purely on a compassionate basis. I will sign papers that you advised antibiotic therapy but that I refused, and that you do not really think that IV therapy can do anything for such large abscesses."

There was no problem with John's thinking, I realized. He had thought the whole thing through — the compassionate use of IV and the consent and release letter. I wondered whether the insurance carriers and folks who sit on the state licensing boards ever learn about such matters.

I relented, and John received his first Infection Control Protocol IV that evening and a second one two days later. There was no sign of abscesses when I saw him a week later. Perhaps he would have healed his abscesses anyway without my IV nutrient protocol. After all, human beings used to heal abscesses before Fleming discovered penicillin.

John was trapped in some drawn-out family legal matters. Neither he nor his sick mother was up to that demanding task. I didn't see him for several months. He returned one day and asked if I could certify his illness. He could not get disability benefits, largely because the disability folks could not understand why he had not applied for such benefits some years earlier. I asked him why he hadn't. "Doc, because I kept thinking it was just a matter of some weeks before I'd get better and resume my work in finance. It never occurred to me that after all these years, my intentions to get back to my work would keep me from getting disability. Ironic, isn't it?" John spoke with a sad smile.

Now I see John occasionally when he totally collapses and requires some urgent medical attention. He suffers from severe and persistent skin rashes, for which he uses sauna therapy. Sometimes I see him when he wants me to write a medical note so that the folks at his sauna do not keep him out because of his skin rash. Sauna is a therapy without which John cannot catch the three to four hours of sleep he does manage to get. John's suffering continues — a victim of his genes, of his environment, of unrelenting fatigue, of universal reactivity, of ever-present muscle pains, of total body skin scaling, oozing and itching and of recurrent abdominal cramps.

"Now I am frightened the way I have never been frightened before. Doc, I can't think now. Now I don't know where this thing is leading me. Where am I going? Doc, do you know?" he asked me the last time I saw him several months ago.

John, above all, is a victim of Star Wars medicine that excels only when people are near death, and it has little to offer in preventing environmental diseases. The irony is that our Star Wars medicine has nothing to offer to people like John even when they stare into the face of death.

Could John's unending miseries have been prevented? I have often marveled at the astounding feats of Star Wars medicine when it deals with people in near-death situations. I have also wondered how utterly ineffective this medicine is in helping people as they *begin* to get ill. Could John's untold suffering have been prevented? Probably — if his genetic handicap had been managed optimally and if his environmental burdens had been alleviated — at least in part, and if he had been nutritionally supported well. Instead, what $N^2D^2$ medicine offered was more and more powerful (and toxic) antibiotics, and other drugs. Whatever damage $N^2D^2$ medicine spared him if any, the politics of disability medicine completed it. John continues to suffer.

M r. Latimer can no longer ride a bike, the *Wall Street Journal* story continued. He has difficulty walking. At night, to combat seizures and nightmares, he takes an anti-epileptic medication. Until recently, he could sleep for only about an hour at a time. The *Journal* continues,

> *"The makers of the pesticide Diazinon, and of Tagamet firmly deny that their products had anything to do with Mr. Latimer's condition. .... When they (Mr. Latimer and his wife) discovered Mr. Latimer's cancer, they accelerated their plans for starting a family, even creating their own sperm bank."*

(parenthesis added)

Could Mr. Latimer's prolonged enzyme damage have been prevented? My answer: The overwhelming probability is that it could have been if he had been managed properly with holistic nondrug therapies. I do not make this statement lightly. It is based on considerable personal experience with such environmentally-induced illnesses. I have had the opportunity of caring for many patients who became suddenly ill after a major chemical exposure. I managed all such cases with intravenous nutrient infusions and carefully looked into all the factors that render persons like Mr. latimer so vulnerable to chemical exposures, including a sharp focus on stress reduction with effective self-regulatory methods. None of these patients followed the course that Mr. Latimer did; his was the common tragedy of environmental illness that is either denied completely — the old all-in-the-head story — or worse, treated with multiple drug therapies that further damage the patient's energy and detoxification enzymes.

I end this chapter with a letter I received from one of my patients.

*"I am encouraged and hopeful beyond words. The paths that once seemed closed now are wide open and beckoning to me. I am coming! The sun is brighter, the music more beautiful, the flowers sweeter — all this because I feel my health returning to me. A gift and a miracle I only imagined a year or more ago. Something I prayed for, cried over, pined for, is at last palpable and real to me. The smallest task accomplished, the most momentary burst of energy — however brief — the unspeakable feeling when I can sing a song — a whole recital — with focus and strength; all these things and many more sit upon me like gold and linger in dark moments. Each day is a new opportunity, a new adventure and a new chance for fulfillment. I am glad, proud, thrilled to be here to experience this growth and transformation.*

*The slow, often painful movement from sickness to health is full of challenge and is ultimately more profound, more resonant and more satisfying than any other*

*I've experienced. I am witness to the undeniable fact that God lives in me — in my body — and he is working with me all the time and guiding me towards that perfection which is my birthright.*

*I let go of the belief in limitation and restriction and instead embrace the faith in the boundless possibility that resides, undaunted, within the human spirit.*

*Amen!!*

**\*\*\*\*\*\*\*\*\*\*\*\*\***

Dear Dr. Ali,

This is the little piece I wrote for our newsletter here at work. (I mailed it to you weeks ago, but apparently it was lost in transit.) I was feeling particularly well that day and felt the urge to express it...

I continue to improve all the time, and I am very grateful for it. Thank you for all your work for the sick.

Your patient,
LN

*In the depth of winter, I fully learned that within me there lay an invincible summer.*

Albert Camus

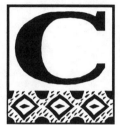

**C**hapter 2

# Pasteur's Sheep and My Canaries

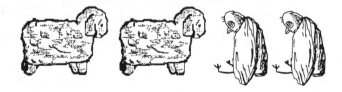

*"I want to go on living. I'm not going to rush it. I love life just too much for that. I think we should all cherish life. There is a wealth within each one of us. I found out I had something rich in me — something special. I don't give a damn if anyone else sees that or not. You know, if someone chooses not to accept the gifts God gives her, it's really her problem. I used to think people should treat me differently—a certain way. Now I don't. It's not important how they feel about me. What is important to me is how I feel about myself."*

A sprightly, gracefully dressed 89-year-old woman spoke the preceding words during her consultation with me. She had experienced some anal symptoms and felt a growth there. The biopsy done a few days later proved what she herself had suspected and what I was sure of during my examination. The anal growth was epidermoid cancer.

The next morning, I went to the hospital. A 31-year-old physician-colleague stood at the emergency department door.

"How are you?" I greeted him with some enthusiasm.
"Tired!" he groaned.
"Were you on call last night?" I asked sympathetically.
"No!" he answered tersely.
"Had a rough night? Someone was very sick?"
"No!" He was still abrupt in his tone.
"Didn't catch enough sleep?"
"No, I slept eight hours."
"Oh, just one of those days." I tried to disentangle myself from a greeting that clearly was turning into a probing.
"Yeah, just one of those days."

As I began to walk on, he relented a little and grinned.

"It's one of those days where you can't just get enough coffee to keep awake."
"Some days are tough, aren't they?" I grinned back at him and quickened my pace.

Chronic fatigue is not a caffeine-deficiency state. Nor is it a matter of advancing age. And it is not about inadequate sleep. Chronic fatigue is the failure of human energy enzyme pathways. It is a state of accelerated oxidative molecular injury. *Chronic fatiguers are different people* — they are an injured people.

## THE FLU AND FOUR FRIENDS

Four freshmen students come down with the flu at their college dorm. One of them is sick with a sore throat for a few days but doesn't miss any classes. The second student also suffers from a sore throat, runs a fever for some days, stays in the dorm and misses some classes. The third student develops fever, rash and enlarged lymph glands in his neck. He is very fatigued and consults his physician. The tests for "mono" — infectious mononucleosis, the kissing disease — come back positive. He is given a steroid shot and advised to go home and rest for a few weeks. At home, he feels unduly tired as weeks pass by. He returns to school, still tired. He gradually regains his usual level of energy over the course of several months.

The fourth student also tests positive for mono and is given a steroid injection. He becomes progressively tired, loses several pounds, develops a hacking cough and runs a low-grade fever. His family physician prescribes more broad-spectrum antibiotics. Weeks go by, but the fourth student doesn't recover. His low-grade fever doesn't let up, and his cough persists. He consults his physician again and is prescribed a course of broad-spectrum antibiotics. His fatigue persists, and he suffers from malaise, headache and muscle aches. His parents are worried now and take him to a rheumatologist. He orders many tests and prescribes yet more antibiotics and some nonsteroidal anti-inflammatory agents. The cough persists and he develops wheezing. His physician orders some more tests and prescribes steroid therapy. He begins to suffer from mood and memory difficulties and becomes depressed. A return visit to his physician earns him a prescription for Elavil. He continues to lose weight and develops joint pain. His parents become very worried and take him to the rheumatologist who orders yet more tests and then prescribes a nonsteroidal anti-inflammatory pain killer. The drug adds stomach discomfort to the long list of his symptoms. The young man's condition continues to deteriorate. His parents panic and take him to a famous fatigue expert who orders over $4,000 worth of immunologic tests and pronounces — in his usual, authoritative tone — that the young man suffers from chronic fatigue syndrome. The young man and his parents have their worst fears confirmed. The fatigue expert then doles out a prescription for acyclovir (an antiviral drug) and changes the antidepressant medication to Prozac.

The fourth student loses more weight, develops "new" allergies, becomes sensitive to perfumes and formaldehyde, and suffers from unrelenting abdominal bloating and digestive problems. He becomes anxious, confused and frightened. A friend gives him a copy of *The Yeast Connection*. The young man begins to read the books and suddenly it dawns on him that the yeast syndrome described in the book fully describes him. He is elated and relieved. At long last, he *knows* what the diagnosis is. He now sees a naturopathic yeast specialist who gives him a load of vitamins and prescribes high colonics. The therapies *really* work and his energy level improves for the first time since he fell ill. His mental functions improve significantly. Weeks go by and his fatigue returns — and with it his worst fears. Deeply disappointed that the relief was just temporary, he now consults another yeast specialist who undertakes another work-up and prescribes Nystatin. Once again, his initial response is very positive. Within a week, there is a recurrence of fatigue and related symptoms. More Nystatin prescriptions are followed by more antidepressant prescriptions. The energy roller coasters persist, each low becoming deeper than the preceding. He continues to waste away.

Deeply anguished and frightened, the parents take the frail body of what was once a well-sculpted figure to an out-of-state fatigue center. A comprehensive work-up this time includes a muscle biopsy that shows injured and split muscle fibers, overgrowth of mitochondria and some dead muscle fibers. A SPECT scan (Single Photon Emission Computed Tomography) shows diminished blood supply to the frontal and temporal lobes of the brain, and a PET scan (Positron Emission Tomography) reveals evidence for impaired glucose metabolism. Cortical evoked potential studies show abnormalities of P3 waveform and reduced amplitudes of some potentials. Many other tests for "biologic immune response modifiers" show evidence of damage to several different components of the immune system. Six months later, the young man is convinced that this "thing" is for life. The parents sadly begin to wonder if this is the end of the dreams they cherished for their son.

An unusual case history? A cheap, sensationalistic attempt at melodrama? Not for those who have suffered the unremitting agony of such devastating journeys. Not for those who will surely see part of their own heart-rending stories in it. All of us who care for chronic fatiguers carry thick clinical charts in our offices that tell and retell such sagas. (The preceding case history, in reality, is a composite of two case histories among my files — findings of SPECT and PET scans and cortical evoked potentials are those that have been described in chronic fatiguers.)

## PROMOTING POOR PROTOPLASM

A senior surgeon-colleague recently told me that he thought the number of children he saw with poor protoplasm had increased markedly during the brief period of his own surgical career.

Protoplasm is the soup of life that makes up each living being. I was introduced to the term "poor protoplasm" in my first year in medical school. This term was used by our teachers for people who were always getting sick — and, in doing so, frustrating their treating physicians. The idea behind this term, of course, was simple: Such individuals were constitutionally weak — genetically destined to be sickly. I didn't see it then, but this model of poor protoplasm comes in handy to us physicians in more than one way. It absolves us of any wrongdoing. Our medical science is sound. We do our part right. Our drugs do what they were designed to do. Now if someone still chooses to be sick, it's really his problem, isn't it?

We medical students learned this lesson well. Unlearning is much harder than learning, and nowhere — it seems to me — is it more so than in medicine. Unlearning is not written into the scripts we physicians follow when we leave medical schools for the "trenches" of clinical medicine. My surgeon friend has been out of medical school for over 30 years. Still, he cherishes the concept of poor protoplasm.

I asked the surgeon why he thought children have poor protoplasm more often than they used to. He shrugged his shoulders.

"Who knows? Maybe you do. I mean you're the one who writes about oxidized fats and denatured proteins and pollutants and increased oxidizing capacity of the planet Earth and the oxidant stress molecules." He chuckled.

My surgeon-colleague left out something important in his brief list of things: the part we physicians play in promoting poor protoplasm.

## HOW DRUG MEDICINE CREATES CANARIES

The prevailing mode of drug medicine creates canaries in two effective ways:

### First,

at the slightest prompting, it feeds little babies broad-spectrum antibiotics (translation: designer killer molecules that have broad powers to kill everything in sight and ruin the delicate bowel ecosystems) and older folks multiple drugs that slowly but most assuredly impair their life span enzymes.

## Second,

it actively withholds from the sick effective, nondrug nutritional and environmental therapies. Chronic fatigue is created by chronic neglect of essential health issues and by shortsighted drug therapies for health problems that can be effectively managed without drugs. It is not only environmental pollutants, poor nutrition and stress that are turning many people into canaries. The tools of drug medicine are contributing their fair share. This sad story does not end here. The champions of drug medicine ferociously harass a handful of holistic physicians who seek to promote health with natural therapies. It may seem a harsh criticism of my profession. But it is well deserved.

## A CLICHE' TELLS THE STORY

*If you treat a cold, it takes three weeks, if you don't it takes 21 days.*

Recently a visiting professor at a hospital conference spoke the above words and grinned broadly to communicate to us how good he felt about his discovery. His comments turned my thoughts to how rapidly human biology is undergoing profound changes as we relentlessly prescribe drugs in pursuit of the glorious dreams of Star Wars medicine.

Of course, we all remember the old cliche': If you treat a cold it takes a week, if you don't it takes seven days. Why did the cliche' change from seven days to 21? Those of us who seek to care for our patients with nondrug therapies know things have changed. Common colds that leave in their wake malaise, muscle aches and a hacking cough for weeks are not uncommon. Such colds not uncommonly turn into pneumonias.

Often I see another facet of this problem of prolonged recovery from common colds: Many chronic fatigue sufferers make painstakingly slow progress with nondrug nutritional, environmental and self-regulatory approach therapies. And then they come down with a cold that is treated with long courses of antibiotics. They nosedive and months of restorative work go down the drain.

The problems caused by the avalanche of oxidative stresses on human biology are very real, though most practitioners of drug medicine still believe them to be imaginary — not something that a little psychotherapy couldn't cure, as a physician powerful in state politics, recently put it.

## A LESSON NOT LEARNED FROM THE GULF WAR

During the Gulf War, many Kuwaiti oil fields went up in smoke — taking massive quantities of toxins with them. It was predictable that all those toxins would come down to the ground as the hot emissions cooled off. Soon after that, at a meeting of the American Academy of Environmental Medicine, none of us had any doubt about three things. First, that many people would

develop environmental sensitivities due to massive exposures —
both among the American servicemen and the native
Mideastern people. Second, that chronic disabling fatigue would
be an essential part of the clinical picture of those who were to
develop such sensitivities. Third, that this illness would be
denied — chalked up to the old all-in-the-head story — by
mainstream medicine as vigorously as it has denied
environmental illness among the civilians. This had to happen.
It was only a matter of time.

And so it did.

*"Congressman Steve Buyer (Indiana
Republican), 34, suffers from a strange,
debilitating illness that, according to the
Texas-based Operation Desert/DesertShield
Association has struck nearly 8,000 of his
fellow Desert Storm veterans. The malady,
for which doctors have not yet fully
identified a cause or cure, takes many forms,
including constant fatigue, memory loss,
blurred vision and, in cases like Buyer's,
chronic respiratory problems ... "*

*People* Magazine; August 30, 1993

*People* went on to report that the Congressman uses a
spray for asthma-like symptoms and carries two bottles of pills
from which he must take six doses of medication daily for sinus

and respiratory  problems.  Where did the Congressman's  malady
come from?  Does he suffer  from poor protoplasm?

> *"His wife, Joni, 35, knew something was*
> *terribly wrong. 'He was a person as strong*
> *as a horse,' she says. 'He was becoming*
> *sick every time I turned around.' ... 'I'm*
> *allergicto everythingthat's green—oak trees,*
> *grass and flowers. It's crazy,' says Buyer. "*

> *People* Magazine;  August  30, 1993

Why did Congressman  Steve Buyer  become  allergic  to
everything that was green?  What's so crazy about it?  Those of
us who practice  environmental  medicine  see  such  cases
everyday. We call it "spreading phenomenon"  — a sequence  of
events by which an environmentally-sensitive  person develops
new sensitivities  as his molecular  defenses  are shattered.

> *"This is a real illness that we don't*
> *understand, " says Maj. Gen. Ronald Blanck,*
> *commander of Walter Reed Army Medical*
> *Center in Washington. "But it's frustrating*
> *because we can't measure the damn thing. "*

> *People* Magazine;  August  30, 1993

Aha, if only we could measure something! Then we could invent a new disease name, and move on to develop a new drug to cure it.

## NUMERICALLY CORRECT!

We Americans, I wrote in *The Cortical Monkey and Healing,* are a numerical people. We love numbers. We cherish them. We live by them. We are sustained by them. When deprived of them, we crave them. We seek safety in numbers. Without our numerical crutches, we are vulnerable.

Modern medicine is a numbers game. Numbers tell us how to label our pain. Numbers define the magnitude of our suffering. Numbers give us our diagnostic labels. Numbers give us our treatment strategies. We conduct research with numbers. To generate numbers, we happily blind ourselves. When simple blinding will not do, we invent methods for "double-blinding" ourselves.

The numbers generated by Star Wars technology in our laboratories should serve as signposts; instead, we joyously submit ourselves to their servitude. In medical school classrooms, we insist that our students become physicians who *care* for the sick and not treat mere laboratory numbers; in clinical medicine, we worship at the altar of numbers. When challenged, we rise to defend our numbers. When no other defense holds up, we invoke defensive medicine, a medicine where the prey is not a patient but the physician, the predator is not a disease but a lawyer.

Why is General Blanck so frustrated? Why should he think fatigue in Gulf War veterans can be easier to understand than it is among civilians? But to General Blanck's credit, he refrained from inventing a new syndrome for Congressman Buyer's chronic fatigue. But then again, perhaps General Blanck and colleagues should learn something from us civilians.

In the third chapter — Lamppost Labels for Human Canaries — I include a long list of diagnostic labels — some more imaginative than others — that we physicians use for chronic fatigue states to hide our ignorance of the real issues. These are labels that we use as crutches as we seek to cure chronic fatigue states with drugs. Actually, I am surprised that "fatigue experts" in the Army have been so slow to come up with a disease label for what ails Congressman Buyer and the other 8,000 Gulf War veterans.

*Reliable sources now indicate that a secret electronic file exists listing 1,521 post-Gulf War veterans that have deceased primarily from congestive heart failure, and to a lesser extent, from cancer. Up till now, this alarming fact has been obscured from public view. ...*

*No tests have been developed to confirm the theory of chemical sensitivity because the VA is convinced the problem is caused by stress or something else, says Dr. Edward Young.*

*Clearly these are not centers of excellence, but centers of "setup," a staged medical charade to create the impression of quality work — how stupid does he think we are?*

Major Richard H. Haines
United States Army, quoted in
*The Environmental Physician* 27:14; 1993

Now let us see what the chronic fatigue experts have to say about the Gulf War veterans who suffer from environmentally induced symptoms.

*In the absence of any diagnosis, the condition has been dubbed 'Gulf War syndrome': a blanket term for one of several illnesses ... Nevertheless, military officials claim that they can attribute only 30 of the 6,000 reported cases of Gulf-War-related illness to chemical exposure. If chemicals were found to cause widespread illness among troops the implications would be enormous.*

*Nature* 364:659; 1993

This is an interesting bit of text from arguably the most prestigious science journal in the world. *Nature* quotes military officials who attribute 30 cases to chemical exposure. That means the military officials now concede that chemical exposure *can* cause illness. That means environmental illness *does* exist. At least we overcame that major hurdle. (I wonder what criteria those officials might have used to accept chemically induced illness in those 30 individuals.) If the chemical were found to cause widespread illness among troops, the journal admits the implication of that would be enormous. That "if" is, of course, the central issue in this matter. For physicians like me who practice environmental medicine, the issue of that "if" has been laid to rest by hundreds of thousands of people who suffer from chemical sensitivities. I see such patients every working day. And so do my colleagues in environmental medicine.

Why did the fourth student become so ill and remain so sick for such a long period of time despite all the glorious tools of Star Wars medicine? Why did the first student recover his infection without missing a day of school? Why did 8,000 Gulf War veterans come down with fatigue? Why did the remaining half a million Gulf War veterans not come down with fatigue? Why did some Gulf War veterans die of a "mysterious illness" while others didn't? Why did the canaries die? Why did the miners live?

## A MOMENTOUS DISCOVERY

Recently, someone discovered something of great importance. He realized people could be safer at home than in a hospital. Fascinating stuff! We understood this as medical students in Pakistan in the early 1960s.

*The result is a war in which humans using refrigerators, sanitation, boiled water, and antibiotics try to kill, starve, and subdue microbes. The microbes fight back by developing new pathways, new proteins, and new strategies for survival that are as ingenious as those devised by humans out to destroy them. It is a war involving millions of lives, causing pain and tragedy. One doctor, interviewed by this editor, said, "When these new drug-resistant strains become endemic in hospitals, you will be safer staying home than going to a hospital, unless you have a truly dread disease."*

*Science*  257:1021; 1992.

Safer at home than in hospitals! Such comments amuse me. Everyone recognizes the chemical risks we all face. And yet when "fatigue experts" of drug medicine lecture on how to treat chronic fatiguers, all they talk about is drugs. They never talk about environmental sensitivities or adverse food responses or allergies. I never hear one word about sugar-insulin-adrenaline roller coasters or about nutrition. Not one word about meditation. Not one word about slow, sustained exercise. Not one word about some spiritual dimensions. All these fatigue experts love to talk about is the Epstein-Barr virus and then they move on to extolling the virtues of their favored antidepressants for treating chronic fatigue.

## CDC DEFINES CHRONIC FATIGUE SYNDROME

Fatigue experts at the Centers for Disease Control, Atlanta, a government agency, have decreed that chronic fatigue syndrome must never be diagnosed if there exists an organic or psychiatric disorder that can explain chronic fatigue.

Government experts often demonstrate a rare streak for making frivolous propositions. Consider the irony of their proposal. They vehemently exclude from chronic fatigue syndrome all organic and psychiatric causes. It is as silly as saying that the chronic fatigue syndrome should not be diagnosed when the fatigue sufferer is either a male or a female. Or when the treating physician is a male and when she is a female. Or when the fatigue sufferer has dark skin and when he has light skin. Or when he is in the Armed Forces and when he is a civilian. Or when the sun is up and when it is down. If fatigue — in their blessed chronic fatigue syndrome — cannot be attributed to organic or psychiatric disorders, what else, may I ask, is there to cause fatigue? Where do they think diseases come from anyway?

## WAITING FOR GODOT

The CDC definition of chronic fatigue syndrome is eminently suited to those who believe drugs are the only legitimate therapies for all diseases. They are quite clear in their heads. They have named the syndrome. That means they now understand the problem. That also means that all that is required now is for some drug company to come up with a drug to cure this dreadful disorder. Waiting for another triumph of synthetic chemistry! Waiting for another miracle drug! Waiting for Godot!

## POLLUTION AND POPULATION GROWTH: THE DOUBLE JEOPARDY

What separates living beings from nonliving objects? The principal threat to life on planet Earth, I wrote in *The Butterfly and Life Span Nutrition*, is that our technology, with some exceptions, is systematically destroying life span enzymes of people and other life forms.

In 1945, the U.S. annual production of chemicals was 8 million tons. By 1985, it had risen to 110 million tons, or 950 pounds of chemicals for every United States citizen. Even the staunchest supporters of the all-in-the-head theory among physicians who ridicule chemically sensitive patients as people with overactive imaginations will have to accept that such massive chemical exposures must have some serious adverse effects on human biology. We cannot drink deeply from these rivers of toxins and not have the chemicals permeate our entire beings.

Global pollution is a much larger problem than is generally recognized. Many pollutants, like dioxins, have half-lives as long as 16 years. That means even after 32 years, 25% of the original amount of a toxin persists in the environment. A second — and equally distressing prospect — is the projected increase of world population from the present number of six and a half billion people to nearly 11 billion people by the year 2025. To feed such an enormous increase in the world population, the use of food technology will have to be increased severalfolds. And, of course, our food processing technology efficiently oxidizes and denatures our foods and destroys whatever live enzymes might exist in them. There are no answers here — except those that arise from the true understanding of biology. The irony is that we physicians who should be at the forefront of this fight are quite forceful in denying that these problems exist. We still embrace the all-in-the-head theory. We continue to believe that any illness that cannot be cured by drugs or surgery simply does not exist.

## HAVE YOU GOTTEN INTO TROUBLE YET?

Recently, a colleague met me at a conference of holistic physicians and said,

"You know, it's so disheartening. Every time I go to a meeting of nutritional medicine or environmental medicine, the first question people ask each other is whether they have gotten into trouble with their state licensing board yet."

"Yes, that's a bad problem," I agreed.

"Do you think it will change?" he followed.

"Yes, I think it will," I responded.

"Oh, well, you were always an optimist."

"Yes, that I am," I conceded.

"I don't see how you continue to be an optimist. Don't you hear the horror stories? Every time you come to a meeting, someone else you know is losing his license." He shook his head and walked away.

This is a time of change in medicine. And in times of

change, the majority opinion in medicine has been wrong more often than not. Some people holding the minority opinion always get destroyed. Their families suffer, often severely and for a long time. Their crime: They think differently. It has always been like this. It probably always will be so.

## WHAT IS MORE IMPORTANT: THE INVADERS OR HOST DEFENSES?

This is the central issue facing those who suffer from chronic fatigue and their caretakers. The battle lines are clearly drawn. On one side are physicians like me who are convinced that the true answer to this problem is in restoring normal energy enzyme pathways with nondrug therapies. On the opposite side are champions of drug medicine who are equally convinced it is simply a matter of time before some drug will arrive at the scene and cure chronic fatigue syndrome once and for all. We have our clinical outcome studies to buttress our case. The drug medicine folks are pregnant with the glorious promise of miracle drugs in the wings.

There is an irony in the battle between holistic medicine and mainstream drug medicine. Hippocrates, the father of medicine, believed in *physis* — the innate healing nature of the human body, and the origin of the word physician — and taught his pupils to look for answers to the problems of sickness in that inner healing capacity of injured tissues. If the injured tissues are allowed to heal, he taught his students, they will do so. Democratus, a contemporary of Hippocrates about 25,000 years ago, thought Hippocrates was nuts. The human body, he pronounced, was made up of tiny particles, which he called atoms. In his theory of *atomism*, sick organs were incapable of healing by themselves. He scorned Hippocrates for his theory of *vitalism*. The battle between atomism and vitalism has raged on in one form or another ever since.

## PASTEUR'S SHEEP AND MY CANARIES

When the French physicians ganged up on poor Pasteur, it marked but one episode in the long saga of a smug majority trying to stifle an enlightened minority of one.

If the French physicians had their way, they would have done to Pasteur what they used to do to criminals in that time: send him away to some distant penal colony to perish. But Pasteur's sheep came to his rescue.

The French gods of medicine in Pasteur's time were vitalists — Hippocrates' notion that diseases healed from within had taken a firm hold in 19th century France. They knew microbes existed within the body as they did in the soil outside. Leeuwenhoeck, the Dutch inventor, invented the microscope in 1719, and looked into the human stool for his initial studies of microbes. The French physicians, of course, knew this. However, they believed that these microbes simply coexisted with human tissues and had nothing to do with human disease. This may appear strange to us today but must have seemed very logical to them. How could microbes cause disease in some people but not in others? they exclaimed. How can environmental pollutants make some people sick and not others? Physicians in drug medicine indignantly ask today.

When Pasteur began to talk about his brand-new idea —
that microbes caused diseases — the French physicians took it
as an affront. What did this mere chemist know about human
diseases anyway? (Louis Pasteur, of course, was not a
physician.) In this, the physicians in the French Academy of
Science were no different from my colleagues in $N^2D^2$ medicine
today. Who are these clinical ecologists anyway? they scream in
dismay. Charlatans! Quacks! Men of dubious qualifications,
using tests of dubious value! If chemical sensitivity was a real
disease, why wouldn't the professors in their ivy league schools
discover that? If chronic fatigue was not an all-in-the-head
problem, why wouldn't our great researchers at the National
Institutes of Health define the disease? If formaldehyde did
cause environmental illness, why wouldn't the whiz kids in our
drug industry find a drug to cure it?

Pasteur's sheep saved him from the silly notions of the
French gods of medicine of his day. The human canaries —
chronic fatiguers of our time — will, I am sure, save us from the
tyranny of the maestros of $N^2D^2$ medicine in the same way.

Pasteur studied tissues of sheep infected with anthrax
bacilli with his microscope. He found large colonies of the
microbes in different tissues of sheep. When he examined
tissues of healthy control sheep, there were no microbial
colonies. He drew the obvious conclusion: Those bacilli were
causing the disease. It is amusing to look back and ask why the
gods of French medicine were so offended by such a simple,
logical conclusion. The story gets more interesting. Pasteur then
proceeded to develop a vaccine against the anthrax bacilli and
immunized healthy sheep against the disease. Here was a mere

chemist — as far as the physicians in the Academy of Science were concerned — who was trying to challenge their sacred dogma. The gods of French medicine were incensed. How dare he? In their rage, they threatened him with everything they could, much like the way our state licensing boards threaten to revoke the licenses of physicians who seek to reverse chronic fatigue without drugs. Pasteur challenged them. Secure in the anonymity of a large professional organization, the individual gods of French medicine accepted the challenge from this heretic.

The story of Pasteur's sheep is well known. In the evening, Pasteur injected two groups of sheep with Anthrax bacilli — one group had been previously immunized with his vaccine, the unimmunized group served as the control. The sheep were put in two separate compartments of a pen. Early next morning, Pasteur and his assistants approached the divided sheep pen from one side and the holy alliance of the gods of French medicine from the other. The immunized sheep were lying on the hay in one compartment and the control group of unimmunized sheep on the other. In the morning mist, there seemed to be no difference between the two groups of sheep. The gods were joyous. A heavy silence fell over Pasteur's group. Louis Pasteur was undaunted. He approached the control group of unimmunized sheep and poked them hard with his long walking stick. There was no movement. The sheep were dead. He then walked over to the immunized group and poked them equally hard. The sheep woke up frightened and ran around the pen. A tumultuous cry arose among the press core. Pasteur's sheep live! So ran the newspaper headlines. Cheap sensationalism! shouted back the unimpressed gods of French medicine.

There is a profound irony here. It took a long time before the medical profession accepted Pasteur's work. (Indeed, some old guards had to die out before the doubts about Pasteur's work in the general medical profession finally dissipated.) And now medicine is firmly — tenaciously and irretrievably for many of my colleagues — incarcerated in the double-blind, cross-over model of drug research. They continue to deny that illnesses such as chronic fatigue states can arise from battered host defenses. For these disciples of Democratus (and Pasteur), where there is no bug, there can be no disease. For the American gods of medicine, the simple concept that food reactions, mold allergy, toxic metal overload, battered bowel ecosystem, and the use of broad-spectrum antibiotics, immunosuppressants and other drugs can lead to chronic states of fatigue is as offensive as Pasteur's idea of microbes causing diseases was for the French gods of medicine.

Now — a century and a half after Pasteur — the gods of American medicine who claim to be Pasteur's disciples and who populate our medical schools and sit on state medical licensing boards think that real diseases can be treated only with drugs and surgical scalpels. Hence, their wrath against those who seek answers to chronic fatigue in Hippocrates' vitalism — in nutritional medicine, in environmental medicine and in medicine of self-regulation. Their venom against holistic physicians today isn't any less lethal than that of French doctors against Pasteur.

The sad truth is that the gods of American drug medicine today are no more enlightened about the real issues in chronic fatigue states than were the French gods of medicine in Pasteur's time. Our American gods of drug medicine know little, if any, about issues of *functional* nutritional deficiencies, adverse bowel responses to foods, battered bowel ecosystems, chemical sensitivities, delayed consequences of toxic metal overload, and the Fourth of July chemistry under the skin of chronic fatiguers. Those are the real issues in restoring normal energy pathways in chronic fatiguers. None of those issues are of any concern to the practitioners of drug medicine because none of them can be truly addressed with the miracles of our synthetic chemistry.

> *If Pasteur were alive today, I know his sheep would have told the same story that my canaries are telling.*

Many champions of drug medicine will snicker at my notions of holistic molecular relatedness in human biology and my canaries. They would want me to put my canaries in two compartments of some cage, too, so that I could follow their prescriptions of double-blinded, crossed-over research models. They would want me to feed one group of my canaries some kind of drug and the other sugar pills. They would insist on that kind of "proof." They do not understand that such a frivolous notion of proof is utterly irrelevant to holistic methods of caring, where the only thing that really matters is whether or not chronically tired people regain their normal energy patterns. From extensive clinical experience I know they do. And I know that from the experience of my colleagues in environmental and nutritional medicine.

Pasteur concentrated on one factor — the Anthrax bacillus — because his sheep were made sick by just that one single agent. I have to think differently for my canaries because my canaries are not made sick by just one thing. They are vulnerable in many ways. They are different from Pasteur's sheep. This the champions of $N^2D^2$ medicine do not comprehend.

## I AM OPTIMISTIC

This is my chance to answer my colleague who doesn't understand how anyone in holistic medicine can be optimistic today.

*Something wonderful happened —and a quiet grass-roots revolution in health care was officially recognized — last week on the sixth floor of government Building C in Bethesda.*

*The something wonderful was the atmosphere of respect and affection accorded to about 90 spokesmen for "unconventional therapies" invited to present their treatments to an unusually eclectic ad hoc panel convened by the National Institutes of Health. ...There is a generosity of spirit manifested here ...In the midst of the optimism and good will, however, was an undercurrent of anger and distrust. There were frequent mentions of unnamed individuals practicing controversial and allegedly successful therapies who didn't dare appear for fear of losing their licenses.*

*Washington Post* June 26, 1992.

I am a realist as well as a dreamer. Within months of this conference, the office of one well-known nutritionist was raided by authorities with drawn guns. They confiscated his supply of vitamins. Some months later, the license of another colleague was summarily suspended because one of his very sick patients developed a complication following an intravenous treatment. How many surgeons do I know whose licenses were suspended because one of their patients developed complications after surgery and died? Indeed, how many surgeons would have still retained their licenses if their licenses were revoked every time a surgical complication developed? Not one! I am sure of that. How many oncologists do I know whose licenses were revoked because the patient died as a result of their chemotherapy and not of his disease? It is not at all uncommon for patients to die of sepsis after their immune defenses have been totally destroyed with chemotherapy. How many internists would still have their licenses if their licenses were to be rescinded every time there was a complication caused by a drug prescribed by one of them?

Then there are times when practitioners of drug medicine turn on holistic doctors, and report them to state licensing boards. I know of physicians whose licenses were revoked because they treated their patients with nondrug therapies. The area practitioners of drug medicine banded together to put them out of business — and did exactly that. Many medical boards take the position that all nondrug, nonsurgical methods of treatment are unconventional, and hence punishable. The holistic physicians who use nondrug therapies have no defense against such tyranny.

Such are the burdens we holistic physicians carry! Such are the risks we take! If you think this is cheap melodrama, please go and listen to the wives of physicians who lost their licenses simply because they tried to care for their patients with nondrug therapies. I know, because I have listened to them. I know many families of holistic physicians that were destroyed by maestros of $N^2D^2$ medicine.

I am not optimistic because I have not witnessed the tyranny of drug medicine or the venom of its high priests. Or because I do not know their capacity for inflicting hurt upon those who choose to think differently. Or because I am not aware of how fiercely the state licensing boards protect the interests of $N^2D^2$ medicine. Or because I do not see the unfaltering devotion of the editorial boards of our medical journals to the double-blind, cross-over. Or because I have not experienced the disdain of disease doctors for those who do preventive medicine.

I am optimistic for different reasons.

*"We are incarcerated in the double-blind, cross-over model," said Majid Ali, a New Jersey pathologist whose clinical practice stresses nutrition, fitness and environmental therapy. "It is not appropriate for holistic therapy, in which there are many variables and neither the practitioner nor the patient can be blinded to treatment."*

*Washington Post*, June 23, 1992

I am an optimist because once we know something, we cannot unknow it. I am optimist because the truth cannot be suppressed forever. And the truth is that the gods of the double-blind, cross-over medicine are false gods. And their disciples who sit on the editorial boards of medical journals and consider all nondrug and nonsurgical therapies quackery are misguided. Their double-blind, cross-over research model is totally and utterly irrelevant to our work with chronic fatiguers. No matter how dictatorial and ruthless the state licensing boards become, holistic physicians are not going to abandon safe and effective nondrug therapies. And the truth is that chronic fatiguers are beginning to see it. They are beginning to see through the folly of hiding behind frivolous diagnostic labels. They are beginning to see through the yarn that practitioners of drug medicine weave for their benefit. They are beginning to see through the false promise of wonderful drugs that are touted to cure chronic fatigue — and only leave them sicker.

The truth is that chronic fatiguers are beginning to stay away from drug trials. They are shunning antiviral therapies that make them more toxic. They are rejecting those megabuck work-ups that only lead to prescriptions for antidepressants.

The truth is that an ever-growing number of chronic fatiguers are not waiting for Godot. By and large, they are looking for answers in their nutrition, environment, self-regulation and in some spiritual dimensions. And by and large, they are succeeding.

These are the reasons I am optimistic. There are yet others.

*Extrapolation to the U.S. population suggests that in 1990 Americans made an estimated 425 million visits to providers of unconventional therapy. This number exceeds the number of visits to all U.S. primary care physicians (388 million). Expenditures associated with the use of unconventional therapy in 1990 amounted to approximately $13.7 billion, three quarters of which ($10.3 billion) was paid out of pocket.*

*New England Journal of Medicine* 328:246; 1993

This is an eye-opening conclusion from a very large

study. It should remove any doubts in anybody's mind as to the preference of American people in health care. Indeed, they preferred nondrug therapies to drugs even when they had to pay for it twice, once as a premium for health insurance and the second time as fee for service. The United States is a democratic society. In a democratic society, the majority opinion determines what the standards are — and what they should be. If we hold as valid the principle of majority opinion, then it is quite evident from the above study what the majority of Americans want: nondrug therapies. Drug therapies must be considered as unconventional — not a bad idea at all, because there is nothing wrong with using unconventional therapies in unconventional (acute, life-threatening) diseases. The conventional health disorders — those caused by problems of nutrition, environment, stress and fitness — should be managed with conventional nondrug therapies.

*"Forget health care reform or reinventing government. The biggest volume of mail being logged in many Congressional offices these days calls on the lawmakers to block action by the Food and Drug Administration to ban the sale of vitamins and other dietary supplements. ... The Hatch-Richardson legislation would lower the new labeling standard to allow health claims for supplements supported only by unconfirmed preliminary studies not subjected to any meaningful scientific peer review ... The*

*fight, in other words, really isn't about keeping supplements on the shelves. It's about the right of unscrupulous companies and individuals to maximize profits by making fraudulent claims. "*

*The New York Times,* October 6, 1993.

This editorial by the *Times* surprises me. The *Times* usually speaks for citizen rights. Why does it choose to act differently in the matter of nutrients? First, it recognizes that Americans are much more interested in protecting their free access to nutrients than they are in Clinton's grandiose plans for revamping the entire healthcare system — in which he cannot succeed unless he makes preventive medicine the centerpiece of his strategy. Next, it moves to defend the regulatory restrictions on nutrients. The *Time's* words against free access to nutrients for Americans do not matter much to me. What is heartening for me is its recognition that Americans consider free access to nutrients more important than Clinton's plans. I continue to be optimistic.

## NIH REFERS A PATIENT TO A HOLISTIC DOC

Blasphemous! Delusive plausibility of an idealogue! Not

really.

Trudy L, a 41-year-old teacher, consulted me for a long list of complaints that included incapacitating chronic fatigue, weight loss, sinusitis, malaise, low-grade fever, skin rashes, daily headaches, arthralgia (joint pains,) myalgia (muscle pain,) neuritis (persistent pins and needles in limbs,) "increased sexuality," mood and memory difficulties and depression.

"I was a teacher. I have a double masters. I had the energy of a butterfly," she spoke fervently. "That was five years ago when I went to Central America. I returned with some kind of parasite. I have had 13 work-ups, with every blood test you can name, and X-rays including CAT scans, MRI scans. The MRI scan showed some bright spots in my brains. I went to Johns Hopkins and Hahnemann. The guy at Hopkins told me it was all depression and gave me a prescription for an antidepressant. The fellow from Hahnemann was honest. He said he really didn't know what my problem was."

I listened to the story. Nothing really new there for me. I thumbed through the heavy chart. In the end, I asked,

"How did you come here?"
"I was referred to you."
"By whom?"
"By NIH."
"NIH?" The words simply escaped my lips before I regained my composure.
"Yes! By NIH." She seemed to sense my surprise.
"That's interesting. Did you ever develop fatigue when you were a teenager?" I tried to change the subject.
"It wasn't easy finding you, Dr. Ali," she returned to the

subject of referral.

"Well! You're here now. Tell me if you suffered fatigue when you were a teenager."

"I wasn't ready to give up," she was intent on telling me more about her journey. "After Hopkins and Hahnemann, I was determined to find someone who could solve this puzzle. I want my life back. So I called NIH, and I called them and I called them. Finally someone there gave me your number."

When the NIH begins to refer patients to holistic physicians, there is hope. I am optimistic.

## CHRONIC FATIGUE IS A STATE OF ACCELERATED OXIDATIVE MOLECULAR DAMAGE

This, in my view, is the essential energetic-molecular basis of chronic fatigue syndrome. I discuss this subject at length and marshall several lines of evidence to support my viewpoint in the chapter, What Is Chronic Fatigue? that follows this brief introduction to the subject of chronic fatigue.

In essence, accelerated oxidative molecular injury to energy enzyme pathways has four causes: 1) nutritional factors, 2) environmental factors, 3) stress-related factors, and 4) factors related to lack of physical fitness.

In the fairly large number of patients I see with chronic fatigue, IgE-mediated mold allergy was present in almost all cases. A large majority of patients also showed adverse bowel responses to foods and tested positive for inhalant allergy. Allergic triggers produce symptoms by oxidant injury. Chronic fatiguers often show evidence of active multiplication of one or more viruses in their bodies. Viruses inflict molecular and cellular damage by oxidant injury. Many of my patients gave histories of extensive antibiotic use during years that preceded the onset of chronic fatigue. Antibiotics are designer killer molecules, even though they are essential for treating life-threatening infections. Nearly one quarter of chronic fatiguers accumulate toxic heavy metals such as aluminum, mercury and lead. Toxic metals act as potent oxidant molecules, both directly and indirectly, by damaging antioxidant enzyme defenses. Serious stressers often play a role in the onset of chronic fatigue. Adrenaline and its cousin stress molecules are some of the most potent oxidant molecules known to human biology. These are the factors that set us up for chronic fatigue and turn people into human canaries. None of these oxidant stresses can be reversed for long with drugs.

## CHRONIC FATIGUE IS PREVENTABLE

As I look back, I cannot remember a single patient who developed chronic fatigue right under my nose. Many of my patients, of course, have come down with acute flu, Epstein-Barr, herpes virus infections as well as other infections such as viral hepatitis and bacterial infections and other problems such as chemical exposure. Although fatigue was frequently a major symptom in such patients, we were able to pursue aggressive nutrient therapies, often with intravenous nutrient infusions, and to support them fully with other nondrug therapies. To date, undue tiredness and fatigue did not turn into chronic fatigue syndrome in any one of these individuals. I recognize that some day it might happen. The important issue is this: Fatigue simply is not a difficult problem to handle when allergies, environmental sensitivities, nutrition, self-regulation and physical fitness are addressed properly, and acute viral infections are managed successfully with effective nutrient protocols, i.e., with intravenous infusions if deemed necessary and without prolonged use of broad-spectrum antibiotics. Such patients overcame their infections and exposure within some days, and recovered their normal energy patterns. *Chronic fatigue is largely preventable.* This is the third core message of this book.

## CHRONIC FATIGUERS DO GET BETTER

The vast majority of chronic fatiguers get better with nondrug therapies within three to six months. *This is the fourth core message.* I relate several case histories to illustrate the patterns of chronic fatigue and associated symptoms that I encounter as a matter of course in my clinical work. I also include data obtained with several of my own clinical outcome studies.

A small number of physicians practice preventive medicine based on molecular and energy concepts of health and disease as outlined in this book. Their experience, in general, is similar to mine. Most people with chronic fatigue respond well to our nondrug nutritional, environmental and other therapies, and are able to regain most of their energy. The exceptions to this are some patients with devastating chemical sensitivity, very high levels of stress arising from extenuating personal life circumstances and very high blood levels of antibodies to Epstein-Barr virus and some other viruses. For optimal results, treatment strategies must be directed to reducing the oxidative stress in the chronic fatigue state with integrated, holistic management protocols.

## CARING FOR CHRONIC FATIGUERS: FOUR ESSENTIALS

From an energetic-molecular standpoint, chronic fatiguers are handicapped . The requirements for their healing processes are different. Others can get better in spite of drugs. Not so chronic fatiguers.

Increased oxidative stress that leads to chronic fatigue states comes from four sources:

1.   Oxidized, toxic and incompatible foods
2.   Environmental oxidants (including allergy and chemical sensitivity)
3.   Stress and stress-related elements
4.   Problems of physical fitness.

These are also the four essentials that must be targeted in the treatment of chronic fatigue. To these I want to add two other sequences of events that are linked to the accelerated oxidative injury that ultimately leads to chronic fatigue states:

1.   *Altered bowel ecology states.* The bowel ecosystem is often

battered in chronic fatiguers because of undiagnosed and unmanaged adverse food responses, mold allergy and yeast overgrowth, stress, and prolonged use of broad-spectrum antibiotics and other drug therapies. I discuss this subject at length in the companion volume *Battered Bowel Ecology — Waving Away A Wandering Wolf.*

2.   *Temperature dysregulation.* Chronic fatiguers are usually very sensitive to cold. There are two main causes for it: 1) injury to autonomic nervous system and 2) injury to thyroid enzymes — oxidative in nature in my view though not yet proven by actual studies — so that metabolically active hormones such as $T_3$ are not produced in a slow, sustained fashion from inactive (such as reverse $T_3$) or less active hormone precursors.

Nutritional support for people who suffer from chronic fatigue has four components: unoxidized foods in the kitchen, avoidance of incompatible foods, nutrition of oral nutrient therapies, and intravenous nutrient therapy in selected cases to "jump start" the cellular life span enzymes.

Environmental strategies focus on pollution-control measures at home and at work, immunotherapy for allergy, and restoration of altered states of bowel ecology.

Self-regulation, with effective methods for desired physiological responses in the body, is essential for good long-term results.

Exercise for chronic fatigue must be slow and sustained. The mind must not be allowed to overdrive the fatigued muscles. I have seen many cases in which dogged determination to pull out of fatigue with strenuous exercise produced disastrous results.

I cover each of these four areas at length in the chapters devoted to the reversal of chronic fatigue.

## DRUGS ARE POISONS THAT SOMETIMES HELP

A psychiatrist-colleague one day limped into my office at the hospital, leaning on a walking stick. He had lost considerable weight since I had seen him last and looked exhausted.

"What happened?" I asked with concern.

"The virus did it," he forced a smile.

"You have lost some weight. Haven't you?" I asked sympathetically.

"Yes, about 15 pounds."

"And you looked tired," I added.

"Tired! You can say that," he strained as he shifted his weight on the stick. "I was very tired to begin with. They put me on heavy doses of antidepressants that make fatigue worse."

"Why?" I asked, surprised.

"I suppose they thought an antidepressant would help. Or maybe they thought the whole thing was in my head and I was simply depressed."

"Did antidepressants help?"

"You really don't know what these psychiatric drugs do to you unless you happen to be the patient." The psychiatrist forced another smile. "The cholinergic side effects were terrible. So I stopped all drugs."

"Hopefully you'll get over it soon." I wished him well.

"I'll tell you something for your next book," he continued. "Drugs are poisons that sometimes help. I don't know who said that, but whoever it was knew something about drugs," he grinned, shifted on his stick and limped out.

He has made the first discovery that drugs do not work for chronic fatigue, I thought. Hopefully he will also make the second: that nondrug, natural therapies do work.

Drug therapies for chronic fatigue are becoming more common among practitioners of drug medicine. Drugs, in my judgment, have no valid place in the care of people suffering from chronic fatigue. Drugs work by blocking, impairing or inactivating enzymes. Almost all drugs increase oxidant stress on tissues. This is the reason why there are no drugs in the PDR that do not have any side effects.

The judicious short-term use of drugs, of course, may be necessary to manage health problems that are often associated with chronic fatigue. I return to this subject later.

## A NEW KIND OF MALADY
## A NEW KIND OF PHYSICIAN

Chronic fatigue will be the *dominant* chronic health disorder of the 21st century. Prophecy is an uncertain business. And perhaps more so in medicine than in any other field of endeavor. Yet, who among us has the wisdom to resist it? I am certain that the epidemic of chronic fatigue states that we witness now will continue to spread among our children, among our adults and among our elderly.

The pandemic of chronic fatigue will also, I am confident, expose the principal weakness of the prevailing mode of drug medicine: Ill-health caused by problems of nutrition, environment and stress cannot be managed with miracles of synthetic chemistry. I do not believe this realization will come from the academia. It will come from the people who suffer from chronic fatigue and who are drugged for short-term benefits and long-term ill health. As the pandemic of chronic fatigue continues to claim new victims in ever-increasing numbers, and as the false promise of drug therapies for fatigue is widely recognized, chronic fatiguers will learn about the real molecular dynamics of such energy, both in health and in states of chronic fatigue.

People who suffer unrelenting chronic fatigue quickly discover that drugs do not work. These people are now forcing their physicians to look beyond the false promise of drugs for a cure. They are learning — and more and more chronic fatiguers will as time passes — the true ·nature of chronic fatigue. They are looking beyond simplistic notions of Epstein-Barr infection, Lyme disease, yeast connection, intestinal dysbiosis, immune-depression syndrome and a host of other diagnostic labels favored by most physicians.

Chronic fatiguers are demanding that their physicians look for the answer to their problems in their *own* host defenses — their energetic-molecular defenses that normally preserve their energy enzyme pathways.

Chronic fatiguers in the future will seek out a different kind of physician — a new kind of physician who understands human biology and the impact of environmental agents on man's genetic makeup. He will be a physician with moral courage to defy the petty platitudes of drug doctors who sit on the state licensing boards and threaten to revoke his license. He will be a holistic physician, someone who understands the metabolism of nutrients, the chemistry of environment, the pathology of immune disorders, the physiology of exercise and the energy dynamics of self-regulation. He will be a new physician for new patterns of suffering. Two things will be important to him: first, the words the patient uses to describe his suffering; and second, the energetic-molecular events that cause that suffering and the natural means of reversing those events. He will have no use for the *scientific vigor* of drug researchers and their obsession with miracles of synthetic chemistry.

These four essential points cannot be stressed enough:

1. States of chronic fatigue are *preventable*.
2. States of chronic fatigue are *reversible*.
3. States of chronic fatigue are caused by *accelerated oxidative molecular injury*.
4. States of chronic fatigue can be managed and the normal energy enzyme pathways restored only through *nondrug therapies*.

Drugs — as necessary as they may be for symptom-suppression in acute distress — cannot be considered legitimate therapies to manage chronic fatigue states.

*Courage is resistance to fear, mastery of fear*
*— not  absence  of fear.*

Mark  Twain

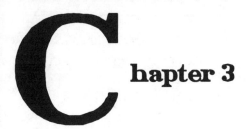

# **C**hapter 3

# Lamppost
# Labels
# for
# Chronic
# Fatigue

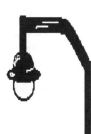

"What is chronic fatigue?" I asked Choua one day.

"Chronic fatigue is what people who suffer from it say it is," he answered absent-mindedly.

"And what is it that fatigue sufferers say it is?" I asked.

"Chronic fatigue is not what those who prescribe drugs for it say it is." Choua didn't answer my question. He put the journal down on the table, walked over to the window and looked out.

Choua had come to my office some minutes earlier. I was at my microscope signing out my surgical biopsies. He picked up a copy of the *P&S The Journal of the College of Physicians and Surgeons* that was on the top of a pile of journals, and was leafing through it when I asked my question. We were silent for some moments. I returned to my microscope. He replaced the journal.

"How is your fatigue book coming?" Choua broke the silence without turning away from the window.

"I try to work at it whenever I can find some time. You know how it is with my schedule," I answered without looking up from the microscope.

Some more minutes passed. Choua walked back, picked up the journal again and started reading. We were silent again. I leaned back from my scope and looked out. It was a clear day, with some thin clouds on the distant horizon. Choua walked back to the window and stared into the sky. When Choua stares into the sky, I learned a long time ago, it isn't very useful to try to pull him back into the conversation. I returned to my scope.

"I want to tell you a story," Choua's voice broke the silence. I looked up from my scope, put the slide back into the slide tray and leaned back on my chair.

"Go ahead, Choua. Tell me the story," I said.

## THE MAN AND HIS LAMPPOST

A man was searching for something at night under a lamppost at a street corner. A passerby looked at the man, stopped, looked at the ground, and asked, "What are you searching for?"

"My money," the man answered.

"Did you drop your coins?" the passerby asked.

"Yes."

"Do you want me to help you look for them?" the passerby volunteered.

"Oh yes! Please do," the man answered.

The passerby stooped low and began searching for the missing coins. Minutes passed, but he found no coins. Finally he stood up and asked, "Where do you think you dropped the coins?"

"There!" The man pointed to a dark area near the middle of the street.

"What?" the passerby's voice rose as his whole body stiffened.

"There," the man pointed to the dark middle part of the street again, without blinking his eyes.

"Are you crazy or what?" the passerby nearly screamed at the man.

"I am not crazy. I am searching for my coins," the man

replied evenly.

"You must be crazy! Why did you make me break my back combing through the dirt here at the street corner when you knew you dropped your coins there in the middle of the street?" the passerby asked in disgust.

"Because it is dark over there. Here, there is light under the lamppost," the man answered matter-of-factly.

Choua finished his story and, without waiting for my response, briskly walked out. That was not unusual for Choua. He often simply walks in, speaks about whatever happens to be on his mind, without ever worrying about what he might be interrupting. Choua's story was an old story. I first heard it from my father when I was a young boy. I saw Choua disappear into the hallway and wondered what might have brought that about. Choua sometimes talks cryptically and leaves the subject abruptly, without bothering to see if he has made his point or not. He then returns sometime later to add to his monologue — and sometimes to simply reverse himself. I don't mind his unannounced visits or his interrupted manner of speech. I guess it gives me freedom to ignore him whenever I want to. Sometimes we engage in two divergent conversations — he with what excites him, I with what interests me. It seems to work well for both of us, at least most of the time.

"You physicians are masters of the art of clouding common language," Choua returned the next day. "It is your treasured legacy from your ancestors of antiquity — the men of spirits who later turned into men of medicine. It becomes an especially high-art form when you confront patients who refuse to conform to your textbook models of diseases. Challenge to your sacred beliefs brings out your most creative impulses."

"Is that the continuation of the lamppost story?" I asked with good humor.

Choua walked over to the window as if he hadn't heard my question, looked out and fell silent. I sensed that beneath his outward calm was some passionate monologue. For several minutes, I waited for it to come out, but he kept quiet. I returned to my paperwork. Choua's presence was distracting. I thought about the subject of the clouding of common English in clinical medicine.

## WE DO NOT UNDERSTAND THINGS JUST BECAUSE WE NAME THEM

During my early days in the clinical wards in Pakistan, conducting morning rounds was a ritual that early Egyptian Pharaohs would not have scoffed at. It was a grand procession, with the professor at the head, assistant professors walking dutifully behind him, and a horde of medical students — their unquestioning disciples — in their tow. When the procession stopped at the head of a bed, the disciples descended upon the poor patient the way I have seen vultures swoon over a carcass. Then we played. We all played the game of words. The purpose: Excel in choosing words that the patient couldn't decipher. The explicitly stated goal was not to let the patient in on what was being discussed. (Patients were regarded incapable of understanding what ailed them.)

"Listen to this!" Choua's voice brought me back from my thoughts. "This is an interesting piece." Choua picked up the copy of *P&S The Journal of the College of Physicians and Surgeons* again and read something there. "This is page 46, volume 13, 1993." Choua looked up from the page, and then started reading again,

> *"Presenting a case could be very traumatic for a lowly student. Case presentations were all at the foot of the patient's bed within his or her earshot, and for this reason complex medical terms were often used for simple conditions, frequently leaving the patient with a bewildered look. We students gloried in the ability to obfuscate ordinary English."*

"Interesting! Isn't it?" Choua asked as he put the *Journal* back and looked at me with anticipation.

"Every profession does that, Choua," I said, without really wanting to defend the prevailing medical terminology.

"How different are things for most medical students today?" Choua asked.

"Not much, I guess."

"How different are they for you now?"

"Different! Very different! You see ..." I replied.

"I know," Choua interrupted me, "I see how you care for your patients. I see how you spend long hours turning meaningless medical jargon into ordinary English so your patients can understand what ails them — in the sense of molecular events, the energy events."

"Do I detect a sarcastic note there, Choua?" I smiled a little.

"No! To each his own. You and your oxygen thing! I have no problems with it," Choua replied flatly.

"This thing about spontaneity of oxidation and molecular duality of oxygen bothers you, doesn't it?" I teased him.

"Will it change?" Choua sidestepped my question.

"Will what change? My ideas about aging-oxidant molecules?"

"No. I am talking about your obfuscated language in medicine," Choua spoke with mild irritation. "Will you physicians ever give up your silly rituals of language?"

"Probably."

"When?"

"Who knows?" I answered with detachment.

"It *will* happen." Choua spoke emphatically. "But it will not happen because you will see the absurdity of it all. It will happen because it will be forced upon you. More and more people are rejecting your *obfussss ... cated* language." Choua minced the word with obvious relish.

"Things are changing." I ignored his word-mincing.

"People read and learn about such matters. They are on to you guys, the meaningless diagnostic labels and empty technical jargon."

"It will take time," I said lamely.

"Well-informed folks are not content with mere diagnostic labels," Choua continued. "People read about the health disorders they suffer from and reflect upon matters of health and diseases. There will be a new class of physicians who will not hide behind diagnostic labels."

"You are the prophet, Choua!" I said sarcastically.

"I have no doubt things will change." Choua ignored the

obvious sarcasm in my voice. "People cannot *unknow* what they once know. Those are *your* words, remember!" Now it was Choua's turn to be sarcastic.

"I know! I know what I wrote," I said in a plaintive tone.

"Enlightened patients simply will not put up with technical jargon that tells nothing but hides much. Molecular thinking — *your* molecular thinking — will free people from the tyranny of medical jargon."

"So what else did you read in the monkey book?" I asked, trying to put up a pretense of irritation.

"The physician of the future will not be into technical jargon. He will be liberated from the suffocating sterility of $N^2D^2$ medicine."

"You know about such things, Choua. At last you are back to your own stuff," I added.

$N^2D^2$ medicine is Choua's favorite expression for the prevailing mode of drug medicine in the United States. I generally do not mind Choua's caustic expressions about physicians. He is a good friend. It's just that he is not always polite in making his assertions.

"So we are back to $N^2D^2$ medicine, are we?" I smiled at Choua.

Choua was silent again. I returned to my paperwork. After several minutes, he spoke again. "Things will change," he began again. "They have to. Two factors will be important in the medicine of the future.

*First, the words that the patient will use to describe his suffering.*

*Second, the energetic-molecular events that cause that suffering. "*

"Today is a day for prophesy, is it?" I looked at Choua, putting my papers back on my desk.

"In the management of chronic health disorders," Choua resumed in earnest, "the names of chronic diseases, as you use them today, will become obsolete. The way you doctors editorialize your patients' words will become irrelevant. This change may seem farfetched and improbable to some, but it is a reality for some people now.

"You call the prevailing drug medicine a tail-end medicine because it bases its diagnostic classifications and therapies on what you see in injured tissues *after* they have been injured. Is anyone listening? You say molecular medicine seeks to address the front-end events — events that initiate disease. That's your front-end medicine. Is anyone listening? You sit here and ..."

"Choua! I thought you were making a prophesy about things that were going to change. What happened? You just changed horses in the middle of the race," I tried to interrupt him.

"Your $N^2D^2$ medical thinking is really nineteenth-century thinking," Choua continued. "You are bringing your nineteenth-century ideas to the problems of the twenty-first century. You look for answers under the lamppost."

"Choua, I don't know what you are saying. One minute you are sure everything will change. And the next, no one is listening to me. Make up your mind, will you?"

Choua looked at me, puzzled, as if trying to figure out whether I was annoyed because I didn't understand what he had said or because I did. We looked at each other for a while, and then he walked out without saying a word. I knew he was not finished. Perhaps he will never be finished with his $N^2D^2$ medicine, I wondered.

## CHRONIC FATIGUE: LOOKING UNDER THE LAMPPOST

People who suffer from chronic fatigue describe their suffering in many ways. Physicians who treat chronic fatigue with drugs use many names for it. Choua is right. There is little in common between the two groups.

Physicians who have written about chronic fatigue have been a creative lot. When we do not understand what ails our patients, we are usually quite ingenious in expressing our ideas — or to be more precise, lack of ideas — in artful language. We physicians are quite good at cloaking our ignorance in elegant but hollow medical terminology.

For chronic fatigue, there is a large menu of terms to suit all tastes: There are terms that say absolutely nothing. There are terms that reflect the writer's preoccupation with one or the other causative factors. Some other terms seek to express uncertainty about the nature of this disorder. Some terms are quite sympathetic to those afflicted by debilitating fatigue. Then there are other terms that are sufficiently insulting to boil the blood of anyone who suffers with chronic fatigue. Most of these terms reflect our desperate attempts to legitimize this disabling lack of energy into a medically acceptable — and *reimbursable* — diagnostic code.

"In the case of chronic fatigue," Choua once said, "it is not a case of one man looking for his lost coins under the lamppost. It is the whole medical profession searching for the answer to a pervasive problem with drugs — searching under a lamppost."

When will chronic fatiguers understand how they lose the power of their energy enzymes. And the efficiency of their detoxification enzymes? When will we physicians stop searching for solutions to the problems of damaged enzymes in drugs that further damage the enzymes? When will we abandon our silly pursuits of solving problems caused by chemicals by prescribing yet more toxic chemicals as drugs? Choua makes a point about his lamppost thing. When will we physicians catch up to him?

## YUPPIE SYNDROME

Yuppie syndrome is a diagnostic label for chronic fatigue that many practitioners of drug medicine adore. I suppose they feel it relieves them of any responsibility to help these people.

This is how some of my patients who were told they suffer from yuppie plague (syndrome) described their problems:

"I am moving on fumes. It seems there is no fuel left there."

"I feel someone has unplugged me."

"I go to bed exhausted, I leave my bed exhausted."

"It is as if all my energy drains into my pillow, my head feels stuck to it. I can't lift my head off the pillow."

"I feel like I am nine-and-half-months pregnant at four o clock in the afternoon all the time."

"I was so energetic. Varsity basketball and all. Now I can barely go to the grocery store."

*************

"I am paper perfect," a young man once told me.

"How do you mean?" I asked.

"I am perfect on paper," he replied.

"What does that mean?" I knew what he meant but asked him anyway.

"I am not anything but tired. I wake up more tired than when I go to sleep. But I am perfect. At least that's what lab tests and scans tell my doctors." He tried to force a smile.

## CHRONIC FATIGUE: A CREATION OF THE MEDIA

By the early 1980s, the problem of chronic fatigue had become so pervasive among the baby boomers that it was thought to be a price one had to pay to be counted among them. Others thought chronic fatigue was an imagined disorder among this overprivileged generation. It is fascinating how many physicians cope with clinical problems they do not understand. An obstetrician I know thinks chronic fatigue among young women is a creation of the media. "My women patients have always been tired," he told me condescendingly once, "but then we never let them celebrate their fatigue."

I do not know who came up with the diagnostic term of yuppie syndrome. Nor do I understand what great insights into human biology led that someone to propose such a meaningless term. It seems safe to deduce from the words that it has something to do with chronic fatigue experienced by young men and women who are considered overprivileged, overindulged and underworked. I suspect the inventor of this diagnosis believed that what these young people think is fatigue is what ordinary mortals know as work.

## SHIRKER'S SYNDROME

Sometime after the label yuppie syndrome became a legitimate medical diagnosis, a problem arose: What do we do when "non-yuppies" complain of chronic disabling fatigue? Some brilliant diagnostician rose to the occasion. He introduced the term "shirker's syndrome." Why not be succinct and clear? If someone shirks work, why not call him a shirker? And why not call the syndrome the shirker's syndrome? Why not call a spade a spade?

The term shirker's syndrome is clearly pejorative — unless of course, the physician using it definitely knows everything there is to know in matters of health, energy and disease, and he is certain that the patient is a liar beyond any shadow of a doubt. Of course, such a claim would be considered ludicrous among all people except among those physicians who use it — and the lawyers on the payroll of some insurance companies who create great legal doctrines out of the words physicians use in their "official" medical reports.

Here is what John, a brilliant financial analyst whose career was abruptly truncated by the condition, who suffered from shirker's syndrome told me:

"I didn't apply for disability all these years in the hopes that I was going to pull out of this thing. I guess I didn't want to because of the stigma of disability."

**************

"My doctor told me I should be grateful. I asked him why. He answered me by saying because my tests were all okay. If that was so, I asked, why was I exhausted all the time?"

"What did he say?" I asked.

"He shrugged his shoulders and made a face."

"And then?"

"And then he wrote me a slip and referred me to another doctor."

"And what did the consultant say?"

"He saw me and ordered a ton of lab tests. In the end, he, too, told me there was no reason for me to be exhausted all the time, and that I should get involved in something, anything."

Here are some more comments from some other shirkers:

"I am not the person I used to be."

\*\*\*\*\*\*\*\*\*\*\*

"I am angry but I don't know why. Maybe I am angry because there are so many things I have to do. And I know I can't if this thing keeps up."

\*\*\*\*\*\*\*\*\*\*\*

"I was drunky, disoriented, groggy, stumbly. I felt like I had a cold in my head all the time."

\*\*\*\*\*\*\*\*\*\*\*

"Oh, I like working, but I just do not have the energy I used to have."

\*\*\*\*\*\*\*\*\*\*\*

And the words of a reformed shirker three months after treatment:

"It's wonderful to wake up in the morning and feel good."

\*\*\*\*\*\*\*\*\*\*\*

I sometimes wonder why shirkers become reformed. Here is what one of them told me recently:

"When I first saw you, I couldn't touch my own arms and legs. I wouldn't let my husband touch them. They used to be so sore."

"And now?"

"Now they feel fine. You know I went back to work two weeks ago. It's part-time, but it's something."

Sometimes, I wonder what my colleagues think of this phenomenon of a shirker's reforming herself. When these people get better with nondrug therapies and resume work, it seems to confirm for some physicians that they were not sick in the first place — i.e., if people can get sick-all-in-the head, why can't they get better all-in-the-head? A patient solved this mystery for me.

"Dr. Ali, when I told my family doctor I was doing well after all those months of fatigue and all those lab tests with negative results, he smiled — a condescending sort of smile. I kept quiet, but I swear I knew what he would have said," she smiled at me.

"What would he have said?" I asked.

"It was obvious," she replied.

"What was obvious?" I persisted.

"He would have said that it proved the point."

"Proved what point?"

"Proved the point that there had been nothing wrong with me to begin with. That my fatigue was a pretense. A way of getting out of work."

"You mean any problems that can be resolved without drugs are not real problems?"

"That's it. That's the whole point." She grinned broadly.

## ALL-IN-THE-HEAD  SYNDROME

"My internist said it was the old all-in-my-head thing. No, he didn't use those words — his medical terminology was quite elegant, but that was what he really he meant."

A young chronic fatiguer

**********

"I was a vibrant health nut until five years ago when I went to Central America. Ever since, I have been getting sicker and sicker. Now I am disabled and drug-dependent. I go from severe fatigue to hyperactivity of nerves and back to fatigue again. I have had all these tests done (she waved a thick pile of reports at me with undisguised hostility) and I am not better."

**********

"I have done the gynecologist. I have done the dermatologist. I have done the allergist. After a while you begin to doubt your sanity."

**********

All-in-the-head syndrome has some interesting aspects. Here is a conversation I had with one of my patients:

"Dr. Ali, the first allergy shot was awful," he said.
"What happened?" I asked.
"It threw me right into deep fatigue," he answered.
"And the next one?" I followed.
"Wasn't so bad."
"And the one that followed?"
"It got better. Maybe a little itching and redness but no fatigue."
"And the next one."
"It was okay from then on."

I wondered about this patient's story. Why would the first allergy injection intensify his all-in-the-head fatigue and the second only moderately so? And why did the subsequent injections not worsen his fatigue? In my experience, all "all-in-the-headers" give clear, undeniable clues to the true nature of their suffering, however, we must take the time to listen to them.

************

Here is another example of a clue given to me by a patient during a follow-up visit nine weeks after I started caring for him: "My arms feel like my arms again. But the allergy symptoms haven't changed much." Why did the arms of this all-in-the-header get better in nine weeks? Why didn't his allergy symptoms improve in that nine-week period? Funny people, these all-in-the-headers!

Choua walked into my office some days later, picked up a draft of this chapter and read a few lines.
"You doctors don't use this all-in-the-head label very often these days, do you?" Choua spoke. "I guess people are on

to you."

"Yeah! It has had so much press of late that we physicians now generally shy away from it," I admitted.

"It used to be a safe diagnosis, wasn't it? I mean among you doctors, it was a nice way of answering awkward questions."

"It had its days."

"You fellows also loved that supratentorial thing. I don't hear that one anymore." Choua smiled a little.

Choua was right. Until some years ago, the all-in-the-head label was a convenient medical term we relied on to disguise our ignorance of the true nature of a clinical problem we didn't understand. The term was especially useful when the patient had the courage to challenge our expertise or judgment. Extratentorial! we would say to each other. Tentorium cerebri is a sheathlike structure in the skull that separates the thinking, cortical brain from what we believe is a subcortical, nonthinking brain. The term supratentorial was absolutely safe. It gave the patient no clues whatsoever, and yet enabled physicians to get the message across to each other comfortably, and in seemingly elegant medical language.

"All-the-head in a way does have some meaning," Choua's voice broke the silence.

"What's that?" I asked.

"Since the centers for perception of fatigue are located in the head, the all-in-the-head label is actually quite factual. It would have been different if ..."Choua stopped in midsentence. He often does that.

"If what?" I asked.

"It would have been different if your centers for perception for chronic fatigue were situated in your big toes," he completed his sentence somberly.

"All-in-the-big-toe! Is that what you have in your mind?" I suppressed a smile.

"Something like that."

"You know how science moves, Choua. Science corrects itself, but sometimes it is a slow process," I offered.

"Science moves slowly!" Choua frowned. "You doctors are some scientists."

## NEURASTHENIA

It's easy to put things into the medical literature. It is extremely hard to take them out when they become obsolete or irrelevant.

Beard, a New York physician, popularized the term "neurasthenia" at the turn of this century. He was a neurologist and his choice of this diagnostic term reflects his intellectual bias. His neurasthenia became a popular diagnosis, and the role of weakness of "nerves" became the prevailing "cause." Beard seemed to have an intuitive sense about the problem. He believed that neurasthenia and associated fatigue — chronic fatigue in our terminology — was caused by the "fatiguing" influence of life in industrial America.

Historically, we physicians are slow to accept new ideas. Beard was a prolific writer and he managed to get his diagnostic label accepted — by the sheer strength of the number of words he put together about his diagnostic entity, it seems. Once we do accept a diagnostic label, we adhere to it tenaciously. So it happened with Beard's neurasthenia. It became an integral part of our sacred diagnostic repertoire.

Here is how some of my patients defined it:

"Fatigue hits me everywhere — in my arms, in my legs, in my neck. Doc, you may think I am going nuts, but the worst thing is when it hits me in my brain."

"A lot of things are going on. I wonder if it is all in my nerves."

"I end up taking naps all the time. Actually, it's more than that. I'm dysfunctional all the time."

We have come a long way since Beard's time. Now we have a fairly good understanding of Beard's "fatiguing" influence of civilization. The basic chemistry of life was not as well understood in Beard's time as it is now. I have no doubt in my mind that what Beard designated as the fatiguing influence of civilization was nothing but increasing oxidant stress, regardless of what the chemical origin of it might be.

## THE DEPRESSION-FATIGUE SYNDROME

Nowhere is the fundamental difference between the treatment approaches of drug medicine and the management philosophy of molecular medicine — as I define here, and in greater detail in *The Ghoraa and Limbic Exercise* — more clearly discerned than when it comes to the so-called depression-fatigue syndrome. It is not critically important whether or not there is a history of depression before the onset of chronic fatigue. First,

I quote some of my patients on this subject:

"My doctor gave me Elavil. I told him I was very tired all the time. 'No, you are depressed.' He smiled knowingly and handed me the prescription."

**********

"I'm not the kind of person who gets depressed. I told my doctor."
"What did he say?" I asked.
"No, you are depressed," he said firmly.

**********

"I asked him why he was giving me Prozac. He replied that it was to prevent depression likely to be caused by the chronic fatigue syndrome."

**********

How can anyone robbed of his natural energy state not become depressed? How can anyone move from a state of energy and vigor to being incarcerated in his house with debilitating fatigue and not be deeply troubled by it? Diseases do not simply arrive from nowhere.

*Merely giving antidepressants for chronic fatigue is intellectual bankruptcy, pure and simple. And it doesn't matter what great gurus of $N^2D^2$ medicine say about it.*

Clearly, antidepressants have a place in the management of chronic fatigue. Of course, it is *never* the real treatment for this disorder. Antidepressants cause fatigue as a major side-effect. Furthermore, such drugs work by blocking certain enzymes or impairing normal neurotransmitter functions in other ways. As much as they are useful for temporary symptom-suppression, they will only compound the problems over the long haul. I describe many of the major disadvantages of drug therapies for chronic fatigue later in the chapter On Restoration Normal Energy Patterns. Worst of all, prescriptions of antidepressants rob the patient of valuable time that must be devoted to the nutritional, environmental and stress-related issues that create massive overload of aging-oxidant molecules. What is required is a holistic approach that is not designed to merely suppress symptoms.

On a positive note, most patients who suffer from chronic fatigue read about such matters and do become enlightened about the real causes of chronic fatigue. They reject antidepressants when they are offered to them as "treatment" for chronic fatigue. At least this is true of almost all of my patients. Chronic fatigue, I wrote earlier, will be the dominant chronic health disorder of the 21st century, and drugs are not going to work for it. Sufferers of chronic fatigue will have no choice but to read up and find the path, no matter how slowly, to restoring their energy patterns. It will become harder and harder for the practitioners of drug medicine to simply dole out prescriptions for antidepressants.

## HYPOTHYROID-FATIGUE   SYNDROME

Hypothyroidism — underactive thyroid in common language — is generally considered as the common cause of chronic fatigue. During the years of my work in tail-end medicine as a pathologist, I accepted the prevailing dogma that hypothyroidism is a disorder of unknown cause — what Choua would call a lamppost diagnosis. My perspective on all diseases in molecular medicine is different, and hypothyroidism is no exception.

The thyroid gland regulates body temperature. Since the functions of energy enzymes are dependent upon the body temperature, this gland is intricately involved in energy status. The evidence for underactive thyroid is usually easy to find in patients with chronic fatigue if only we look for it. In my experience, the common mistake in this area is this: We dismiss the possibility of underactive thyroid status when the laboratory tests come back negative. In many such instances, a two- to three-day record of body temperature clearly reveals temperature dysregulation. The final proof of this comes from clinical benefits that such patients receive from low-dose thyroid replacement therapy.

Thyroid gland dysfunction can cause fatigue, and I am careful in evaluating thyroid function for every single patient who consults me for chronic fatigue. I want to emphasize that in my clinical experience, thyroid disorders rarely are the primary causes of chronic, persistent, disabling fatigue.

What are the energetic-molecular basis of hypothyroidism? What causes the thyroid gland to slow down and add to the problem of low energy? In my view, there are three principle reasons for this:

## First,

many viruses and other microbial agents are known to cause inflammation of the gland that eventually leads to thyroid damage and funtional impairment.

## Second,

injury to thyroid hormone receptors in tissues caused by certain molecules belonging to dioxins, DDT and related families of chemicals. These molecules are structurally very similar to thyroid hormones, and hormone receptors are "blocked" by them, so excluding thyroid hormones.

## Third,

excessive oxidative damage to de-iodinases — and possibly other enzymes that convert metabolically inactive thyroid pro-hormones to active thyroid hormones.

I propose the last element as a hypothesis, but it is my strong sense that future research will fully validate it. Oxidant injury can be predicted to damage de-iodinase enzymes that convert inactive thyroid hormone precursors into active hormones — as well as convert $T_4$ hormone to metabolically much more active $T_3$ hormone. The concept of oxidative injury to thyroid enzymes is entirely consistent with oxidative injury to several other enzyme systems that are inactivated or destroyed by oxyradicals.

## DIOXINS IN MOTHER'S MILK INJURE INFANT'S THYROID GLAND

As for thyroid toxicity of chemicals, Dutch researchers investigated the effects of dioxins present in the mother's milk fat on the thyroid gland function of 38 breast-fed infants. The study showed how dioxins in the breast milk cause thyroid dysregulation. Blood levels of the thyroid stimulating hormone of the pituatry gland (TSH) were higher in group of infants fed breast milk containing higher concentrations of dioxins than those given milk with lower levels (Pluim *et al. Environ Health Perspectives* 101:504; 1993). Dioxins and related chemicals, furans, block thyroid hormone receptors in cells (Environ Health Perspectives 1989;82:323-336.)

How do dioxins and furans cause thyroid dysregulation? Because of their structural similarity with $T_4$ hormone, these chemicals can be expected to: 1) block $T_4$ receptors; 2) impair entry of $T_4$ into cells; 3) interfere with conversion of metabolically less active $T_4$ to metabolically more active $T_3$ hormone; 4) impede binding of $T_3$ to nuclear receptor; and 5) increase TSH production in the pituatry gland by reducing nuclear $T_3$ receptor occupancy in the gland.

The use of DDT was banned in the United States over 20 years, but it is still manufactured by U.S. companies for export to Third-World countries. It is also produced as a byproduct —up to 10%—of manufacture of other pesticides such as trichlorophenoxyacetic acid. A part of DDT that we export to Third-World countries comes back to us as fumigant on fruits and vegetables that we import from them.

Sometimes I see physicians prescribing large doses of thyroid hormones to treat chronic fatigue syndrome, clearly a poor strategy. I quote a patient: "My doctor kept increasing the dose of synthyroid. My hands and feet were like a furnace and my heart was racing, but I was still very tired."

## LYME DISEASE

There is no question that Lyme disease can cause chronic fatigue. In my clinical experience, however, this has been a very rare occurrence and happens mostly when people with Lyme disease are loaded up with potent (and toxic) antibiotics in the absence of restorative therapies.

An interesting aspect of this problem is best illustrated by the following conversation that a patient had with a Lyme disease specialist before she consulted me:

"Do I have Lyme disease?" she asked.
"Yes!" the specialist asserted.
"Are the tests positive."
"No!"
"If all the tests are negative, how do you know I have Lyme disease?"

"The tests are not reliable."
"How accurate are they?"
"At best, less than fifty percent of the time."
"Then how do you diagnose Lyme disease?"
"By my clinical judgment."

Here is how my conversation with her went:

"Did you have food sensitivity tests done?" I asked.
"No!" she replied.
"And mold allergy tests?"
"No!"
"And pollen and dust?"
"No!"
"Toxic metal tests?"
"No!"
"Did you fill out any questionnaire about environmental sensitivities?"
"No!"
"About stress-related factors?"
"No!"
"Past history of antibiotic therapy?"
"No!"
"Past episodes of fatigue?"
"No!"
"Past episodes of severe viral illnesses?"
"No!"

How does a Lyme disease specialist go about diagnosing Lyme disease when Lyme disease tests are negative and when he does not perform any of the tests that might give him some clues as to the nature of the true problem? I wondered about this as I sat listening to her tell me about several important events that took place before she developed chronic fatigue for which the diagnosis of Lyme disease was made and heavy doses of antibiotics prescribed.

Here are some illuminating quotes from the August 24, 1993, issue of *The New York Times:*

*"I'm concerned that there are people who are marketing very long courses of antibiotics to treat Lyme disease without a good prospective study, and I am very concerned about profiteering," said Dr. Klempner. Hoffman-Roche Inc, the maker of ceftriaxone, an intravenous drug marketed as Rocephin that is commonly used to treat advanced Lyme disease, has underwritten teaching videos about Lyme disease, featuring doctors who believe in extended treatment ... On the other hand, some of the doctors who advocate only limited treatment have become consultants to insurers.* This is a terrible area, and people are being treated with prolonged courses of antibiotics without any attempt to find out what's going on."

So the battle lines are drawn sharply. There are drug makers who profit richly from selling antibiotics and there are insurers who do not wish to pay for the benefits. Lost in this battle are the patients whose bowel ecosystems are devastated by prolonged use of broad-spectrum antibiotics, often for long periods of time.

"Without any attempt to find out what's going on!" the physician quoted by the *Times* laments. That's the crux of the matter. What's wrong in chronic fatigue is clearly injured molecular defenses. What is needed is an approach to restore those damaged molecular defenses — a *holistic* approach to the problems of chronic fatigue. And this, of course, is utterly unacceptable to the champions of $N^2D^2$ medicine.

---

## MYALGIC ENCEPHALITIS
## MYALGIC ENCEPHALOMYELITIS

---

Choua assigns these two diagnoses to his list of *lamppost-labels for diseases-from-Mount Olympus.*

"For you doctors, to name something is to understand it," Choua said one day. "To classify it is to conquer it," he continued. "You physicians come up with such elegant words for complex disorders that you do not understand. You simply name them and move on to search for drugs that can cure them. There are few things you love more tenderly than tongue-twister names derived from obscure Latin and Greek words."

"What are we angry about today, Choua?" I mused.

"Do you think your patients have inflamed brains," Choua asked me once.

"How could anyone suffer so much and not have inflammation in his brain," I replied with good humor.

"No! No! I don't mean that," Choua spoke impatiently.

"Do they have inflamed brains? Inflamed the way you see them with your microscope when people have encephalitis?"

"No, I don't think so. I have personally never seen that," I replied seriously.

"Has anyone ever described that?"

"I don't think so. Well, I don't know if anyone has ever done so." I tried to be precise in my response.

"What is encephalitis?"

"Inflammation of the brain."

"What is myalgic?"

"Choua, I don't use this term, but myalgic refers to something about the muscle."

"So what does myalgic encephalitis mean?" Choua asked.

"Well ... well, literally it means ... or should mean something about muscles that has something to do with inflammation of the brain," I answered tentatively.

"Good! Now tell me what is encephalomyelitis?" Choua continued.

"Is this thing going to take us anywhere, Choua?" I asked with annoyance.

"Nowhere! That's the point." Choua smiled. "Put it this way in your fatigue book, so people know how absurd this diagnosis is for those who suffer chronic fatigue."

Choua's words come to me as I write about these two diagnostic terms. Choua is so right. The term myalgic encephalomyelitis is deceitful, plain and simple. It implies inflammation of the brain and the spinal cord. This has not been documented. I suspect that this term was invented to provide a basis for administering certain drugs to these unfortunate people. Since there would be no need to coin such a tongue-twister of a term just to justify the use of simple nutrients, it was probably chosen by someone interested in using some heavy pharmacologic artillery, say something like acyclovir (a drug that interferes with DNA synthesis and can be expected to do some serious long-term damage). The use of drugs with a high potential for toxicity, Choua often says, must be defended by the use of disease names that carry equally high potential for intimidating the patient.

Why would any physician think of brain inflammation when he cares for a patient with chronic fatigue? I have wondered about this. This is how some of my patients have described their problem:

"I hear the words, but I cannot make out what they mean."

********

"I feel directing difficult. I used to enjoy directing. Now, I simply want to be directed."

********

"I run an office. Now I look at stuff on my desk and don't know what to do."

********

"I pick up the phone to call Joyce, and I hear myself saying, "Joe, you have my ... and then I realize I want Joyce and not Joe."

********

"It's as if I have to think through fog."

**\*\*\*\*\*\*\*\***

Here is a husband describing an event concerning his wife who suffered from chronic fatigue: "I was in the living room and I noted a strong smell of gas. I ran to the kitchen. There she stood cooking, completely unaware of the intense gas odor. It is frightening what this thing has done to her sense of smell."

## THE LIMBIC ENCEPHALOPATHY SYNDROME

The limbic system includes some parts of the brain generally thought to be involved with integration of affect and experience (intuitive functions), feelings and passions, memory, and higher regulation of hormonal and autonomic functions. It includes the hippocampus, amygdala, substantia innominata, piriform cortex and septum.

There is strong clinical and experimental evidence that there is limbic system dysfunction in chronic fatigue states. Mood, memory and mentation difficulties are very common among chronic fatiguers. I illustrate some of these symptoms with direct patient quotes. I believe these symptoms result from oxidative injury to neurotransmitter and nerve cell receptor molecules although this has not been documented with actual research studies to-date.

Some chronic fatigue experts believe that chronic fatigue is the result of damage to this system in the brain. Indeed, some have postulated that there is a "fatigue receptor" in the medial temporal lobe of the brain. In support of their theory, they cite studies that show the presence of specific viral receptors for herpes simplex virus-I in that part of the brain. (Such receptors are present in many other tissues of the body, but that doesn't distract the believers in this syndrome). To lend additional support for their viewpoint, they cite PET scan studies of the brain that show reduced blood supply to the parts of the brain included in this system in patients with so-called chronic fatigue syndrome. High-density lesions in the hippocampus and amygdala have been observed in 10% of children and 90% of the elderly who suffer from chronic fatigue. Exercise decreases blood flow to the limbic system. What should we expect? The fatigue experts further propose that inadequate blood supply to the limbic system causes cognitive and perceptive disorders, and leads to changes in personality. I agree that many patients with persistent, debilitating chronic fatigue do suffer from serious personality changes. Indeed, in some cases, changed personalities literally produce *changed* people.

To treat limbic encephalopathy, the proponents of this lamppost diagnosis recommend "altering cognitive states with cognitive behavioral therapy," modification of limbic function with biofeedback, and stimulation of limbic neural activity by extracranial electrical stimulation. Fascinating stuff! From imaginative folks!

This is how some of my patients who suffer from chronic fatigue describe their suffering:

"It's as if I am driving in the rain at all times."

**********

"Often I have no knowledge of where I am going or what I am doing."

*********

"I'll look at you and you will seem a mile away. Then I'll forget what I was talking about. I used to dance. Now I can't focus."

*********

"I am a nurse and I teach nurses. I have a wonderful husband and a gorgeous little boy. Last year we moved to a new house. I thought all my dreams had come true. I had everything I ever wanted. But I am angry most of the time because I want to do so much, but I cannot do anything."

*********

"It's hard when no one listens, no one understands."

## POST-VIRAL SYNDROMES

Choua returned two days later.

"Here is an interesting paper you should discuss in your book," he said.
"What is it about?" I asked.
"Viral problems."

"What kind of viral problems?"

"The kind that lead to chronic fatigue," Choua read a passage:


*The post-viral fatigue syndrome has been observed in epidemics and sporadically throughout the world during the past 50 years. Various names have been used to describe it. They have included epidemic neuromyasthenia, epidemic myalgic encephalitis, Iceland disease and Royal Free disease, to name a few. Investigators have failed to incriminate a virus or toxin, and the absence of objective abnormalities has led others to propose that the illness is psychogenic.*

*Journal of Infection* 10:211;1985.


"So?" I shrugged my shoulders when Choua finished reading.

"What does it tell you?"

"Whatever it says, Choua. I have read such articles before. I don't quite know what's on your mind," I answered.

"It says nothing. That's the point. Your journals are full of such texts that reveal nothing about the true nature of chronic fatigue but hide much with lamppost diagnoses."

"You're back on labels again, are you?" I shook my head.

"Actually, the authors of this article follow that introduction with a report of their extensive data for fifty patients with this problem."

"What are they saying?" I asked.

"Here, I'll sum it up for you:

## First,

a severe decrease in suppressor lymphocytes in early stages.

## Second,

a significant decrease in helper lymphocytes later in the course of this syndrome.

## Third,

immunoglobulins G, A and M were present in normal concentrations.

## Fourth,

immune complexes were present in nearly two-thirds of patients.

## Fifth,

complement activation was observed in nine out of 50 patients.

*Sixth,*

> antibodies to smooth muscle were present in 18
> patients.

*Seventh,*

> antibodies to insulin and insulin receptors were not
> found in any patients.

*Eighth,*

> a mild increase in the HLA-B8 haplotype was found,
> though numbers were considered too small for
> significance. And,

*Ninth,*

> Ninth, 35 of the 50 patients had high antibody titers to
> Coxsackie B viruses."

"That's a pretty good study. What are you grumbling
about, Choua?" I asked when he finished his litany.
"Now listen to this:

*We have not yet measured their IgE
concentrations. Our clinical impression,
however, is that there is a high incidence of
atopic illness in patients with this syndrome.*

Remarkable! Isn't it?" Choua grinned.

"They should have done allergy tests," I responded.

"You don't see it! Do you?" Choua's eyes narrowed.

"See what?"

"These are two most extraordinary statements. IgE antibodies cause the hay-fever type of allergic reactions. They spent vast sums of money to do such extensive and expensive tests. You know those tests for antibodies for insulin and insulin receptors are awfully expensive. How often do you do such patients for your fatigue patients? How important are the test for insulin receptors to the management of chronic fatigue? And yet they failed to do the simple tests that would have given them useful information. Do you know what is most remarkable about all this? They did all those fancy tests that told them little but didn't do allergy tests even though they recognized the high incidence of allergy in their patients."

"No one can do everything," I remarked lamely.

"Bullsh ..." Choua stopped in midsentence.

"Don't bullsh me, Choua! No one can do everything in any research," I said firmly this time.

"When did you last see a patient who suffered from chronic fatigue and whose micro-elisa IgE assays were all negative?"

"I don't remember."

"Did you ever?"

"No! Okay, you are right. I have never seen that," I relented.

Choua walked over to the window and fell silent. I felt some relief. Minutes passed. I knew he couldn't resist returning to the subject, that day or some other day.

"This story doesn't end here," he spoke after a while.

"Where does it end?"

"What these *researchers* did *not* do was much more important than what they did. They did add good data to several earlier studies that showed evidence of an injured immune system in chronic fatigue. But they didn't do any of the real stuff."

"Pray, tell me Choua, what didn't they do that was so unforgivable?" I poked him a little.

"They didn't look for any of the important factors that damage the molecular defenses *before* such people develop chronic fatigue after viral infections," Choua answered, without taking note of my provocation. "They did not look into the use of antibiotics that damage the normal bowel ecosystem, steroids that suppress the immune system, and other drugs that block energy and detoxification enzymes. They did not look for chemical sensitivities and heavy metal overload. They did not look for environmental toxicants. They did not look for major emotional, personal and financial stressors. Indeed, they did not look for any of the factors that would have told them why their patients couldn't cope with their viral infections and regain their normal energy patterns the way other people do."

"Why didn't they?" I asked when Choua finished his monologue.

"Because they are practitioners of $N^2D^2$ medicine," Choua spoke curtly and shifted uneasily on his feet.

"If mankind were going to be extinct, what would be the likely cause?" Choua asked.

"You are the one in the prophesy business, Choua. You tell me," I answered.

"No! No! I'll give you four options," he said sternly.

"Okay, what are the options?" I decided to play along.

Not that I ever have a choice in conversations with Choua.

"First, some global geologic events bring forth climactic changes that man cannot survive. Second, some terrorist group succeeds with what the Russians threatened to do but couldn't. Third, environmental pollutants do you in. Fourth, viruses take over human genetic machinery." Choua stopped and leaned forward to hear my response.

"You are the prophet! You tell me," I taunted Choua.

"Would you cut this sh ...Cut this nonsense of prophesy out, will you!" Choua's voice rose in anger.

Choua is one of the coolest beings I know. It is so rare for him to lose his calm like that. I relished the moment.

"Those are tough options. How do I know how mankind is going to end?" I tried to hide my amusement.

"It will be viruses," Choua looked like the cat that swallowed the canary.

"Choua, you know such things. And God knows about such things. I surely don't." I tried to irritate him further.

"Lederberg thought viruses were the only real competition left." Choua didn't bite this time.

"Who is Lederberg?" I asked.

"He is a professor at Rockefeller."

"Another one of those Rockefeller professors who win Nobel Prizes."

"Yes! Another one of them." Choua seemed relieved at my straight question.

"Oh! So what competition was he talking about?" I asked.

"Competition for dominance on planet Earth," Choua replied.

"And you agree with him."

"Sort of."

"Explain, Choua. Explain! 'Sort of' is not enough." I

feigned anger.

"Yes, viruses are the main competitor for humans. He is right."

"So you want me to say that if mankind becomes extinct, viruses will have done us in," I tried to summarize.

"Yes!"

And then Choua was gone.

******** 

Viruses are nothing more than some strands of DNA wrapped in protein envelopes. They are living organisms, and yet they do not eat, breathe or move. These bits of DNA strands — some are composed of the other type of nucleic acid called RNA — cannot breed except when they can enter a living cell and steal some of its life soup. And still, these seemingly hapless bits of DNA or RNA are tenacious commandos — skillful in deceit and masters of sabotage. How do they do that?

*We are not defenseless against them (viruses) ... We know their tactics and where they live. One way would be to establish an international disease-surveillance network.*

Choua read me the above lines from a popular magazine a few days later.

"These fellows really think an awful lot of themselves, don't they? I guess they don't read too much about the flu virus, and the herpes virus, the Epstein-Barr virus and the AIDS virus!"

"Today is a virus day," I concluded.

"You haven't been humbled yet," Choua didn't acknowledge my attempt at making conversation.

"In 1981 alone, over 340,000 Cubans contracted dengue fever. Just in one country. And what can you do against dengue virus?" Choua frowned.

"Try acyclovir?" I asked meekly.

"Oh yes! Oh yes! Acyclovir! Why not?"

"Sometimes it works against some viruses." I knew that was a weak statement but made it anyway.

"And how does this great miracle drug work, may I ask?" Choua spoke tersely.

"It blocks viral replication," I answered.

"How?" Choua was adamant.

"By interfering with the viral DNA synthesis."

"Yes, it messes up viral DNA. It also messes up your own DNA."

"So what's the answer?"

"Learn to coexist!" Choua spoke the words slowly but firmly.

"Learn to coexist with viruses?" I asked in disbelief.

"Yes! Learn to coexist. Strengthen your own defenses so you can coexist without one destroying the other."

"Easier said than done."

"What choice do you have. One day you have a migraine attack and the next day you develop fever blisters. Doesn't that tell you something about the herpes virus?"

"Yeah, but ...?"

"Let me ask you a question," Choua interrupted me. "Tell me what is the difference between love and herpes?"

"What?"

"Herpes is forever."

Even in humor, Choua can be schizoid.


Viruses have evolved complex and cunning methods of infecting their preferred hosts. Carr and Kim of Whitehead Institute in Cambridge, Massachusetts, described in the May 21 issue of *Cell* how certain peptides — short chains of amino acids — normally hidden well within the viral membrane are "sprung" into action when the virus decides to invade the target cells. When I read reports like these I am sobered by how viruses have humbled us for decades, and how their inventiveness always seems to be several steps ahead of us humans as we design clever strategies to control them. The flu virus has defied us and so has the AIDS virus. Indeed, to date we have no effective drugs against viruses. The few we do use are toxic not only to viruses but also to human tissues.

I don't know if and when we will prevail over viruses. I have serious reservations about our chances when I consider the effects of the potent antibiotics used to combat bacteria. I do recognize how essential broad-spectrum antibiotics are for treating life-threatening infections. Still, I cannot ignore the devastation wreaked by clearly avoidable use of antibiotics in a huge number of patients I have seen. We pay a huge long-term price for short-term gains with the use — and mostly abuse — of antibiotics.

## WE HAVE TO LEARN TO COEXIST WITH VIRUSES

This is the main lesson I have learned from my patients who have suffered from chronic viral infections. The notion that we can eliminate viruses from our internal environment is both simplistic and dangerous — simplistic because it is inconsistent with whatever we do know of viruses, and dangerous because therapies designed for destroying viruses are destroying us much more effectively than they do viruses.

Choua walked in one day, waving a magazine. "Put this in your book: 'I feel like damaged goods'."

"*New England Journal of Medicine* again. Is it?" I chided Choua.

"No. It's *New Woman,* June 1993. This quote is by a young woman who suffers from herpes infection."

"So?" I asked.

"Remember you developed fever blisters once after a migraine attack."

"That was a long time ago." I remembered telling Choua about it.

"How long after the headache did the blisters appear?"

"A few hours if I recall correctly."

"So tell young women who feel damaged by the herpes virus what that is all about," Choua counseled.

"What's there to tell? Herpes virus lives in everyone."

"So why did she feel *damaged*?"

"Because some $N^2D^2$ doctor told her so. Is that it?" I taunted Choua.

"Tell them viruses have as much right to share this planet Earth as we do. And that it's a foolish dream of $N^2D^2$ doctors to sterilize people of all viruses. And that drugs that hurt viruses hurt them by messing up their DNA, and that which messes up the DNA of a virus also messes up the DNA of people. And that..." Choua stopped in midsentence and began to shuffle some journals on my desk. He picked one up, thumbed through the pages, and then read:

*On the basis of the results of this study we postulate that there is persistent enteroviral infection in the muscle of some patients with postviral fatigue syndrome and that this interferes with cell metabolism and is causally related to the fatigue.*

"This is *British Journal of Medicine,* March 23, 1991, issue." Choua closed the journal and put it back on my desk. "These people did some muscle biopsies on some chronic fatiguers and found specific enteroviral RNA in more than half of patients with chronic fatigue syndrome and in only fifteen percent of controls."

"So what's the message? Do we ..." I began.

"The viruses are here to stay," Choua interrupted me. "Unless you decide to cook all the muscle fibers in chronic fatiguers the way your oncologists cook the whole immune system before they try to revive it with their bone marrow transplants, you have to learn to live with viruses."

"How?"

"Somehow!" Choua brushed my question away.

"How, Choua? How? How do people learn to live with viruses?" I moaned.

"By strengthening their own defenses, that's how! Why is that so very difficult for you to understand? All those millions who see holistic practitioners know that. Why can't you?" Choua spoke the words slowly, as if trying to mitigate his distress at my thick-headedness.

## CHRONIC EPSTEIN-BARR SYNDROME

There are three important things to know about the Epstein-Barr virus.

### First,

this virus affects almost all people in all countries. In the underdeveloped countries, it usually spreads by water and food contacts. Since the immune systems of children in such countries are usually not as violated by antibiotic abuse, they cope with this virus well and resulting chronic immune damage appears to be uncommon. In developed countries, EBV infections usually occur as the "kissing disease" in high schools and colleges and, cause significant chronic illness.

### Second,

EBV is not a dangerous virus for adults who have strong

molecular defenses.

## *Third,*

EBV is reactivated, replicates aggressively, and deals devastating blows to the immune system when a person's molecular defenses are broken by various factors such as allergy, chemical sensitivity, extensive antibiotic abuse, multiple drug therapies, altered states of bowel ecology, viral and bacterial infections, parasitic infestations, and stress.

The story of Epstein-Barr virus began on March 22, 1961, when Dennis Burkitt, a little known surgeon from Africa, described his experience with cancer in African children at the Middlesex Hospital Medical School in London. In the audience was Epstein, a virologist at the medical school, who was searching for viruses that might cause certain cancers in humans the way they do so in animals. Epstein obtained biopsy tissue from Burkitt and, along with his co-researchers, Achong and Barr, succeeded in isolating a virus belonging to the herpes group of viruses from the cancer cells. The virus was named Epstein-Barr virus. Within several years it was recognized that this virus is ubiquitous in human populations in all parts of the world, and most likely is present in all.

The infatuation of many physicians with the so-called chronic Epstein-Barr syndrome began some years ago with the simplistic hope that acyclovir or other antiviral drugs could be used to cure this infection — and hence, chronic fatigue caused by it. Another triumph of drug chemistry. In a careful study, acyclovir was found to be ineffective for patients who suffer from chronic fatigue and who have high levels of Epstein-Barr antibodies (*N Eng J Med* 319:1692; 1988.) This, however, did not deter the Epstein-Barr enthusiasts who kept looking for more potent — and toxic — antiviral drugs.

There is some value to doing Epstein-Barr antibody tests in the management of patients who suffer from persistent, debilitating chronic fatigue. In my clinical experience, very high levels of these antibodies indicate extensive replication of the virus, and patients with such levels require restorative oral and intravenous nutrient therapies for longer periods of time than those who do not show high levels of antibodies against Epstein-Barr, retroviruses or other viruses.

## THE CHILDHOOD VIRAL INFECTION ACTIVATION SYNDROME

Some physicians prefer the theory that chronic fatigue states result from reactivation of viruses that first invade human tissues during childhood viral infections. Next, they move on to the second part of this theory that reactivated viruses cause the production of lymphokines (hormone-like substance produced by immune cells called lymphocyte) that give chronic fatiguers tired muscles and bruised spirits. Finally, such researchers return to their favorite subject of the use of drugs to combat reactivated viruses.

Why are the childhood infection viruses being reactivated in our children, adults and the elderly? Why didn't they get reactivated in the past decades? Chronic fatigue states were seen so uncommonly as late as 1960s. Why do they get reactivated now? Why is such viral reactivation spreading like a pandemic? The proponents of this theory are not concerned with such questions.

I suspect that the real origin of this theory has something to do with the ability of some chronic fatigue "researchers" to measure lymphokines in their laboratories. This phenomenon, of course, is not uncommon at all. We physicians love to invent diseases in our laboratories. It matters little whether or not such diseases have any relevance to real people.

## THE ENVIRONMENTAL ILLNESS SYNDROME

Sometime ago I saw a seven-year-old boy with hyperactivity syndrome and attention deficit disorder who was assigned to a special class because of behavioral problems at school. He responded extremely well to our allergy management and selection of food choices based on an electrodermal conductance food profile. After a few months, I received a call from his very distressed mother. She told me it seemed as if her son had reverted to the old behavior problems, even when she and her son had been extremely careful in following the food choices we had established. Of course, he had been diligently following my allergy immunotherapy schedule and taking his nutrient supplements regularly. I was at a loss to explain why this happened. There had been no birthdays and no picnics — no clear reason why he should have relapsed. I asked one of our nurses to spend some time with the mother and carefully go over all the management details. There were no clues. I asked the mother to be patient and keep looking for answers to this puzzle. She called me a couple of days later.

"We've finally figured it out," she exclaimed with excitement.

"What did it turn out to be?" I asked with relief.

"We have figured out why Joe was totally out of control." She could barely contain herself.

"What was it?" I repeated my question.

"The paint!"

"You had your house painted? Why didn't you tell me when I asked about it?" I asked.

"No! It wasn't our house. We would have figured that out. He visited his grandparents two days before his relapse. We didn't realize it until yesterday."

"What happened yesterday?"

"He went there again, and again his symptoms returned, but not to the same degree as before. I guess the paint had outgased a lot by yesterday."

We are in the midst of the largest and most dangerous experiment in human biology. It has been estimated that Americans are exposed to about 65,000 chemicals in their daily lives. In 1945, the U.S. annual production of chemicals was 8 million tons. By 1985, it had risen to 110 million tons, or 950 pounds of chemicals for every United States citizen. Even the staunchest all-in-the-header will have to accept that such a massive chemical avalanche must have some effect on human biology. We cannot drink deeply from this fountain of chemicals and not get hurt.

I once asked Choua what he thought of the problem of chronic fatigue in environmental illness. He shrugged his shoulders, and then smiled and said,

"You know environmental illness causes chronic fatigue. Clinical ecologists have known this for years. People with environmental illness get better when they are properly managed. Now it's different. There is a lot of grant money available to use drugs to treat fatigue, and fatigue experts are sprouting everywhere."

## THE FOOD ALLERGY SYNDROME

"I saw an allergist. He did his tests and told me I was not allergic."

"How did he do the tests?"

"With the skin tests."

"And all the tests came out negative?" I asked with surprise.

"Yes! But do you want to know what was so funny?"

"What?"

"The more skin tests he did, the sicker I became. I got flushed. My heart raced. I had muscle spasms and abdominal bloating."

"Did you tell him about that?" I asked.

"Yes! He could also see I was sweating."

"What did he say?"

"He said all the food tests were negative."

"All negative?" I asked with disbelief.

"Did you tell him about your past history of food allergies?"

"Yes, I did, but he was not impressed."

"And he insisted you do not have food allergies?"

"All negative. He insisted all tests were negative because of ..."

"Because of what?" I blurted out and then recovered. "I'm sorry. Why did he think all the tests were negative?"

"I guess because my skin lumps didn't measure up to his calipers," she smiled knowingly.


Food allergy — along with mold and other types of inhalant allergies and chemical sensitivities — *is* what sets people up for chronic fatigue. It is also one of the most misunderstood areas in medicine.


"Do you know the problem with your $N^2D^2$ doctors when it comes to allergy and environmental sensitivities?" Choua asked me once.

"What?" I asked back.

"They suffer from attention deficit problems," Choua grinned.

"Physician-bashing again, eh!" I teased.

"No! Simply stating the truth," Choua replied seriously.

"Pray, Choua, tell me what is the truth?"

"If people don't get very sick right before them — or preferably don't die before them — these practitioners of $N^2D^2$ medicine can't see any harm in anything. They are quite content. Diseases come from Mount Olympus. And that's that!"

"You have a one track mind, Choua," I complained.

"Oh yes! Tell me how else would an allergist tell a patient he is not sensitive to foods when his patient suffers right before him as he puts needles into her flesh?"

"Because for the skin test to be positive, the wheal of the skin test must expand from four millimeters to a minimum of seven millimeters," I tried to explain.

"Four millimeters to seven millimeters, eh! See how quickly even you lose your common sense. Allergy symptoms are what the patient who suffers from them says they are. Not what your champions of $N^2D^2$ medicine say they are," Choua reproached.

"That's absurd. You have to have some objectivity."

Choua looked at me, his eyes brimming with ridicule. "Chronic fatigue is what people who suffer from chronic fatigue say it is. It is not what your maestros of drug medicine say it is." Choua shook his head and walked out.

## THE CANDIDA-RELATED COMPLEX

"Dr. Ali, will I ever get rid of my yeast?"

"I hope not," I answered.

"No?" She was taken aback.

"Because ..."

"Because what?" she quickly cut me off." I'm sorry, I didn't mean to interrupt you so rudely." She slumped back into her chair.

"Because if you did get rid of your yeast, you wouldn't live for long."

"You aren't serious, are you?"

"Yes, I am. The only way you can get rid of the yeast in your bowel is to sterilize it. And I know you wouldn't live more than a few weeks if I did that."

A well-known commercial declares that more doctors

recommend their XYZ vaginal cream for candida problems than any other cream, that more women use XYZ cream than any other cream, and that more yeast infections are cured by that cream than any other cream. As for the first claim, it may be true. It simply represents the fact that the manufacturer of the XYZ cream has the most money to hire its "experts" to lecture at our hospitals or to spend on its sales force that invades physicians' offices. Physicians generally have a poor understanding of the fact that yeast overgrowth and infections are problems of altered bowel ecology, and that vaginal yeast problems are a spill-over phenomenon — yeast invades the vaginal tract only as a secondary event. They will prescribe most what is most talked about. The second claim of that commercial may also be true. It means they have the most money for glittering TV commercials. The third claim, however, that their cream *cures* more yeast infection than any other is simply absurd. *No vaginal cream can ever cure yeast infections.* Yeast overgrowth and infections can be properly addressed with good long-term results only when they are seen as *ecologic problems* of the gut and not as diseases to be cured with drugs.

I'm afraid chronic candidiasis is as much a lamppost diagnosis for some of my colleagues in alternative medicine as is chronic Epstein-Barr infection with practitioners of $N^2D^2$ medicine.

*Candidiasis should never be considered the root problem for anyone with chronic fatigue.*

Candida species of yeasts are clearly of importance in any discussion of normal bowel ecosystems. In my experience, however, the clinical importance of this yeast is grossly exaggerated. I submit the following data for the detection of antibodies against four different types of yeast and six other allergens in the blood of 200 consecutive patients with chronic fatigue states in one of my studies. These data throw some light on the relative importance of these common yeasts.

| INCIDENCE OF IgE ANTIBODIES with specificity for yeast allergens in 200 patients with chronic fatigue | |
|---|---|
| Cephalosporium | 97% |
| Alternaria | 96% |
| Aspergillus | 95% |
| Candida | 83% |
| Milk | 83% |
| Egg | 75% |
| Ragweed | 78% |
| Bermuda grass | 63% |
| Oak | 62% |
| Cat | 50% |

The above data indicate that as far as IgE antibody response to yeast is concerned, antibodies to candida species were less common than three other types of yeasts that we studied — cephalosporium, alternaria and aspergillus.

Altered states of bowel ecology are of central importance to any discussion of chronic fatigue. Persistent, disabling fatigue cannot be understood without understanding the ecology of the bowel in health and how it is disrupted in the "predisease" states. In my experience, chronic fatigue cannot be managed — and normal energy patterns restored — without successfully addressing all the elements concerning the normal bowel ecology. Simple-minded efforts to *cure* "yeast syndromes," "intestinal dysbiosis," "leaky gut syndrome," "autobrewery syndrome" or other similar syndromes that focus on one or the other aspects of bowel ecology are of limited value. I discuss this essential subject in the chapters Battered Bowel Ecosystem and Chronic Fatigue. For an in-depth discussion of this essential subject, I refer the reader to the companion volume *Battered Bowel Ecology — Waving Away A Wandering Wolf.*

## THE NATURAL KILLER CELL DEFICIENCY SYNDROME

This is the name Japanese and some other people favor for chronic, persistent fatigue. It is true that a decrease in the number of the natural killer cells in the blood is common in chronic fatigue states. However, the critical issue is this: The deficiency of natural killer cells is a *consequence* rather than the cause of chronic fatigue. As Choua would say, this is another one of the lamppost diagnoses that tell people who suffer chronic fatigue nothing and hides much from them.

## STIFF-MAN SYNDROME

Here is an excerpt from *Family Circle* (Sept. 1, 1993):

*"But the tests continued, and the neurologist eventually suggested that Chris' symptoms might be related to "stiff-man syndrome," a chronic progressive disorder characterized by painful muscle spasms and stiffness. During the next two months, Chris and Wayne experienced thrilling highs when an explanation made sense, and the symptoms subsided. But within a few days of taking (in turn, and in varying combinations) Valium, Dilantin, Klonopin, Depakote, Lioresal and Catapres, each drug would suddenly stop being effective. The spasms would return.*

*In her journal, Chris described her suicidal state of mind while taking Klonopin: The winter darkness oppresses me. ...My life seems meaningless, hopeless. I terrified my family yesterday..."*

Chris' story of painful muscle spasms and stiffness is a common story for physicians like myself who devote most of their professional energy to the problem of chronic fatigue. Failure of multiple drug therapies, again, is an entirely expected outcome in this setting. Indeed, such drug therapies can be *counted* upon to worsen the fatigue problem. Drugs, I write earlier in this volume, work by impairing, blocking or outright destroying enzymes. Drugs further damage the injured the injured energy enzymes in chronic fatigue states. What amused me in the above excerpt — and I include it here for comic relief — is the neurologist's brilliant diagnosis of the *stiff-man syndrome*. Where can anyone find a more glowing testimonial to the intellectual bankruptcy of practitioners of drug medicine. The commonly made diagnosis of *restless leg syndrome* is equally absurd, though all textbooks of internal medicine describe it a legitimate medical entity. Such is the currency of silly thinking in $N^2D^2$ medicine.

---

## THE OVERCHARGED (OR DYSFUNCTIONAL) IMMUNE SYSTEM SYNDROME

*After years of dismissing chronic fatigue syndrome as yuppie hypochondria and little more than a figment of the imagination, doctors in growing numbers are coming to believe that it is a distinct condition and one that may reflect an overcharged immune system.*

*The New York Times*  Dec. 4, 1990

We physicians had a pretty good handle on this messy problem of chronic fatigue syndrome. After all, it was a problem created by the irresponsible, headline-seeking media. We were quite content being aloof. It didn't behoove the men of "scientific" medicine to indulge the charlatans of cheap news media. And now this. The *Times* has decided to join the *National Enquirer*. How awful! Where is it all going to end?

It was very heartening for many sufferers of chronic fatigue to finally see *The New York Times* come to their defense. After all the *Times* cannot be wrong. Or can it be?

"If my immune system is really overcharged, how come I am so sick?" a chronic fatiguers asked me once. My patient is right and the *Times* has been mislead by its sources. In reality, the immune system in chronic fatigue states is not overcharged but badly damaged. My colleagues and I have conclusively shown that the capacity of the immune system for producing protective (antigen-specific IgG) antibodies in chronic fatigue is severely impaired (Ali et al., *Am J Clin Pathol* in press). In the chapter On Reviving Injured Energy Enzymes, I describe two case histories of a mother and her son that clearly illustrate this phenomenon.

Some people use the term IL2 syndrome for chronic fatigue — in view of excessive production in fatigue patients of IL2 — a hormone-like substance produced by activated immune cells. Excessive production of IL2 — and of several other similar substances — is a consequence and not the cause of immune injury seen in chronic fatigue. I consider such phenomena parts of the last-ditch effort of the damaged immune system to recover. Parenthetically, I might add here that a subset of chronic fatiguers do not develop flu-like viral illnesses. This protection may be due to the excessive production of IL2 and related hormones. Such patients often develop viral infections as their health is restored with nondrug therapies.

## DRUG OVERLOAD AND CHRONIC FATIGUE

Janet P, a severely overweight woman in her late sixties, returned for her first follow-up visit about 10 weeks after I first saw her and started her on our protocols of environmental and nutritional medicines. She complained of severe fatigue and reported no signs of improvement. That doesn't happen often in my practice, and almost always I am able to dig out the reasons why no clinical benefits were observed with our management protocols.

"Have you been taking the immunotherapy injections?" I asked.
"Yes," she replied.
"And nutrient protocols?"
"Yes, except when I was in the hospital."
"Why did you have to go to the hospital?"
"Heart palpitations."
"What drugs are you taking now?"

She pulled a list of drugs from her handbag. I reproduce accurately below what I saw on that list.

| | |
|---|---|
| Triavil 2/10 | 2/daily |
| Calan SR 240 mg | 2/daily |
| Tagamet 400 mg | 2/daily |
| Clinoxide (Librax) | 2/daily |
| Nortriptyline 75 mg | 1/bedtime |
| Lorazepam 1 mg | 1/bedtime |
| Mevacor 20 mg | 1/bedtime |
| Ansaid 100mg | 2/daily |
| Voltaren 75 mg | 2/daily |
| Quinaglute Duratab | 2/daily |
| Vasotec 5 mg | 1/daily |
| Enteric Coated Aspirin | 1/daily |
| Thyroid 60 mg | 1/daily |

I returned to her chart when she left the office.

"How do drug companies conduct their drug research?" Choua surprised me. I hadn't realize he had slipped in sometime after Janet left the room.

"You know how!" I wasn't in the mood to engage Choua.

"By taking one drug at a time and comparing its effectiveness and toxicity with a placebo or another drug." Choua answered his own question. "Do drug companies ever conduct research with the concurrent use of two drugs — or of three drugs?"

"For chemotherapy protocols they do," I interjected.

"How do two drugs react with one other?" Choua ignored my comment. "How do they affect a person when taken together? How do three drugs interact with one another? How do they affect a person when taken together? What happens when a person is prescribed thirteen drugs at one time?"

"You tell me, Choua," I shrugged my shoulders.

"Why would anyone prescribe thirteen drugs at one time

in the first place?" Choua asked.

"Beats me!"

"This is how it happens," Choua continued. "The patient goes to one doctor and leaves his office with one or two or three prescriptions. A few days later, he visits another doctor with some different symptoms and leaves that doctor's office with another one or two prescriptions. Your lip service to the true cause of disease notwithstanding, you prescription pad-toting warriors of $N^2D^2$ medicine are basically in the drug business — you are into mere symptom-suppression — the more the symptoms, the larger the number of prescriptions you dole out. Except ..."

"Except what?" I asked.

Choua studied my face for some moments and then walked out without answering my question. Except what? I wondered what Choua had in mind, and why he left me hanging like that.

---

**CFIDS:**
**Chronic Fatigue Immunodeficiency Syndrome**

---

"I wandered from doctor to doctor until I finally saw one who had read about the Incline Village, and he finally diagnosed me with CFID syndrome."

"They did six-thousand dollars worth of tests. They told me I had CFID syndrome. Then they gave me a Prozac prescription."

*CFID Research Vaults Forward: Convincing*
*Evidence  of  Retroviral  Infection  and*
*Immune  Activation  Found  in  CFIDS*
*Patients.*

*The CFIDS Chronicle  Fall 1991*

"Choua, what do you think of CFID syndrome?" I once asked.

"It's okay!" Choua  surprised  me.

"Okay?"

"Yes! Those folks did some good work. At least they recognized that chronic fatigue is real and that it has something to do with the immune  system."

"How about those claims that they solved the mystery of CFID by detecting  retroviral  sequences  in patients  with CFID?"

"Science moves  like that."

"Whaa..at?" I was baffled. "What did you say, Choua?"

"I said science moves like that. Sometimes there are missteps. Then it corrects itself," Choua answered calmly.

"Ah, such tolerance for other people's point of view! What am I witnessing, Choua? A new day! A new Choua!" I provoked  him.

"Their hearts are in the right place. That's why!"

"So that's it! When holistic folks make a mistake, we must look the other way. But when the mainstreamers  drift away, no matter for how short a period of time, they must be castigated.  Is that  it, Choua?"

"Their hearts are in the right places," Choua  repeated.

## CDC'S CHRONIC FATIGUE SYNDROME

In 1985, a group of investigators at the Centers for Disease Control, in Atlanta, proposed the following three sets of two major criteria (considered essential for diagnosis), eleven minor criteria (six required for diagnosis), and three physical signs (two of three required) for the diagnosis of chronic fatigue syndrome[2].

A) Major criteria: 1) new-onset fatigue lasting longer than six months; and 2) no other medical or psychiatric conditions that could cause symptoms.

B) Minor criteria: low-grade fever, sore throat, painful cervical or axillary lymphadenopathy, generalized muscle weakness, myalgia, fatigue lasting 24 hours or longer after moderate exercise, headache, migratory arthralgia, sleep disorders (hypersomnia or insomnia), neuropsychiatric complaints (one or more of the following: photophobia, visual scotomas, forgetfulness, irritability, confusion, difficulty concentrating, depression).

C) Physical signs: 1) low grade fever (99.5° to 101.5°); 2) pharyngitis, nonexudative; and 3) cervical or axillary lymphadenopathy.

It is evident from the preceding discussion of the molecular dynamics of chronic fatigue that these criteria are not usable in our model of accelerated oxidative molecular injury.

There are two important issues here: 1) How much fatigue interferes with the individual's life?; and 2) What are the molecular basis of chronic fatigue and how can fatigue be alleviated? The CDC criteria hold that chronic fatigue syndrome may not be diagnosed when there exists any organic or psychiatric disorders that can cause fatigue. If chronic fatigue is not caused by organic or psychiatric disorders, how else, one may ask, can chronic fatigue be caused? It is akin to saying that chronic fatigue should not be diagnosed when the treating physician is either a male or a female.

The next time I saw Choua, I asked if he had any opinion on CDC's chronic fatigue syndrome.

"Reductio ad absurdum," he deadpanned.
"Absurd! Is that what you think of CDC criteria?" I asked.
"Yes!" Choua answered emphatically.
"Com'n, Choua, the whole world uses their criteria and you call it reductio ad absurdum," I protested.
"Why don't you see how meaningless their criteria are?" Choua snapped back. "They hold that chronic fatigue syndrome should be diagnosed only when all organic and psychiatric causes have been excluded. Now if that's not absurd, I don't know what is! Where do they think chronic fatigue syndrome comes from? Mount Olympus! Is that what you believe?"
"Choua, you do have a point, but CDC criteria were put together as a working formulation," I said defensively.
"And that's the problem! A silly working formulation can only take you to silly conclusions. Tell me, if they continue to deny that fatigue can be caused by organic lesions — by some of *your* events — what chance is there that anyone can ever find out what the nature of the problem is?"

"Yes! There is that problem," I admitted meekly, ignoring Choua's sarcastic reference to my molecular ideas of disease.

"You don't see the absurdity in this, do you? The government officials are usually experts at making frivolous propositions. But this one wins the award."

Choua abruptly left, and within minutes he was back with some medical journals. "Here!" he spoke scornfully, "listen to this:

*Chronic fatigue syndrome: Is it real? ....The major reason patients fail to meet research criteria is that nearly 70% have a psychiatric disorder. ... A carefully taken history, physical examination, and simple laboratory testing are usually sufficient to establish the diagnosis. Therapy with antidepressants or nonsteroidal anti-inflammatory drugs may be effective in selected patients.*

This is your *PostGraduate Medicine,* volume 89, page 44, 1991. These fellows still do not know whether chronic fatigue syndrome is real or not." Choua finished reading.

"I know, most physicians are still unsure whether this syndrome exists or not," I remarked.

"See, what your prescription pad-toting champions of $N^2D^2$ medicine are saying. Antidepressants and nonsteroidal drugs. That's it." Choua spoke scornfully.

"It's changing." I didn't know what else to say.

"Load them up with antidepressants. They will be too fogged out to protest what your heroes of Star Wars medicine are doing to them. And if that is not enough, give'm steroids. It will destroy their immune systems but they will feel better for enough weeks so you can write your papers. Right?"

"It will change," I said timidly.

"And listen to this," Choua said, putting the first journal back and picking up another. "This is your *Annals of Internal Medicine*, volume 109, page 554, 1988. They are saying, and I quote,

*'Less than 5% of highly selected persons presenting at a specialized fatigue clinic met strict criteria for chronic fatigue syndrome'."*

"You can't expect ..."

"Expect what?" Choua interrupted. "Some common sense from these warriors of $N^2D^2$ medicine?"

"You have your opinions," I said, throwing my hands up.

Choua picked up the third remaining journal.

"This is the *American Journal of Medicine,* volume 90, page 730, 1991," he started.

*The chronic fatigue syndrome (CFS) was formally defined in 1988 to describe disabling fatigue of at least 6 months duration of uncertain etiology. Reports of CFS have emerged from the United States, Canada, the United Kingdom, Australia, New Zealand, Israel, Spain, and France. The disease primarily affects individuals between 20 and 50 years of age, and there is a preponderance of females. Although a triggering infectious illness is reported by most patients with CFS, there is no convincing evidence linking any currently recognized infectious agent to CFS. Multiple minor immunologic aberrations are frequent but are inconsistent and of uncertain significance. There is no consistent evidence of myopathy nor of physical deconditioning. Depression is found in approximately 50% of CFS patients, with depression preceding the physical examination in half of the cases. No therapy has been proven effective in controlled clinical trials with prolonged follow-up, although antidepressants have not been formally evaluated. The long-term prognosis of patients with CFS has not been well studied, but CFS appears to be a disease of prolonged duration with considerable morbidity but no mortality. Further research into the pathogenesis and treatment of CFS is necessary.*

"Notice there is not a single word in this scholarly dissertation about nutrition." Choua put the copy of the journal down.

"Mainstream docs don't believe in nutrition. You know that, Choua." I agreed with him.

"Not one word about environmental toxins!"

"You know what they think of environmental medicine."

"Not one word about allergy."

"And that, too."

"Not one word about energy dynamics. Not one word about energy enzymes. Not one word about self-regulation. Do you see how stupid that is? How incredibly stupid?"

Choua looked at me and then out the window. And then he was gone.

---

## I AM NOT HERE FOR A DIAGNOSIS, I AM HERE TO FEEL BETTER

Here is a conversation I had with a patient during her initial consultation with me:

"What do you think is wrong with you?" I asked.

"What does it matter?" she replied.

"What does it matter?"

"Yes! What does it matter? What do I care?"

"What do you care?" I asked incredulously.

"Dr. Ali, all I care is to get better. You are the eleventh doctor I have seen. They told me I had a positive ANA test and I might have lupus. Then they said I had a positive rheumatoid factor so I might have rheumatoid arthritis. Then they said the Epstein-barr test was positive and that I had chronic fatigue syndrome. One doctor was sure I had candida. Someone else was equally sure I had CFID. Then ..."

She stopped and looked at me. I kept quiet.

"They did many lab tests and gave me several different diagnoses. It's all in my file I gave you."

"Yes, I have thumbed through it," I reassured her.

"They gave me antidepressants and antibiotics and immunoglobulin shots. And I got sicker and sicker."

"And now?" I asked.

"And now!" She looked surprised. "Now I don't care what's wrong with me. I am not here to ask you for a diagnosis. I just want some relief. I simply want an end to this suffering. I ask you for some help. Do you think you can help, Dr. Ali?"

I sat in silence for some moments as she searched my eyes for some response. "I just want some relief. I simply want an end to this suffering," she spoke finally.

## HE MUST REALLY BELIEVE IN FATIGUE

In a medical conference, a surgeon complained of tiredness and how he couldn't get rid of a cough and muscle aches that he had for about six months. He spoke about how he had used antibiotics on three different occasions and taken cough suppressants and expectorants, each time with limited benefit. "But you know me, I don't believe in vitamin therapy," he said to another surgeon in the room as he winked at me. I chose not to respond.

"He must believe in sickness," Choua spoke as he joined me on my way back to the laboratory.

"What do you mean?" I asked.

"Didn't he say he has been tired for six months and can't get rid of his cough?"

"Yes! But that might be due to allergy. In fact, it probably is," I ventured.

"Or perhaps a persistent viral infection," Choua suggested.

"That's a distinct possibility," I agreed.

"Do you know what I think he believes in?" Choua asked.

"What?"

"Fatigue!"

"Far out!" I couldn't resist a smile. "Tell me, Choua, how did you arrive at such a brilliant diagnosis?"

"Didn't he say he tried antibiotics but they didn't work?"

"So?"

"And antibiotics and drugs didn't work."

"So?"

"And he doesn't believe in nutrients."

"So?"

"He has found out drugs don't work for fatigue and muscle aches. But he doesn't believe in nutrients."

"So?"

"What else is there? He can't believe in drugs, because he found they didn't work. He doesn't believe in nutrients. There is nothing else there. He really must believe in chronic fatigue."

## THE IT SYNDROME

Sometime ago, a woman in her mid-forties came to see me. She looked very distraught. As she sat before me, with my eyes fixed on her completed general history and chronic fatigue questionnaires, I sensed considerable tension in her as she restlessly fidgeted with her fingers and shifted her position in the chair. Patients tell their physicians a great deal with such body language. I observed her thus for some moments while I finished reading her history of multiple symptoms of sinus allergy, headache, muscle aches, abdominal cramps, yeast infections, PMS and mood swings, and incoherent repetitions of the parts of her story. This is how part of my conversation with her during the first visit went:

"Things were okay before *it* happened," she said testily.

"The anxiety?" I tried to translate *it* for her.

"I was working. I was doing things at home. And then *it* happened." She ignored my suggestion.

"Did you suddenly become depressed?" I made another

suggestion.

"The pressure. I couldn't do anything when *it* happened." She clenched her teeth as she uttered *it.*

"Pressure of what? Panic attacks?" I asked another leading question.

"*It* was all over. Stomach cramps and bloating and diarrhea." She again ignored my lead.

"Did you ever have colitis before that?"

"I have always had these problems. My doctor said it was irritable bowel syndrome. Another one said it was spastic colitis. But *it* was never like this. *It* really turned me inside out." Her jaw muscles quivered again when she mentioned *it.*

"Did you suffer from fever? Sore throat?" I resisted one more time the temptation to ask her what that *it* was.

"I frequently get sore throats. You know the allergy sore throat and bronchitis. But not like this. This was different!"

"Do you have difficulty remembering things?" I asked.

"Remembering things! Oh, yes. My memory is awful. I go to one room and when I am there I forget why I went there."

"Do you sometimes wake up tired?"

"Dr. Ali, this *thing* doesn't let me sleep. I turn and turn in my bed until morning. Then I doze off. Then I wake up. *It* is killing me." Her lips trembled a little.


## *Fourth of July Chemistry*


I do not know what my colleagues in obsessional psychopathology industry make of that *it.* I know what *it* meant to me — molecular fireworks, i.e., millions of sparks of electron transfers, zillions of electrons turning, twisting, colliding, setting off zillions of explosions. *It* was the relentless agony of riding unrelenting molecular roller coasters — an agony of riding the chemistry of the Fourth of July.

I wondered  how I was going to explain all this to her. I had seen such under-the-skin  fireworks a thousand  times. I had also seen them subside — turn into calm, sustained energy patterns — a thousand times. But would she understand  all that while her whole inside convulses with the shock waves of *it*?

I told her I was going to call *it* a state of molecular burn-out, and that we were going to try to down-regulate  her whole chemistry. Next, I outlined  our total program: I insisted that she attend  my next three weekly autoregulation  workshops. We drew some blood samples. Then I prescribed Ativan to buy some time. What did I observe when I saw her at my six-month follow-up visit? The same thing that I almost regularly observe after patients  with recent-onset  chronic fatigue are managed with integrated  treatment  protocols of self-regulation, oral and intravenous nutrients, allergy, bowel ecology restoration,  and slow, sustained, limbic exercise. The demon of *it* succumbs to the angel of *knowing*.

---

## AOE SYNDROME

Here  is my conversation  with Robert  Y., a young man in his early thirties,  who consulted  me for chronic fatigue.

"What's wrong with me?" he asked.
"You're tired! Very tired!"

"Is there a name for this thing?"

"Yes."

"Do you know it?"

"Yes! I do most assuredly."

"You mean you know what ails me?" He leaned forward in his chair.

"Yes."

"You are the ninth doctor I have seen for this thing. Six of them gave me five different diagnoses. The other three said they didn't have any clue. Tell me, what is it?"

"It's AOE Syndrome," I said with clinical authority.

"AOE syndrome!" He gazed at me, intent, hard. I looked back at him impassively. Suddenly his face broke in a smile.

"You just made it up, didn't you?" He grinned.

"Yes!" I replied.

"Just like that!"

"Yes, just like that," I added calmly.

"Can you do that?"

"I just did! Didn't I?"

"No, I mean is it legal?" He looked puzzled now.

"I don't know if it's legal." I shrugged my shoulders.

"You mean it is legal for any doctor to invent a diagnosis whenever he wants?"

"I can't speak for others, but I just did. Didn't I?" I asked with a gentle smile.

"I don't believe this." He chuckled.

"Everyone else makes things up. What's so terrible if I make something up."

"Nothing! I guess there is nothing wrong with it." He smiled again. "But tell me what does AOE stand for?

"Absence of energy," I answered in a matter-of-fact way.

"Absence of energy, eh!"

"Yes! Absence of energy," I rejoined.

"What *scan* do you use to make this diagnosis?" He flashed a broad smile this time.

"The scan of your words," I replied and then added, "I mean I scan your words."

"That's it?"

"That's it."


He studied my face for some long moments as if to determine what to make of me.

"You're not serious, are you?"

"Yes, I am."

"Are you saying I have chronic fatigue just because I said so?"

"Is there a better way for me to know that?" I answered his question with a question.

"No blood test?" His face bore a quizzical expression now.

"Yes! We will do some micro-elisa tests for inhalant allergy and electrodermal conductance tests for a food sensitivity profile, and then we will do some tests for temperature regulation and some others for toxic metal overload."

"How about all the expensive immune tests that everyone talks about?"

"Only if that becomes necessary. I already know your immune system is damaged."

"And for chronic fatigue? Any tests for that?"

"Tests for fatigue?" I repeated his question. "None!"

"Then how do you know I am not simply lying? How do you know how I tired I am?"

"There isn't a blood test around that can measure fatigue

in blood or tissues yet."

Fatigue measured by a blood test? Expressed as milligrams of tiredness per milliliters of blood? Or as grams of fatigue per 100 grams of dried muscle tissue? Or should it be grams of desiccated brain tissues? I mean that's what it's about, isn't it? The old all-in-the-head story? I suppressed a smile as the thought crossed my mind. That would make my life so much easier, wouldn't it? I mean I could quantify chronic fatigue — or absence of energy — or health for that matter — in such an objective way, I could then give my nutrients in an equally objective way, couldn't I? And my colleagues in drug medicine could use their drugs in precise quantitative ways. Our numbers would have been so precise, our research so scientific! We would have taken biopsies of tissues affected by the state of absence of energy — and absence of health. We could see tissue tiredness with a microscope. We love biopsies, don't we? I mean, it doesn't much matter whether the biopsies tell us anything or not. We pathologists always use such elegant language to prepare our reports. The less we know about what we see with our microscopes, the more erudite we are in writing our reports. The longer the pathologist's report, the surer you can be of the pathologist's ignorance about what he is describing. It would have been so much easier to publish papers. Editors of our journals love blinded numbers. It would have been so lovely. I could have published my papers so easily. I could have been so *scientific.*

In actuality, almost all parts of the classical immune system show evidence of damage in chronic fatigue states if we do the right tests. The reason I do not order such tests is that the test results only tell me what I already know, and more importantly, such tests do not help me much in designing my therapies for restoring energy and detoxification enzymes. So I focus on the type of laboratory tests that are clinically most useful.

My eyes fell upon Robert's face. He looked obviously puzzled. I smiled sheepishly, trying to suppress my errant thoughts.

"Okay, I accept the diagnosis. Now what's the treatment?" Robert asked me somberly.

"Bring back the energy." I made light of my own words.

"Presence of energy," Robert mocked my words.

"Yes! Presence of energy! That's it. We are into rejuvenating enzymes — energy and detoxification enzymes."

"And how do you plan to do that?" Robert frowned for the first time.

"By doing as many natural and nontoxic things as we can do to bring back your old level of energy."

"How?" he asked intently.

"With nutritional therapies!" I answered evenly.

"And what might they be?"

"Food choices in the kitchen, oral nutrient therapies, and, if necessary, intravenous nutrient therapies."

"And?"

"Environmental controls."

"And?"

"Environmental therapies."

"What would they be?"

"Diagnosis and management of allergies."

"And what else?"

"Self-regulation and slow-sustained exercise," I completed the outline of our programs for chronic fatigue.

*Thou canst not stir a flower*
*without troubling a star.*

A poet

*A butterfly flutters its wings in Dallas*
*and changes weather in Denville.*

A physicist

*In biology, if we change something in one*
*way, we change everything in some way.*

A biology observer

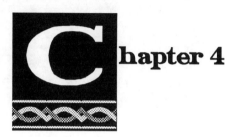

**C**hapter 4

# What is
# Chronic
# Fatigue?

## Chronic Fatigue
### Is a Failure of Energy Enzymes

My viewpoint — chronic fatigue is a state of accelerated oxidant molecular injury — evolved as a natural extension of my theoretical interest in the aging process and of my clinical work with patients with chronic fatigue. For some years now, I have tried to reduce several, complex issues involved in chronic fatigue to two basic questions:

*First, what is the energetic-molecular basis of chronic fatigue?*

and

*Second, how can normal energy enzyme pathways be restored in patients who suffer from chronic fatigue?*

What separates a grain of sand from a sandpiper? Or a stone from a sunflower? Or a mound of dirt from a mosquito? Or a mountain from a man? The answer: enzymes. Enzymes are organic molecules that sustain the physicochemical processes of life — by facilitating metabolic pathways that generate energy and those that are involved in detoxification pathways. Enzymes are what living organisms use to protect themselves from toxic molecules that are produced within them as waste products of metabolism and those that exist in their environment.

How is it that a sunflower can bloom only for a few days? And a mosquito can live only for about 18 days? And a man perhaps for 110 years? The answer to all three questions is the same: The length of the life span of an organism is determined by the ability of its tissues to produce enzymes that generate energy and assist the body in ridding itself of toxins. The longer an organism can produce such enzymes — life span enzymes, in our language — the longer its life span.

Chronic fatigue is the chronic absence of energy. Energy, in turn, is an enzyme function. It follows that chronic fatigue is a failure of energy enzymes.

Such simple reasoning led me to the reasonable conclusion that if I were to seek the cause(s) of chronic fatigue, I must direct my inquiry to energy enzymes. But this raised the expected question: What is the energetic-molecular basis of the failure of energy enzymes? This question proved to be quite tedious for me initially.

## SPONTANEITY OF OXIDATION IS THE TRUE CAUSE OF THE AGING PROCESS

Spontaneity of oxidation in nature — in my view — is the true cause of the aging process in humans and in all other aerobic lifeforms — that is, living beings that utilize oxygen as the basis of their survival.

Two principal theories have been put forth to explain the chemical nature of the aging process. In the mid-fifties, Bjorksten proposed his theory of aging. The centerpiece of this theory holds that tissues age when proteins are denatured by cross-linking — types of chemical reactions in which some parts of the long, threadlike protein molecules are clipped, bent out of shape, and reinserted back into the molecules in such a fashion that abnormal, cross linkages are formed between the protein molecules. Cross-linked proteins are obviously damaged proteins and so are unable to perform their various metabolic functions. Enzymes of human energy pathways, I might add here, are also proteins and may be expected to fail in their energy roles if they are cross-linked. Some years after Bjorksten proposed his theory, Harmon put forth his theory of free radical damage as the root cause of the aging process. Since Bjorksten and Harmon proposed their theories, a huge body of research reports have presented several lines of evidence that support these two theories of aging.

The questions that remained unanswered for me for several years as I reflected on these two theories were simply these: 1) What triggers free radical formation? and 2) What initiates the process(es) that lead(s) to protein cross-linkages?

My interest in the nature of the aging process in man derives from my years of work in research and in the clinical practice of pathology. Over a period of about 30 years, I have had the opportunity to examine close to 100,000 biopsies and surgical specimens. No pathologist can look at damaged tissues day after day for decades and not wonder where the tissue injuries begin. The causes of diseases, as they appear in medical texts, are almost always based on our view of how tissues look *after* they have been damaged or destroyed. Medical texts rarely, if ever, discuss the energy and molecular events that occur *before* the tissues are damaged. In general, the discussion of the cause of degenerative and immune disorders usually ends with a simple comment like "cause unknown." *Nature, Science* and other science journals regularly publish reports of the physical phenomena in biology that result in tissue injury, decay and death. Such reports often focus on energetic-molecular events that initiate the processes eventually culminating in clinical diseases as we see them. But such journals are rarely read by physicians. Medical journals usually carry only those segments of such knowledge of biology that serve physicians in prescribing drugs or approaching diseases with their surgical scalpels.

In the chapter, Ten Lessons Learned From Patients in *The Cortical Monkey and Healing*, I describe how I followed my interest in the beginning of disease processes through my journey in the fields of general surgery, orthopedic surgery, trauma, surgical pathology, clinical pathology, immunology, allergy, environmental sensitivities, nutrition, fitness, self-regulation and planes of consciousness.

In this context, one conversation that I had with my research colleague in allergy and immunology, Madhva Ramanarayanan (Dr. Ram), Ph.D., stands out vividly in my memory. During the late 1970s and early 1980s, Dr. Ram and I developed the IgE micro-elisa assay for the diagnosis of inhalant allergy and the IgG micro-elisa assay for monitoring the efficacy of immunotherapy for such disorders. During this time, we often had long discussions about where and how such allergies might begin. One day, Dr. Ram and I were going out for lunch when he abruptly stopped and asked me to wait for him while he quickly changed the buffer for a research project that we were engaged in.

"Ram, what would happen if you didn't change the buffer?" I asked without really looking for an answer.

"It wouldn't work that well," Ram answered without hesitation as he walked to his refrigerator.

"Why, Ram, why wouldn't the old buffer work well?" I asked.

"Because old buffers become stale," Ram replied.

"So? What's the problem with stale buffers?" I asked absent-mindedly.

"The stale buffers don't work well."

"Why, Ram, why don't the stale buffers work as well?" I pressed. I still don't know why on that day of all days did I ask for answers to such mundane questions. Every child who has ever conducted a science experiment in school knows the answer. Everyone knows stale buffers don't work well, just like everyone knows fresh fruits taste better than those that are overripe and spoiled. I didn't expect Ram to answer my question, and he didn't.

---

**FRESH FRUIT SPOILS WITH TIME,
WHY DON'T SPOILED FRUITS
GET UNSPOILED WITH TIME?**

---

Sometime during lunch, Ram suddenly asked me if I was serious about my questions about buffers.

"Yes, I am. Tell me why stale buffers don't work as

well?"

"Because they get oxidized," Ram answered.

"Why do buffers get oxidized?" I asked, still not knowing where my questions were going to take me.

"They just do!" Ram shrugged his shoulders.

We both forgot about what obviously seemed like a trivial conversation about the buffering capacity of buffers and why stale buffers do not work very well. Some days later, Dr. Ram casually asked me if I wanted to know why buffers get oxidized.

"Oh yes! Tell me, why do buffers get oxidized?" I asked.

"Because oxidation in nature is a spontaneous process," Ram answered calmly.

"What? What did you say, Ram?" I felt a jolt.

"Oxidation is a spontaneous process," Dr. Ram repeated in his usual tone.

Buffers become spontaneously oxidized with time. Why don't oxidized buffers become spontaneously unoxidized with time? Fresh fruit spoils spontaneously with time, everyone knows that. Why doesn't spoiled fruit spontaneously get unspoiled with time? Why are the chemical changes involved in the oxidation of buffers and spoiling of fruits unidirectional? Fish hooked out of water rots within hours at room temperature. Why doesn't the rotting fish spontaneously become "unrotting"? Cut, wet grass decomposes spontaneously in some days. Why doesn't the decomposed grass spontaneously get "undecomposed" in some hours? Butter turns rancid spontaneously. Why doesn't rancid butter later become "unrancid" spontaneously? And, for that matter, how is it that the word "un-decompose" doesn't exist in the English language?

At least, I don't remember anyone ever using it in spoken language or in writing. These thoughts hit me with the force of a lightning bolt. These simple questions had never risen in my mind during all those years of biology classes in high school and college. Nor did they take form during years of my search for the cause of disease as I spent long hours studying microscopic slides. Now for the first time, I suddenly saw the possibility of an answer to that most fundamental of all questions. Oxidation is a spontaneous process — that meant it required no outside clues nor any external programming. Fresh fruits get spoiled because they get oxidized. Spoiled fruit doesn't get unspoiled because it cannot spontaneously get unoxidized. Rancid butter cannot turn unrancid because it doesn't have the reserve of energy to do so.

Oxidation is a loss of electrons — those tiniest packets of energy that are in perpetual motion within atoms and molecules, restless, and bursting with a desire to break loose. Whenever I see young people rebelling, I wonder how can it be any different! It is the nature of living things to want to break loose — in this, electrons are no different from teenagers. In this fundamental equation of life, an amoeba is no different from a dinosaur, nor a lowly shrub from the loftiest of all giant sequoia trees. At atomic and molecular levels, life reduces itself to this simple pattern. Living things age — and die and decay — because they cannot forever control this loss of electrons and energy contained within them. What would be expected if the rate of the energy loss were accelerated? Fatigue! This, indeed, is what happens when a world-class sprinter literally collapses at the finish line. And then he recovers, usually within minutes, because of his conditioning. What would be expected if this rate of energy loss were accelerated *chronically*? Chronic fatigue! What would be expected if the normal oxidative pathways were relentlessly overdriven by allergic triggers, chemical sensitivities, designer killer molecules in our antibiotics and pesticides, oxidants in pollutants, metabolic roller coasters of sugar and neurotransmitters and the powerful oxidant molecules of stress? Unrelenting fatigue — chronic fatigue!

These questions and answers swirled in my mind's eye in flashes of images. Then there were other images. Images of damaged cells, decaying tissues, decomposed organs. The images of rancid butter merged with those of lipid peroxidation of fats in the cell membrane, and the images of decomposed cut grass mingled with those of decaying cells and dead tissues with pockets of pus. It was a high-speed kaleidoscopic motion of injured things.

So, my interest in the basic cause of chronic fatigue, in reality, was a continuation of my search for the initial energetic-molecular events that turn a state of health into a state of absence of health, and then finally into a state of disease. During this period, I diligently searched the medical as well as biology journals for any information that would disprove my evolving concept that spontaneity of oxidation in nature is the true cause of the aging process in man — and for that matter — all other life-forms capable of aerobic (oxygen-utilizing) metabolism.

With time, I became convinced of the theoretical validity of my viewpoint about the essential link between spontaneity of oxidation in nature and aging in man. I also recognized that the experimental and clinical data from diverse fields of inquiry in medicine and biology was entirely consistent with my viewpoint. It was now just a matter of time before I would recognize the essential oxidative nature of the injury to the energy enzyme systems of human energy pathways. *It couldn't be anything other than oxidant molecular injury*. It was *that* simple.

Here, then, was a possibility for me to reduce the many complex issues of chronic fatigue to the two simple manageable questions: 1) What is the energetic-molecular basis of chronic fatigue?; and 2) How can the normal energy enzyme pathways be restored in people who suffer from chronic fatigue?

I relate here for the reader one other image that is still as sharp in my mind as the day I first saw it.

Sally M., a woman in her early forties, consulted me for disabling fatigue. She'd led an active, energetic life except for some allergy symptoms. However, following an attack of a "virus infection that did not clear up for weeks," she developed persistent fatigue. When she consulted me, she suffered from intractable abdominal bloating, muscle aches, joint stiffness, headaches, severe PMS symptoms, and difficulties of mood, memory and mentation. On the second visit, when I reviewed her laboratory results and prepared to start my nutritional and allergy treatment protocols, she complained of "wormy"feelings in her breast, "electric shocks" in her left flank before eating and a "sinking feeling" in the pit of her stomach after meals. Sometimes she felt "blue" and sometimes "angry and hostile." Conscious of the fact that such symptoms are often dismissed by physicians with the old all-in-the-head label, she hesitantly asked me if I thought she were losing her mind. Two of the three physicians she consulted before seeing me had found nothing wrong with her, and had advised her to see a psychiatrist. Indeed, medical texts have no disease labels that fit these symptoms.

I saw Sally's molecular rage one day during one of my ghoraa runs — my morning limbic run. In a flash image I saw Sally lying curled up on the ground, consumed by a fire of "molecular rage." Her body heaved as she struggled to sit up and then it collapsed. I saw her body quiver with bursts of adrenaline, cholinergic fly balls, and neurotransmitters turning and twisting upon themselves. I saw molecular fireworks. I saw oxyradicals in a feeding frenzy, poking gaping holes in her cell membranes. I saw a hemorrhage of magnesium and potassium molecules through the leaky cell walls. I saw calcium molecules flooding the cell innards and suffocating their life span enzymes. I saw violent whirlpools of energy waves. There were cortical electrical sparks all over her body, as if all her tissues were being shorted. Bursts of adrenaline. Pools of lactic acid. Spiking potentials of membrane phospholipids. Feeding frenzy of oxyradicals. Sally's body chemistry was in a pyrotechnic state. Her cell membranes were shot full of holes.

Sally made another attempt to rise, convulsed and collapsed. So that is it. That is what severe fatigue is. It is lacerated cell membranes. It is violated cell innards. It is the hemorrhage of magnesium and of potassium. It is mitochondrial enzymes within the cells drowning in a calcium flood. It is the agony and death of cells. But first and foremost, it is a state of a high oxidative turmoil — a Fourth of July chemistry.

> **OXIDATION IS NATURE'S GRAND DESIGN TO MAKE SURE NOTHING LIVES FOREVER**

I wrote the above line in *The Butterfly and Life Span Nutrition* because this simple insight provided me with the scientific basis for my model of aging-oxidant and life span molecules. Aging-oxidant molecules exist to make sure no life form lives forever and — when not counterbalanced — cause premature aging and disease. Life span molecules promote health and prevent accelerated aging by holding in abeyance the aging-oxidant molecules. I included this statement in *The Ghoraa and Limbic Exercise* for the same reason — it allowed me to put my own experience with different types of physical exercises that are necessary for optimal health within the larger perspective of energy dynamics in human physiology. I include it here for the third time because this statement more than any other provides the sound scientific framework for my clinical work with chronic fatiguers.

## OXYGEN: THE MOLECULAR DR. JEKYLL AND MR. HYDE

The problem of chronic fatigue cannot be understood without understanding the molecular duality of oxygen. Oxygen is a molecular Dr. Jekyll and Mr. Hyde. Oxygen ushers life in. It terminates life. It sustains life by building essential molecules. It ends life by becoming reactive and destructive to living molecules, cells and tissues. Life in the world of oxygen is fresh and clean; oxygen disintegrates the dead material. A world without oxygen would be a world full of stench; proteins in rotten eggs produce foul-smelling gases such as ammonia and hydrogen sulfide in the absence of oxygen.

Dr. Jekyll oxygen is molecular oxygen — atmospheric oxygen that sustains life. Mr. Hyde oxygen is nascent oxygen — atomic, toxic oxygen that kills life. The essential tragedy of our time is this: Our technology is rapidly turning life-sustaining, molecular oxygen into life-destroying, nascent oxygen. To solve the health problems caused by unbridled nascent oxygen, we use drugs that further increase its oxidant effects.

## THE GREAT KILLER MOLECULE

Oxidation is nature's grand prescription to make sure nothing lives forever. Oxidant molecules are like little matches, ready to put things on fire when lighted. A match can burn out the whole forest. How? It is ignited by oxygen, and the oxyradical formation triggered by this process perpetuate the process of burning. Nature designed life span molecules to provide a counterbalance to the oxidant molecules. These molecules prevent ignition by oxygen and hold in check other types of oxidant molecules. Living things generate these molecules so they can save themselves from immediate destruction by oxidant molecules.

## REDUCTION REQUIRES EXPENDITURE OF ENERGY

The opposite of oxidation is reduction — a process by which atoms and molecules gain electrons. The "loss" by oxidation is balanced with the "gain" of reduction during life.

Living things live because they can expend energy. It is

the energy of reduction that provides a counterbalance to oxidant stress, the essence of the aging process. How long can the reduction arm of the redox reaction hold in abeyance the oxidative arm determines how long a rose will bloom and how long an elephant will live. How effectively the reductive arm restrains the oxidative arm determines how fast we recover from a viral infection or from an incision made by a surgeon. The success of our antioxidant energy dynamics determines how well we cope with the progressive oxidant stress of environmental pollutants, allergic triggers, toxic metal overload, metabolic roller coasters, musculoskeletal stresses that arise from physical inactivity, and the potent oxyradicals released by the "fight or flight" stress response. This is the beginning of the state of chronic fatigue.

## HOW CAN NORMAL ENERGY PATHWAYS BE RESTORED IN CHRONIC FATIGUERS?

The second basic question that I set out to answer, at least in part, was how to restore normal energy patterns in people who suffer from chronic fatigue. It is one thing to theorize about the true beginning of the aging process — and by implication — the beginning of disease. It is altogether a different matter for anyone to put such notions into clinical practice without knowing what the possible outcomes might be.

When I returned to the practice of environmental medicine after many years of full-time work in pathology, I mostly drew patients with complex, unrelenting immune disorders and environmental illness who had received little if any benefits from standard drug therapies. It didn't take long to identify a common denominator in their clinical symptomatology: a disabling defect in their normal energy patterns. Within a short time, it became clear that I should focus my clinical and research interests on energy patterns in health and disease — and, of course, what everyone was calling the chronic fatigue syndrome.

Over the years, I have had the opportunity to care for a large number of patients who suffered from chronic, persistent, fatigue, most of whom recovered to return to active lives. I spent several thousand hours listening to their plight in order to define what chronic fatigue is. I also spent long hours reflecting on what the energetic-molecular basis of chronic fatigue might be. I have conducted several studies to test my hypothesis that chronic fatigue is caused by accelerated oxidative molecular injury and, in turn, to prove the clinical efficacy of therapies that eliminate or reduce such oxidative injury, thereby alleviating chronic fatigue.

> **ENERGY ENZYMES FAIL**
> **WHEN THEY ARE DAMAGED BY**
> **ACCELERATED OXIDANT MOLECULAR INJURY**

Chronic fatigue, in the context of human energy dynamics, cannot be grasped without a clear understanding of the essential nature of the basic redox equation of life:

Oxidation occurs spontaneously in nature and causes decay and death. Reduction prevents decay and death but requires active expenditure of energy. For the professional reader, I have written at length about the molecular duality of oxygen, and its impact upon human biology in my review articles entitled *The Agony and Death of a Cell* and *The Molecular Basis of Environmental Illness* published in the course syllabi by the American Academy of Environmental Medicine, Denver, Colorado. Specifically, I presented the scientific evidence for my viewpoint in a paper published in the *Journal of Advancement in Medicine* (1993; 6:83-96). That paper is reproduced in the Appendix by permission of its publisher, Human Sciences Press, Inc. In this chapter, I summarize that evidence.

## *Chronic Fatigue*
### *Is Accelerated Oxidative Molecular Injury*

I propose that chronic fatigue is a state of accelerated oxidative molecular injury. Evidence for this viewpoint — though clearly not complete at this time — is sufficiently strong to provide us with a reasonable framework for formulating nondrug therapies for successful clinical management of chronic fatigue. Equally important, in my view, is the fact that no significant clinical nor experimental data exist that would invalidate the core point of my theory.

The evidence that I marshal to support this hypothesis includes the following:

1. The spontaneity of oxidation in nature is the basis of the

aging dying processes for all life forms that depend on oxygen for respiration, and redox (oxidation-reduction) dysregulations are the initial events that lead to clinical diseases. I elaborate this core aspect of my hypothesis in later chapters of this book.

2. The incidence of chronic fatigue in the general population is increasing, as is the oxidant stress in the Earth's atmosphere.

3. Molecular evidence for oxidative cell membrane injury in chronic fatigue is furnished by changes in the ions — electrically charged metal molecules — that are normally present within and outside the cells.

4. Immune dysfunctions that occur in chronic fatigue are consistent with initial oxidative injury.

5. There is a genetic similarity among patients who suffer from immune disorders such as rheumatoid arthritis, systemic lupus erythematosus, pemphigus vulgaris, and patients who suffer from chronic fatigue (HLA-DR regions).

6. Direct morphologic evidence of increased oxidative stress on the cell membrane is shown by:

> A high frequency (up to 80%) of erythrocyte membrane deformities in chronic fatigue.
> Reversibility of these deformities is effected by intravenous antioxidant therapy with vitamin C.

7.  Changes in electro-myopotentials observed in chronic
    fatigue are consistent with intracellular ionic and
           membrane changes seen in chronic fatigue.

8.  Clinical entities commonly associated with chronic fatigue
    are known to increase oxidative molecular stress; and

9.  Normal energy pathways are restored and the related
    muscular and neurological symptoms are relieved with a
    global strategy to reduce oxidant stress — including
    optimal food choices, oral and intravenous nutrient
    protocols, management of allergies and chemical
    sensitivities, self-regulation, slow, sustained (limbic)
    exercise, and management of coexisting disorders.

From a clinical standpoint, this model of the molecular
basis of chronic fatigue is useful for managing chronic fatigue
without drug regimens.

My colleagues and I are conducting several research
studies with our patients who suffer disabling chronic fatigue. In
one series of 100 consecutive patients, we found mold allergy in
all and pollen and food allergy in most cases. Allergy increases
oxidant stress. About 80% of the patients gave a history of
extensive antibiotic therapy. Antibiotics are designer killer
molecules and are powerful oxidants, both directly and
indirectly. About one-quarter of our patients had elevated blood
levels of toxic metals such as aluminum, mercury, lead, nickel
and others. Toxic metals are potent oxidants. They both
paralyze life span enzymes and activate oxidant enzymes. Many
subjects in this study suffered from unusual degrees of stress
*before* they developed a state of chronic fatigue. Adrenaline and
related stress molecules are virulent oxidant molecules. Viral

and bacterial infections in most cases seemed to play only contributory roles. These microorganisms damage tissues by producing oxidant molecules. In one of my recent studies I observed direct microscopic evidence of oxidant injury of the red blood cell membrane in about 80% of cells (Am J Clin Pathol 94:515; 1990).

## CHRONIC FATIGUE IS FAILURE OF ENERGY ENZYMES

The state of chronic fatigue, in a sense, is molecular quicksand — an entrapment of energy and detoxification enzymes within whirlpools of misdirected electromagnetic and electron transfer events that deplete the sufferer of all his energy. This is the essential nature of this syndrome. The tissues are being beaten like the proverbial dead horse. Treatment with drugs buries the unfortunate patient deeper into this quicksand.

It seems highly probable that in the state of chronic fatigue, there exists also a direct oxidant injury to neurotransmitter receptors and other receptors at the neuromuscular junctions. Such injury would be expected to further disrupt the cell membrane potentials and the electromagnetic impulses that govern muscular activity in health. This is speculative on my part, but I have a strong sense that further research into the modes of oxidant injury will document such evidence.

Most important, people who suffer from chronic fatigue, and develop multiple immune deficits that almost always precede chronic fatigue, need to become aware of the unrelenting state of metabolic burn-out of their energy and detoxification pathways. Tissues are severely fatigued because they are being relentlessly punished.

## *Experimental and Clinical Evidence in Support of the Hypothesis*

Below I summarize for the general reader an enormous body of experimental and clinical data that led me to my theory that chronic fatigue is caused by accelerated oxidative molecular injury. I recognize my theory is lacking sound scientific support in some areas; however, these missing pieces of evidence, in my view, do not substantially weaken the essential strength of this theory: It allows formulation of rational and effective nondrug therapies for restoring damaged energy enzyme pathways and for relieving related symptomatology.

## FIRST, SPONTANEITY OF OXIDATION IN NATURE, AGING AND CHRONIC FATIGUE

The spontaneity of oxidation in nature, I wrote earlier, is where all injury to living things begins. Chronic fatigue begins when oxidant injury is persistent and the body's antioxidant molecular defenses are unable to cope with it.

This is not a mere theoretical construct. Extensive clinical experience has convinced me that this must form the centerpiece of all therapeutic strategies for limiting the excessive oxidant injury and restoring normal energy enzyme pathways. This will become clear as I continue presenting evidence in support of my theory.

## SECOND, INCREASING OXIDANT CAPACITY OF THE EARTH IS INCREASING OXIDANT INJURY TO HUMAN ENZYME SYSTEMS

Recent reports published in *Nature* and *Science* give frightening evidence of an enormous increase in the oxidizing capacity of planet Earth. Comprehensive studies predict that tropospheric $O_3$ (ozone in the upper layers of the atmosphere) will decrease by up to 1% per year over the next 50 years. The ozone layers in some parts of the atmosphere were reported to be 20% less than the expected value for spring 1993. On a more personal level, all we need to do is look out the window and see the clouds of pollution hanging in the air on most days. Acid rains are leaching toxic metals like aluminum and mercury from the soil and dumping them into our water supply. We design efficient ways of killing life and then pour these chemicals as pesticides by hundreds of thousands of tons into our soil. Over 99% of pesticides enter the soil directly, the remaining less than 1% indirectly. Pests do not metabolize pesticides, and almost all of what they take in they put back into our Mother Earth. In synthetic chemicals, we have unleashed an avalanche of oxidants that our antioxidant defenses cannot cope with.

A human face was put on this problem recently by a colleague who was returning to Newark, New Jersey, after a short visit to Florida with her only child, a five-month-old boy. As her plane descended, she looked out the window and cringed at the thought of immersing her five-month-old into the awaiting avalanche of chemicals and filling up his little lungs with toxic pollutants. But, then, what choice is there? *Where else can I take this innocent soul?* she wondered. *Phoenix, Arizona? Denver, Colorado?* Those cities once were regarded as safe havens for people with asthma and other respiratory problems. That was then! Now both cities, because of the regional topography that holds stagnant air, are more polluted than metropolitan New York.

What is the clinical relevance of these projected increments in the oxidizing capacity of Earth? We hear about more skin cancer caused by sunlight and we mumble about loss of ozone and what it will do to our future generations. As for me, that future is here: Chronic fatiguers — our human canaries — are now telling us, in unmistakable terms, what the shape of those things in the future will be. Recent reports of vague, ill-defined symptoms and fatigue among many veterans of the recent Persian Gulf War was another reflection of the images of the future. The chronic fatigue "scholars" will forever debate about what does and what doesn't constitute chronic fatigue. This much is certain — whatever criteria anyone uses for the diagnosis of chronic fatigue, it is evident that the incidence of chronic fatigue reported in the closing decades of the 20th century far exceeds that reported in the opening decades of this century.

## THIRD, OXIDANT INJURY POKES HOLES IN CELL MEMBRANES

A cell looks at the world around it through its

membrane. Thus, the cell membrane is the true interface a cell has with what surrounds it. All events that take place within a cell are in some way or another related to energy dynamics at the cell membrane. Tiniest structures within a cell are called cell organelles, and, like the parent cell, these organelles look at the world around them through their plasma membranes. I have been fascinated by the goings-on at the cell membrane and plasma membranes for over two decades.

As far as a single cell is concerned, the rest of the body belongs to the world outside. The total energy of a cell is devoted to keeping internal order and protecting itself from external disorder. This simple statement need not be ascribed any profound metaphysical meanings. It simply says what I mean. For example, cells from experimental animals cultured in petri dishes grow and flourish with internal clues, with no direction from outside.

## 49 SISTER-BRIDES KILL THEIR 49 BROTHER-GROOMS

"The gods of Mount Olympus," Choua once said to me, "knew something about this problem of chronic fatigue."
"Tell me about it. What did the gods of Mount Olympus know about energy enzymes?" I braced myself for one of Choua's flights.
"The gods knew about your stuff — your theory of aging-oxidant molecules and oxidant injury to cell membranes. You know, the stuff about what's inside the cell hemorrhaging out

and what's outside the cell flooding the cell innards."

Then Choua told me the following story:

*The twins Aegyptos and Danaus each had fifty children — Aegyptos had 50 sons, and Danaus, 50 daughters. The twins fought for inheritance and Aegyptos won. Soon thereafter, Danaus fled with his daughters to Argos where he became the king. The 50 boys came to woo the 50 princesses. King Danaus schemed to revenge himself, and pretended to agree to give his 50 princesses in marriage to Aegyptos' 50 sons. In secret, he advised all of the brides to murder their respective husbands on the wedding night. All obeyed their father except Hypermnestra who helped her husband escape. He later returned, slew his Uncle Danaus, and founded the famous line of Argive kings. The murderous 49 Danaus sisters were condemned to live in Tararos — and as eternal punishment — were required to fill a cask with a hole in the bottom. The vessels given to them to fetch water were sieves.*

"So you think chronic fatiguers suffer the way Danaus's daughters did? Is that the idea?" I asked when Choua finished his tale.

"Isn't that what happens in chronic fatigue?"

"What happens in chronic fatigue?" I asked.

"Why do you give your chronic fatiguers IV drips of magnesium and potassium and taurine and stuff?"

"Because they lack it."

"Why IV drips? Why not just by mouth?"

"Because with IV drips, I can force an awful lot of stuff through the cell membrane, all at once and all in balance. Nutrients taken by mouth usually do not work as well as IVs do."

"What results do you see after IV infusions?"

"They feel better!"

"For how long?"

"In the beginning, it is usually for just a few days."

"Why do you think those fellows feel better for a few days and then go downhill?" Choua continued.

"I guess because the cells lose it through the holes in their membranes. Potassium and magnesium leak out and excess sodium, calcium and water flood the cell innards."

"And then?" Choua pressed on.

"Well! Then ..."I stuttered a little.

"Why do your friends in $N^2D^2$ medicine dole out calcium channel blocking drugs by the ton?" Choua exaggerated.

"Because these drugs block the influx of excess calcium into the cells?" I went along.

"And why do you suppose that works?"

"By preventing flooding of mitochondrial energy enzymes with excess calcium."

"And?"

"And excess calcium within the cells is a poison for mitochondrial ATPase and other energy enzymes!"

"Why do you use taurine in your IV drips?" Choua asked.

"It stabilizes cell membranes."

"How?"

"It is an antioxidant."

"How do antioxidants stabilize cell membranes?" Choua pressed on.

"By preventing oxyradicals from poking more holes in cell membranes," I replied.

"By plugging those gaping holes in cell membranes," Choua added.

"In a way that's true," I consented.

"How do drug doctors treat chronic fatigue?"

"Some use acyclovir. Some others antidepressants and gamma globulin shots," I answered.

"How does acyclovir work? Does it repair the cell membrane?"

"Acyclovir works by interfering with the viral DNA synthesis. I don't think it has anything to do with the cell membrane or the holes in them."

"Do antidepressants close those holes?" Choua asked.

"No! Well, maybe indirectly. I mean they might if depression increases oxidant stress."

"What does IV therapy have to do with Greek gods?" I returned to where Choua had begun.

"The forty-nine killer brides." Choua looked out of the window.

"What do the killer brides have to do with IV therapy?" I persisted.

"The cask with the leaky bottom. The hole in the vessels, the brides in Tararos," Choua snapped and walked out.

## LEAKY CELL MEMBRANES

Human cell membranes normally show a physiological

potential — negative electrical charge — of -60mV to -90mV. This potential and the enzymes such as NADPH located at the cell membrane normally maintain the structural and functional integrity of the membrane. When the cell membrane is stimulated by internal or external stimuli, it depolarizes (loses it negative surface charge). This process of depolarization makes the membrane more permeable — or leaky. The result: What's inside the cell hemorrhages out and what's outside floods the innards. To cite one specific example, in health, sodium is predominantly an extracellular mineral while potassium is largely intracellular. This partition is maintained by the so-called sodium-potassium pump. The leaky cell membrane results in sodium influx and potassium efflux. Both events, unless quickly reversed, lead to serious cellular malfunction. Similarly, in health, the cell membrane works hard to keep its magnesium in and extra calcium out. Oxidant injury allows the extracellular calcium to flood the cell innards and intracellular magnesium to leak out.

Neural therapy for chronic pain and immune disorders is based on the principle that abnormal cell membrane potentials create illness and clinical relief can be obtained with simple, nontoxic therapies that restore the membrane potential dynamics. Such therapies are much favored by European physicians. Among the casualties of our infatuation with drugs and surgical scalpels in the United States are those European researchers whose work in neural therapy is almost completely ignored by physicians in this country.

The cell membrane distinguishes what is "self" for the cell and what is "un-self." How does it do so?

1. It protects the cell innards from oxidant injury by

employing a sophisticated arsenal of antioxidant enzymes.
2. It turns information into physical change.
3. It admits what is needed: food and oxygen.
4. It allows escape of what is not needed anymore: waste and molecular debris.
5. It autoregulates its own form and functions.
6. It adjudicates the conflicts among the cell innards.
7. It receives signals for replication and decides when to act upon those signals and when to reject them — it separates noise from music.
8. It *thinks* for itself.

Within the cells are cell organelles, each having its own plasma membrane. Each such plasma membrane also *thinks for itself* to protect its internal order from external disorder.

What does accelerated oxidant injury do to cell and plasma membranes? It pokes holes in the cell membrane — what's within the cell hemorrhages out, what's outside floods in. This is how chronic fatiguers become magnesium- and potassium-depleted. This is how calcium flooding their mitochondrial enzymes weakens them, and this is why my colleagues in drug medicine are so infatuated with calcium channel blockers for symptom suppression.

The cell membrane separates internal order from external disorder by generating, propagating and integrating electrical signals from within as well as without. It has tiny tunnels in its structure through which pass minerals, nutrients and waste. Some of these tunnels are called membrane channels. These channels are proteins that fold upon themselves to make conduits that allow the passage of molecules through them. In such gating function, a portion of protein molecule folds upon itself to serve as the lid that opens or closes as the need arises. Clever beings, these proteins! The transfer of electrically charged minerals (ions) across these protein conduits (ion channels) is regulated by voltage sensors.

Recent studies clearly demonstrate how oxidant injury molests and mutilates these channel proteins. The form and function of these proteins have been intensively studied. Evidence points to a five-fold symmetry for the multitude of channels activated by the neurotransmitters acetylcholine, glutamate, glycine, and GABA, and four-fold symmetry for the voltage-gated potassium, sodium and calcium channels, and probably for the related cyclic nucleotide-activated channels as well. The function of subunits of multi-subunit gating proteins is finely orchestrated, and is very vulnerable to oxidant injury.

Magnesium and calcium stabilize the myocyte cell membrane and play a critical role in all energy events occurring in the myocyte. Sodium, potassium, calcium and magnesium are all life span minerals, and are of great interest to us in our understanding of the problems of molecular and cellular health, fatigue, weight gain and the development of catabolic maladaptation. Mitochondrial fatigue is caused by many factors.

The principal threats posed to mitochondrial health today arise from supermarket foods, environmental toxicants, molecular roller coasters triggered by bad eating habits and stress molecules. Mitochondrial fatigue is also caused by physical inactivity.

Supermarket food is making us Americans sodium toxic. It is also making us magnesium deficient and potassium poor.

Common use of diuretics (water pills) and other drugs compound these problems. These are some of the essential reasons why I use liberal supplementation of minerals such as magnesium, potassium and molybdenum in the management of my patients with chronic fatigue states.

Some brief comments about calcium, a closely related mineral, may be included here. The primary problem concerning calcium is that of maldistribution. Calcium is deposited in soft tissues and blood vessels where it does not belong and it is not delivered to bones where it is needed. At autopsy in elderly individuals, I regularly observe how calcium in arterial plaques destroys the elastic tissue of the vessel wall, and yet their bones are mushy with osteoporosis. Calcium deposits in the vessels lead to blockages that suffocate our tissues and give us heart attacks and strokes. Calcium in ligaments and joint capsules robs us of the fluidity of motion and gives us painful joints. Concurrently, lack of calcium in bones gives us osteoporosis.

---

## FOURTH, OXIDANT INJURY DAMAGES ENERGY ENZYMES AND MUTILATES GENES THAT ENCODE FOR SUCH ENZYMES

---

This is one area where some essential evidence to support my theory is lacking. This is also where — and I am as confident of it as I am of anything in human biology — future research will clearly and unequivocally establish the link between oxidant injury and the state of chronic fatigue.

Enzymes are proteins, and proteins are very vulnerable to denaturation by oxidant injury. Earlier in this chapter, I write how threadlike protein molecules are clipped by proteinases and peptidases and by oxidant stress. When these proteins repair themselves by finding the clipped-off segments — or synthesize new ones — mismatching mistakes occur. Mismatched, or cross-linked molecules are different not only in form but also in function. This is where the trouble begins.

Chronic fatiguers almost always have low body temperatures that can be normalized with a combination of self-regulatory methods for warming body tissues and low-dose thyroid replacement. It is known that in many such cases conversion of inactive thyroid prehormones to active thyroid hormone $T_4$ is slowed down due to impairment of enzymes that facilitate such reactions. More important, conversion of $T_4$ to much more metabolically active $T_3$ is inefficient due to impaired action of de-iodinase enzymes. The central question for me has been this: What impairs such enzyme functions? I am certain it will be proven to be oxidant injury.

Chronic fatiguers almost always experience chronic abdominal bloating, cramps, episodes of diarrhea and constipation and other related bowel symptoms. Such digestive-absorptive functions in the bowel ecosystem, of course, are enzyme functions. The question for me has been this: What impairs such enzyme function? I am certain it will be proven to be oxidant injury.

Chronic fatiguers frequently suffer mood and memory difficulties. In the last few decades, we have learned much about the neurotransmitter changes that cause such problems. But how are neurotransmitters produced in the body? By enzymes!

The question in my mind, again, has been this: What impairs such enzyme functions? I am certain it will be proven to be oxidant injury.

Muscle weakness, of course, is the symptom chronic fatiguers know most about. Oxidant injury to essential energy enzymes in the muscles plays a key role in the cause of chronic fatigue. Mitochondrial ATPase is a primary energy enzyme in the heart and other muscles. Antibodies against this enzyme sometimes develop after inflammation of the heart muscle caused by viral infections. Deficiency of some other essential muscle energy enzymes, such as myoadenylate deaminase, occurs after viral infections. These observations, scant as they are, furnish strong indirect evidence that failure of muscle energy enzymes occurs after oxidant injury to muscles. Oxidant injury denatures and alters the structure of such enzymes; the immune system then sees them as alien molecules and produces antibodies to destroy them. It seems certain to me that further research into these areas will substantiate this.

Intracellular acidosis — increased acidity within the muscle cells — is associated with muscle fatigue in health. Nuclear magnetic studies have shown a marked increase in such acidity in chronic fatigue syndrome. Such studies also point to excessive glycolytic (sugar-burning) activity in the muscle rather than inadequate oxidation as the cause of increased acidity within muscle cells — strong, though indirect, evidence of oxidative dysregulation.

How is energy generated in the muscles? By mitochondrial enzymes! What impairs such enzymes? I am certain it will be proven to be oxidant injury.

I can sense the growing impatience of some readers with my line of reasoning. But how do you know all that? the purists will frown. I know because each week my copies of *Nature* and *Science* carry reports that oxidant injury mutilates genes that encode for such enzymes. I cite two examples.

Protein-tyrosine phosphatase is an enzyme that plays a role in muscle energy generation. Recently, oxidant injury to a gene that encodes for enzyme creatine phosphokinase has recently been documented (*Nature* 359:644; 1992).

ACE (angiotensin-converting enzyme) plays a major role in regulating blood pressure and thereby in regulating some aspects of heart function. Indeed, ACE-inhibitors make up a class of drugs for controlling blood pressure that are making handsome profits for their makers. Recently, injury to a gene that encodes for angiotensin-converting enzyme — deletion polymorphism in technical jargon — has been shown (*Nature* 359:641; 1992). This report fascinates me. Could such gene injury have been caused by increased environmental oxidant stress? Heart attacks were very infrequent at the beginning of this century. Today, heart attacks are extremely common. We associate heart attacks with high stress, processed foods and oxidized lipids such as cholesterol and others. We should recognize the common denominator in all these factors: oxidant stress.

Can oxidative damage to ion channel proteins in the cell membrane increase membrane permeability — poke holes in the membrane? Can that lead to the efflux of magnesium and potassium and the influx into the cell of calcium? This, in my view, does happen, and I believe future studies will document it fully. Lowered levels of intracellular magnesium and potassium are seen in a host of clinical disorders including chemically-induced cell membrane injury, chemical sensitivity, food allergy and viral infections. Additional proof that gating derangements occur in chronic fatigue states is furnished by studies that use intravenous magnesium and potassium infusions. Patients with chronic fatigue respond well to such infusions in almost all cases.

The oxidizing capacity of the Earth is increasing at a frightening rate. It is not a gentle trend; it literally represents a seismic shift. So I have a strong sense that future research will document oxidant injury to genes that regulate essential enzyme functions in human energy pathways. That will confirm my position on accelerated oxidative molecular injury.

## FIFTH, OXIDANT INJURY MUTILATES IMMUNE MOLECULES AND CELLS

In clinical medicine, many physicians talk about the immune system as if it is made up of several discrete pieces that interact with each other only in limited ways. Thus we talk about humoral (antibody) deficiency disorders, cellular (lymphocyte) disorder, immune complex diseases and complement deficiency disorders. Nothing could be further from the truth. The immune system is a molecular mosaic, an ever-changing kaleidoscopic motion of an enormous number of immune molecules. During the late 1970s, early reports appeared about an unusual immune disorder — the disorder that we later came to recognize as AIDS — it was quite evident to me that with time all known and many unknown immune deficits would be encountered in patients with that disorder. This indeed did happen.

When the term CFID — chronic fatigue immunodeficiency syndrome — gained popularity in the mid-1980s, it was equally evident to me that with time each and every known and many unknown immune deficits would be described in patients with debilitating, persistent chronic fatigue. I was certain that the simplistic ideas of identifying a specific immune deficit, by incriminating one or more viruses such as Epstein-Barr virus or coxsackie viruses, would be proven to be just that — simple-minded notions of "researchers" who look for some laboratory tests to "establish" the diagnosis of the so-called chronic fatigue syndrome so that they can treat this syndrome with this or that drug. This has also come to pass.

Below I list salient immune deficits that I have observed in patients with chronic fatigue or that have been described by others:
1. Depression of cell-mediated immunity
2. Structural and functional deficiencies of natural killer lymphocytes
3. Diminished ability of immune cells to respond to challenge (mitogenically stimulated mononuclear cells)
4. Variable changes in CD4 and CD8 types of lymphocytes
5. Depletion of CD4 CD45RA lymphocytes
6. Changes in the body's ability to produce antibodies against viruses, bacteria and various types of yeasts.
7. Alterations in humoral response such as mild IgA deficiency

8. Elevated levels of immune complexes
9. Presence of autoantibodies such as rheumatoid factor, antinuclear antibodies and cold agglutinins
10. Increased number of B cells
11. Evidence of T-cell activation furnished by studies showing elevated blood levels of IL-2 and T8 receptors and increased number of CD3, CD20 and CD56 cells
12. Blood levels of enzymes 2'5'A synthetase and RNAse are elevated indicating activation of lymphocytes by viruses or exposure to interferon. These changes appear to represent polyclonal B-cell activation.

The above immunologic deficits and abnormalities have led some investigators to consider chronic fatigue syndrome an acquired immunodeficiency state caused by one or more viruses belonging to the herpes or the enterovirus families. Indeed, in a very small subset of patients with chronic fatigue, strong circumstantial evidence suggests an important initial role of viral infections. In my viewpoint, these immunologic changes are consequences of the state of accelerated oxidative molecular injury that results in chronic fatigue, rather than primary causes of the so-called chronic fatigue syndrome or the CFID syndrome.

## SIXTH, SOME GENES RENDER US VULNERABLE TO OXIDANT INJURY

My theory that chronic fatiguers are human canaries

evolved from my work with such patients. Over and over again, I saw a clinical pattern of undiagnosed and unmanaged allergies in childhood, extensive use of broad-spectrum antibiotics for recurrent infections and acne, slow recovery from viral infections, recurrent episodes of vaginitis in young women, frequent use of drugs for anxiety, stress and depression, increasing sensitivities to foods, abnormal bowel responses, and, finally, chronic fatigue states.

For several years, I searched for the common denominator among such patients that I could use to identify such patients. To-date, I am convinced the best genetic marker for chronic fatiguers is IgE antibodies. There have been occasions when patients with chronic fatigue vehemently denied having a history of allergy symptoms. Invariably, a careful and diligent search brought out history of hidden or neglected allergies, such as long-forgotten eczema of infancy, episodes of remote sinusitis or reactions to foods.

The clear proof of allergy, however, is in the detection of IgE antibodies with sensitive and specific micro-elisa assays. The commonly performed RAST assay is not nearly good enough for this purpose. Indeed, many of my patients with clear allergies were told they did not have allergies just because the RAST test was found to be negative. To date, I have not seen a single patient who developed chronic fatigue of over six months duration who could not be unequivocally proven to be allergic with sensitive and specific micro-elisa tests for IgE antibodies. I am convinced that an allergic genetic makeup sets people up for chronic fatigue. Cumulative oxidant injury caused by allergic triggers, extensive antibiotic therapies, drug abuse for mere symptom suppression, viral and bacterial infections, chemical exposure and the powerful oxyradicals of "fight-or-flight" stress lead to chronic fatigue states. Genes are what set people up for chronic fatigue.

In support of my viewpoint, I cite studies that show common genetic patterns between chronic fatiguers and patients who suffer from a host of autoimmune disorders such as lupus, rheumatoid arthritis, pemphigus vulgaris, IgA and gold nephropathies (kidney diseases), and other related disorders. Specifically, patients in these groups share genes on the HLA-DR4 region antigens. In one recent study, over 40% of patients with chronic fatigue syndrome were positive for antigens of HLA-DR3 region. This common association may be seen as the evidence of genetic predisposition in individuals with these HLA antigens for oxidant, and at later stages, immune injuries. As I discuss later in this chapter and in the chapter Where Does It All Begin?, there is strong enzymatic evidence that abnormal autoimmune responses are associated with — and most likely triggered by — induction (too much of) or inactivation (not enough of) of certain enzyme systems.

## SEVENTH,
## OXIDANT INJURY DEFORMS CELL MEMBRANES

In one of my research studies, I examined red blood cells of patients with chronic fatigue with a high-resolution, phase-contrast microscope. I observed deformities of the red cell membrane and loss of normal plasticity of cell walls in up to 80% of cells (Am J Clin Pathol 94:515;1990). The cell membrane deformities included sharp angulation, spike formation and saw tooth-like irregularities. These changes were most marked in patients who suffered from acute and chronic food, mold and pollen allergy reactions.

A surprising finding in this study was how readily such deformed cells regain their healthy, round appearance and become invigorated and pliable after the oxidant stress upon them is relieved with 15 grams of vitamin C given as an intravenous drip. Thus, the oxidant nature of the observed deformities was made clear. Vitamin C, of course, is the quarterback water-phase antioxidant in human tissues.

## EIGHTH, OXIDANT INJURY DISRUPTS PATTERNS OF ELECTROMAGNETIC ENERGY IN MUSCLES

A consistent pattern of markedly diminished galvanic skin responses and increased electromyopotentials is observed in patients with chronic fatigue as compared with patients with essential hypertension and healthy subjects (personal unpublished observations.) Evidence of diminished perfusion and decreased glucose utilization in certain parts of the limbic system of patients with chronic fatigue associated with psycho-neurologic symptoms has been recently reported. These observations are consistent with the consequences of oxidative injury to the neurones (nerve cells) in parts of the limbic system. Parenthetically, it may be added that during training sessions in effective self-regulatory methods, more than half of these subjects show moderate to marked reductions in their electromyopotentials, albeit for short periods of time. With long-term training in slow, sustained breathing patterns with prolonged unforced expiration, reduction in muscle potentials is achieved by most patients with chronic fatigue.

## NINTH, STRESS CAUSES CHRONIC FATIGUE BY OXIDANT INJURY

Stress causes oxidant injury, and unrelenting stress causes unrelenting oxidant injury.

We all have seen nature movies where a gazelle is chased by a leopard. In those few moments when the fate of the gazelle is determined, both the prey and the predator are in a frenzy of energy — their muscles are taut even as they go through frenetic motion, their hair on end, their eyes bulge with dilated pupils, their lungs hyperventilate, their entire bodies quiver. Where does all that energy come from? For this theater of life and death, both the hunter and the hunted put out their "oxidative best." How?

## OXIDATIVE FRENZY

In scientific jargon, this "fight-or-flight" response represents adrenergic peaks — rapid bursts of stress molecules such as adrenaline, nor-adrenaline and their cousin molecules. The purpose of these molecules is to maximize the energy response, both for the gazelle and the leopard. Adrenaline and its cousin catecholamine molecules, I wrote earlier in this chapter, are some of the most destructive oxidant molecules in human biology. What we consider "fight-or-flight" response is in reality an oxidative frenzy. It can only last for brief periods of time. Either the prey escapes or the predator feasts.

What happens to these molecules after the oxidative frenzy is over? Or in the conventional language, the "normal" receptor roles of adrenaline are played out? This question is rarely addressed in our medical school classes. Adrenaline and its cousin stress molecules are turned into powerful oxidant molecules by a number of different molecular transformations. Specifically, these molecular permutations include:

A.  Auto-oxidation of adrenaline and its cousin stress molecules (dihydroxyphenols) to oxyradicals
B.  Oxidation of adrenaline and related molecules to organic free radicals by superoxides
C.  Dehydrogenation of their degradation products to tetraisoquiniline to isoquiniline-redox cycle

In *The Cortical Monkey and Healing,* I wrote that stress is an integral part of human biology. Stress can trigger, mimic or exaggerate almost all disease processes. In biology, the stress response is an essential element of an organism's physiology. Knowledge of the causes of stress is essential for prevention of stress. But this knowledge, by itself, cannot dissipate the stress. Extensive clinical work with patients devastated by chronic stress has convinced me that the so-called mind-over-body approach to stress is but a cortical trap set by the cortical monkey who, in reality, loves to recycle misery — and when that is not sufficient, it precycles the feared, future misery. *An energy-over-mind strategy gives far superior clinical results.*

## TENTH,
## VIRUSES INJURE CELLS BY OXIDANT INJURY

Until recently, chronic fatigue was considered by many to be caused by a chronic Epstein-Barr infection. However, laboratory evidence of certain retroviral sequences in the blood of patients with chronic fatigue has since been reported.Yet, the occurrence of viral infection in patients with chronic fatigue cannot be accepted as evidence that fatigue is caused by such viral infections. The development of persistent chronic fatigue after viral infections is well-documented, and this is fully consistent with the present hypothesis. Viral infections have been shown to increase oxidative stress, and mortality from acute influenza infection in mice can be drastically reduced with the use of antioxidants such as superoxide dismutase (*Science* 244:974;1989). A clinical correlate for such experimental observation is the ability to prevent the development of chronic fatigue following acute viral infections, including those caused by hepatitis B and Epstein-Barr viruses, with the use of oral and intravenous antioxidant nutrient therapies (personal unpublished data). Viral infections in my own clinical practice, in general, did not lead to chronic fatigue when aggressively managed with oral and intravenous antioxidant therapies and with other necessary supportive measures. It appears that viral infections culminate in chronic fatigue states only when molecular defenses are suppressed due to food and mold allergy, chemical sensitivity, toxic metal overload, extensive use of antibiotics, stress, anxiety and depressed states. These infections prove to be the straw that broke the camel's back of molecular defenses.

Recently, several cases of chronic fatigue have been shown to meet the diagnostic criteria of idiopathic CD4 T-lymphocytopenia (ICL) — commonly known as AIDS-like illness in HIV negative individuals — adding to the long list of many known and some as yet unknown viruses that have been suspected to cause chronic fatigue. In one of my own studies of chronic fatigue, I observed serologic evidence of past Epstein-Barr virus infection in over two-thirds of the patients and very high titers of IgG antibodies (presumably reflecting ongoing viral replication) in about one-third of the patients. A single patient from Australia suffering from severe, persistent chronic fatigue showed serologic evidence for HTLV-III infection. She responded extremely well to our nondrug therapies and obtained near-complete relief within eight weeks.

## ELENTH, ALLERGIC TRIGGERS AFFLICT US BY TRIGGERING OXIDANT INJURY

How do allergic triggers cause a runny nose, itchy eyes or abdominal cramps? In the classical type of hay fever allergy, the symptoms of allergy reactions are triggered by the release of histamine and related chemical mediators of the allergic response. These mediators are released by events that occur at the cell membrane receptors. What is the basic nature of such events? At the root of such events are oxidative mechanisms involving NADPH and related enzymes. The cell membranes of cells involved in allergic reactions are literally bathed in oxidative soup.

It is well-recognized that allergies can cause short-term

fatigue; however, the prevalence of specific IgE antibodies in patients with chronic fatigue in this study suggests that an underlying IgE-mediated allergy may play an important, if not pivotal role, in the causation of chronic fatigue.

The results of my own published and unpublished studies described later in this volume have convinced me that an IgE genetic marker is, at this time, the most important — and clinically useful — marker of the subset of people who are vulnerable to disabling chronic fatigue. I discuss the clinical implications of this important fact fully in the section on management of chronic fatigue.

## TWELFTH, CHEMICALS INJURE CELLS AND MOLECULES BY OXIDANT INJURY

Chemical toxicity is largely a dose-dependent phenomenon. Chronic fatigue associated with exposure to industrial toxins is well established. Chemical sensitivity, by contrast, is dose-independent; chronic fatigue associated with it is clinically well recognized, though the mechanisms involved have not been fully elucidated. Both chemical toxicity and sensitivity, as discussed earlier, result from the oxidizing potential of these agents. I discuss this subject further in the chapter Where Does It All Begin?

## THIRTEENTH, TOXIC METALS INJURE MOLECULES AND CELLS BY OXIDANT INJURY

Fatigue is a well recognized symptom of anemia, and is considered a consequence of the lowered oxygen-carrying capacity of blood. However, anemia as the major or a contributory cause of fatigue was not observed in a single case of 100 consecutive cases of chronic fatigue in one of my studies. Diminished blood levels of oxyhemoglobin were observed in a majority of patients with mercury toxicity and chronic fatigue, and a lack of oxygen was proposed as a possible molecular basis of chronic fatigue. Is this observation inconsistent with my theory? Mercury and other heavy metals are known to bind with the reducing potential and/or with the reducing function such as the sulfhydryl group of enzymes and other proteins, thereby inactivating them. As a consequence of this, the natural reducing mechanisms are impaired and oxidative mechanisms potentiated. Indeed, this mechanism is likely to play a role in the etiology of chronic fatigue in patients with heavy metal overload in the study cited above.

## FOURTEENTH, SUGAR INJURES MOLECULES AND CELLS BY OXIDANT INJURY

Sugar is the principal antinutrient in the United States

today. Evidence from diverse lines of scientific research are beginning to unravel the story of sugar ravages. To cite one example, until recently we considered hypertension in the vast majority of Americans essential i.e.,of unknown cause. Now we know that up to 80% — the real number is probably higher — of the so-called essential hypertension is associated with high blood insulin levels. In other words, insulin dysregulation appears to be related to the incidence of high blood pressure. How does that happen except through sugar dysregulation? These data bring much consternation to practitioners of $N^2D^2$ medicine because they fully validate the theory and practice of nutritionist physicians who have talked and written about the role of sugar for years. I wonder if this will bring any regrets to any of the medical licensing boards who revoked the licenses of some practitioners because they treated hypoglycemia when it was considered to be a phantom, all-in-the-head disorder.

Recently, professor Dillman, the Russian endocrinologist, Pavlo Yutsis, M.D., of New York, and others have proposed that sugar dysmetabolism can lead to immunodepression, and that such metabolic immunodepression can lead to impaired cell-mediated immunity and chronic fatigue. The factors that lead to such metabolic immunodepression include:

1. Disturbances of carbohydrate and lipid metabolism that include glucose intolerance
2. Post-prandial hyperinsulinemia (abnormal insulin peaks after meals)
3. Raised serum levels of free fatty acids and LDL cholesterol
4. Accumulation of oxidized lipids in the plasma membranes of T-lymphocytes and monocytes.

Many clinicians like myself recognize chronic fatigue as an important aspect of the clinical syndrome of rapid hyperglycemic-hypoglycemic shifts that are followed by similar peaks of insulin and adrenaline. Adrenaline and its cousin molecules, I wrote earlier, are powerful oxidizing agents. Furthermore, glucose autoxidation causes oxidative protein damage in the experimental glycation model of diabetes mellitus and aging; both factors support the proposed hypothesis.

## FIFTEENTH, MUSCLE BIOPSIES IN CHRONIC FATIGUE SHOW OXIDATIVE INJURY

Muscle tissue can be oxidatively injured, pathologically, as a result of crushing injury, viral myositis, myalgia and myopathies or physiologically, as a result of long-distance running or heavy weight lifting. Indeed, some well-meaning but poorly informed fitness "experts" even advise their elderly subjects to undertake strenuous physical exercise in the hope that such exercise will first damage the muscle fibers and then lead to muscle buildup by repair reaction. Of course, all such muscle injury is oxidative in nature.

A large number of structural changes have been observed in the muscles of chronic fatiguers. These include:

1. Cellular degenerative changes (vacuoles, cytoplasmic bodies, misplacement of nuclei, basophilic (blue) discoloration, etc.)
2. Fiber splitting
3. Fiber atrophy

4. Increased muscle lipid and glycogen content
5. Single muscle fiber glycogen depletion
6. Mitochondrial hyperplasia (overgrowth)
7. Deficiency of enzymes such as myoadenylate deaminase
8. Cell necrosis (cell death)

Several chronic fatigue researchers have tried to discover the cause of the so-called chronic fatigue syndrome by performing muscle biopsies. Predictably, these researchers have returned empty-handed, because all muscle injury is oxidative in nature, and one can predict with great confidence that oxidative injury in chronic fatigue syndrome will not be fundamentally distinguishable from that which is caused by other types of muscle injuries.

*Degenerative and/or regenerative features were seen in 32 (43%) CFS patients. There was no correlation with a history of viral infection. Necrosis was an uncommon finding and other abnormalities occurred in only a few biopsies. ... Since, necrosis can be seen in asymptomatic individuals, it is unlikely to be a significant abnormality in CFS.*

*Chronic fatigue syndrome.* Wiley, Chishester (Ciba Foundation Symposium 173) p 107, 1993

Translation: Damage to muscle cells in chronic fatigue

is the same as is seen in healthy persons after muscle injury.

Some other researchers have reported a higher number of microscopic abnormalities in chronic fatigue syndrome (up to 75% of patients). The essential element in this discussion, however, is that the patterns of muscle cell injury in chronic fatigue syndrome are no different from those observed in other forms of oxidative muscle cell injury.

## MUSCLES ADAPT TO OXIDATIVE STRESS

There are two major types of muscle fibers (cells): the Type I, or slow-twitch, and Type II, or fast-twitch fibers. In *The Ghoraa and Limbic Exercise,* I wrote how fast-twitch, Type II muscle fibers generate energy by burning sugars, much like the burning of dry paper — there is a flash and there are ashes. We need such bursts of energy for activities such as sprinting or lifting heavy weights. Slow-twitch, Type I fibers, by contrast, generate energy in an even, sustained fashion — much like a candle burns, slowly but over a long time. In health, groups of muscles that are called upon to furnish rapid bursts of energy, such as calf muscles, predictably have a larger population of fast-twitch, Type II fibers. By contrast, muscles that are required to generate energy in more sustained fashion — such as the tibialis anterior muscle on the front of the leg — have a larger proportion of slow-twitch, Type I fibers.

Studies with muscle biopsies in chronic fatigue syndrome have uncovered two important lines of evidence that support my oxidative hypothesis:

1.  Mitochondria overgrow in the muscle cells in chronic fatigue states. In *The Ghoraa and Limbic Exercise*, I describe mitochondria as the tiniest, sausage-shaped structures that function as cell powerhouses. Mitochondria are composed of a large number of shelflike cristae that provide spaces for oxidative energy enzymes within the mitochondria. The overgrowth — hyperplasia in scientific jargon — of mitochondria furnish one of the strongest evidence that muscle cells in chronic fatigue states are subject to accelerated oxidative molecular injury.

2.  The number of slow-twitch, Type I fibers decreases in comparison with fast-twitch, Type II fibers. This change has been considered of uncertain significance by the researchers. To me, however, it suggests an additional bit of evidence to support the oxidative hypothesis: Overdriven, oxidatively damaged muscles adapt to accelerated oxidative molecular injury by favoring those fibers that utilize oxygen more efficiently (fast-twitch) over those that utilize oxygen less efficiently (slow-twitch.)

---

## SIXTEENTH, PREVENTING DISEASES BY PREVENTING OXIDANT INJURY

---

The strongest evidence for my hypothesis derives from my clinical outcome studies of successful reversal of chronic fatigue states with nondrug, antioxidant therapies. This is where the proverbial rubber meets the road. In addition to my rather extensive work with chronic fatigue, I have had the privilege of evaluating clinical results with such therapies obtained by many of my colleagues using nondrug antioxidant therapies.

I cite here data obtained with one of my own studies. Of the 100 consecutive patients with the chief complaint of chronic fatigue who were treated at the Chronic Fatigue Clinic at the Institute, 46 met the CDC criteria for chronic fatigue syndrome. IgE antibodies with specificity for at least three mold antigens were present in all 100 patients. Eighty-eight patients gave a history of extensive antibiotic therapy and reported symptoms indicative of altered states of bowel ecology. Elevated blood levels of one or more heavy metals (Pb, Hg, Al, Cd and As) were found in 37 patients. Serologic evidence for active viral replication was not detected in the majority of patients. Major stress (as assessed by the patient) preceded the onset of chronic fatigue in less than 10% of patients. All patients were managed with integrated treatment protocols of oral and intravenous nutrient therapies, antigen immunotherapy for IgE-mediated allergy, training in effective methods for self-regulation and a program for slow, sustained exercise. The intravenous nutrient protocol was formulated to provide a strong nutrient antioxidant support, and not to correct any putative nutritional deficiencies. The outcome data for these 100 patients with chronic fatigue was as follows: Excellent response (symptom relief > 80%), 68%; good response (symptom relief between 60% and 80%), 12%; modest response (symptom relief between 40% and 60%), 8%; and poor response (symptom relief between 0 and 40%), 12%.

In later chapters of this book I give detailed recommendations for restoring the energy enzymes and reversing the state of chronic fatigue with nondrug antioxidant therapies. In those chapters, I furnish additional outcome data obtained with some of my other studies.

## SUMMARY

*On the principle that science is the art of the possible, in Medawar's phrase, the attribute of a physical model that matters most is that it should be tractable, not that it rigorously embody what is known of the real world.*

Nature 359: 359; 1992

The strength of my theory that the state of chronic fatigue is a state of accelerated oxidative molecular injury is that it represents a synthesis of many known facts of biology, certain aspects of the impact upon genetic makeup of environmental factors, several astute observations made by clinicians who manage patients with chronic fatigue, and some personal clinical observations. It derives its principal merit from the clinical outcome of studies that show successful results obtained with therapeutic strategies that seek to reduce oxidative molecular stress by integrating *all* the relevant aspects of applied clinical nutrition, environmental control and desensitization for IgE-mediated disorders, effective self-regulatory methods and programs of slow, sustained exercise combined with methods of meditation.

---

The emerging pandemic of incapacitating chronic
fatigue — and its partial expression in easy fatiguability among
people who otherwise appear in good health — cannot be
understood by the prevailing model of one-disease-one-etiology
model of research in medicine. Nor is the model of
investigating the therapeutic efficacy of a single pharmacologic
agent with the double-blind cross-over model relevant to the
problem of chronic fatigue. Indeed, the notion that one or
more pharmacologic agents can be developed to reduce
excessive oxidative stress that arises from a host of
environmental, nutritional, microbiologic and stress-related
factors seems highly improbable and inconsistent with the
general hypothesis proposed.

*Serenity is not freedom from the storm but peace amid the storm.*

Anonymous

*Chronic fatigue carries with it life-changing possibilities—whether we change or not is determined by the choices we make.*

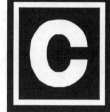

# Chapter 5

# How Does It All Begin?

"How does chronic fatigue begin?" I asked Choua one day between patient visits in my Denville office.

"How does it begin?" Choua tilted his head, "You see chronic fatiguers all day long and you don't understand how it all begins."

"I have some ideas. But tell me how you think it all begin."

Choua looked at me with quizzical eyes, shook his head but said nothing. Then he walked over to the window, and, with his back turned to me, looked out. I knew I had lost him. I looked at the back of his head and wondered what thoughts might pass through it. After some moments Choua stepped out and I picked up the chart of my next patient.

It was close to midnight when I finished with my last appointment that day. I began to stuff my papers into my briefcase to leave when I heard the door move. I looked up. Choua stood in the door holding a blue folder. "Oh no, not now!" I mumbled to myself. In the office, the staff keeps clinical charts of male patients in blue folders and those of female patients in canary folders. Choua obviously wanted to say something about some boy or man, and I sensed it had something to do with the question I had asked him earlier. He must have searched for a chart that he thought made his point in a telling way, and having found one to his liking, he now wanted to say his piece.

"Long day!" I tried to persuade Choua to postpone his comments to some other time.

"This is where it begins!" Choua waved the blue chart at me, ignoring my hesitation.

"Can we look at it tomorrow?" I suggested.

"Hear this," Choua said, opening the chart while ignoring my suggestion.

"It's kind of late, isn't it, Choua?" I pleaded, this time directly.

"No one could put it better!" Choua was exuberant with his find.

"It's very late," I repeated.

"This is little David's chart. There is a letter in it from his allergist to his pediatrician that says it all. It tells you exactly where fatigue begins," Choua chirped.

"Okay! Let's make it quick," I said with resignation.

"It says it all." Choua pulled a sheet of paper from the folder and started reading:


### Dear Dr. General Practitioner,

#### Re: David Hives

Thank you for referring David Hives to me. He presented as a two-and-half - year old with chronic urticaria and occasional wheezing since October of 1992.

His urticaria is possibly exacerbated by eating hot dogs, peanut butter and tomato sauce. He has no history of rhinitis or food allergies and has a history of an allergic reaction to Amoxicillin. He lives in a 50-year-old home, with no pets, no smokers, but with wall-to-wall carpeting. His past medical history is significant for recurrent tonsillitis.

RAST testing to trees, grass, English plantain, ragweed, cat, dog, dust mite, Alternaria was negative as well as to milk, soybean, eggs, peanut and tomato. His CBC showed a white count of 6.8 with 67 polys, 24 lymphs and 1 eosinophil. His ESR was 7. Hep screen, monospot and immunoglobulin levels are pending.

It is not clear what the etiology of his urticaria is. It may be secondary to a chronic infection. He is currently being treated with Benadryl prn but may require a short course of Prednisone if his symptoms become more severe.

I hope this information will be of help to you in managing his case.

Sincerely Yours,

Allergy Specialist, M.D.

Diplomate, American Board of
Allergy and Immunology

Doesn't it say everything?" Choua looked up as he finished reading. I remembered the letter. David's mom had asked me to read this letter when she first consulted me. Choua had read the letter verbatim except where he substituted "Dear Dr. Pediatrician" for the name of the pediatrician and "David Hives" for David that appeared in the beginning of the letter and "Allergy Specialist, M.D." for the name of the allergist at the bottom of the letter. So considerate of Choua, I mused.

"Let's go. We'll talk about it some other time. It's getting very late, past midnight." I wanted to end the conversation.

"It's a revealing bit of medical letter writing, isn't it?" Choua was not deterred.

"Yes! That it is. Let's go." I picked up my briefcase as I tried to pass Choua standing in the door.

"Dumb! But revealing!" Choua let me pass and then followed.

"What's dumb about it?" I looked at him sternly. "It's a sort of boiler-plate letter that physicians write to each other."

"You are tired! Aren't you?" Choua asked sympathetically.

"No, I am not tired," I softened my tone, "but I have to leave now if I am to catch some sleep before I go to the hospital in the morning." I quickened my pace.

"This letter doesn't grab you?" Choua seemed a bit disappointed.

"No! It doesn't grab me!" I gave a curt answer.

"The letter begins by recognizing that little David suffers from chronic urticaria and wheezing," Choua went on as he moved faster to keep pace with me. "Urticaria is skin protesting with hives and wheezing is bronchial tubes protesting with spasms. Right?" Choua began to interpret the allergist's letter.

"Right! Right! Choua." I didn't want to let him engage me in this discussion that late at night.

"So this allergist takes what little David's skin is telling everyone who cares to listen and turns it into his medical diagnosis. And then he ...."

"So what's wrong with that?" I interrupted Choua with frustration.

"Then he goes on to say," Choua continued, either not noticing or deliberately ignoring my frustration, "that David's urticaria 'is possibly exacerbated by eating hot dogs, peanut butter and tomato sauce.' "

"So?" I said with irritation.

"You didn't hear this letter well when I read it to you, did you?" Choua asked with a grin.

"I heard you," I complained, "but I don't see why you are making so much fuss about it."

"Amazing! It's amazing!" Choua exclaimed. "You don't see the utter stupidity of it all, do you?"

"You are always seeing things, Choua," I taunted him.

" 'His urticaria is possibly exacerbated by eating hot dogs, peanut butter and tomato sauce. He has no history of rhinitis or food allergies'. Amazing! Isn't it? I mean that the allergist didn't see the inconsistency in his words. You don't either. In one sentence the allergist writes about reactions to hot dog, peanut butter and tomato, and in the same sentence he declares — with overriding authority — that David has no food allergy." Choua chuckled.

"He did use the word 'possibly,' didn't he?" I countered.

"Then the letter gets more interesting," Choua didn't seem to find it necessary to respond to my objection. "The allergist next goes on to write that David is allergic to

Amoxicillin."

"What's so interesting about a two-and-half-year-old boy being allergic to Amoxicillin?" I asked with annoyance.

" 'RAST testing to trees, grass, English plantain, ragweed, cat, dog, dust mite, Alternaria was negative,.." Choua calmly resumed reading the allergist's letter, " 'as well as to milk, soybean, egg, peanut and tomato'."

"So?" I shrugged my shoulders. "The RAST tests were negative, and the allergist interpreted that to mean that David is not allergic. That happens all the time."

"All the time!" Choua repeated after me. "What type of blood test do you do to diagnose allergy?"

"Micro-elisa test," I answered.

"Why don't you use the RAST tests?" he asked.

"You know very well why!" I answered with irritation, "because the RAST tests misses out on more than fifty percent of allergies."

In the late 1970's and early 1980's, my colleague Madhava Ramanarayanan, Ph.D., and I developed micro-elisa assay IgE antibodies for diagnosis of allergy. Early in its development, we were pleasantly surprised to observe that our micro-elisa assay was far more sensitive than the RAST test. Specifically, we discovered that in the blood of patients with clinical mold allergy, our micro-elisa assay detected IgE antibodies with specificity for molds in twice as many samples as the RAST test. Our assay was also clearly much more sensitive than the RAST test for grass, tree and weed pollens and for cat and dog allergens. During the several months that followed, we repeated our experiments on several occasions to make certain that we were not making any mistakes. We published our data in a series of papers in *The American Journal of Clinical Pathology, Annals of Allergy, Clinical Allergy* and some other journals. In these papers, we included procedural details and furnished reasons why micro-elisa assay was superior to the RAST test. In our simplistic thinking, we had hoped that micro-elisa would replace the RAST test within some years. Immunology researchers are not good judges of what is or is not profitable for the industry. The RAST test prevailed despite its poor diagnostic efficiency. Almost 12 years after we published our results, researchers at a major American diagnostic company presented results with their version of micro-elisa assay — that, in reality, was our assay in a different garb and gave almost identical results. *Maybe now things will change, we hoped. Maybe now our allergists will discontinue using the obsolete RAST test and will begin to diagnose allergies more accurately with the superior micro-elisa assay.* We were again wrong. New methods in medicine gain rapid acceptance only when there is money in them for some group.

"Do you do hepatitis screens and mono spot tests to diagnose allergy?" Choua's words brought me back.

"Not for allergy diagnosis," I answered.

"This allergy specialist did!" Choua spoke derisively. "He didn't do the right tests for allergy diagnosis, but did hepatitis screen and mono spot tests and immunoglobulin tests. What do you make of it?"

"It's late, Choua! Let's call it a day."

"The best part comes next." Choua continued reading the letter, brimming with energy. "It is not clear what the etiology of his urticaria is. It may be secondary to a chronic infection. Now does that make any sense at all?" Choua wailed.

"Actually, Choua, people do develop allergy to bacteria," I said in defense of the allergist.

"My foot!" Choua suddenly raised his voice.

"Your foot or no foot, that does happen," I responded

calmly.

"C'mon! What kind of silly defense is that? An allergist who cannot diagnose common inhalant allergy talks about bacterial allergy! What did your micro-elisa test show?"

"You are carrying the chart, not me, Choua! You must have looked at those results. Those tests were positive. There is no question the boy is allergic," I admitted.

"That allergist is looking for justification for using antibiotics to treat allergy. He isn't thinking of desensitizing the kid for bacterial allergy," Choua taunted. "Bacterial desensitization is not where his head is. I'll bet he has never desensitized any child for bacteria."

"You know what populates people's heads, I don't," I snapped back. "Antibiotics is not what she ..."

"Oh yes! I forgot. She glossed over Amoxicillin allergy. The drug doctors don't dwell on adverse effects of drugs. I mean, you have to have faith in the tools of your trade, don't you? The drug doctors can't say too much against drugs. Can they? I mean what kind of PR would it be if they spoke against their drugs?"

"That's ridiculous! Choua, you cannot help it. Physician-bashing is in your bone marrow. Isn't it?"

"'He is currently being treated with Benadryl prn but may require a short course of prednisone if his symptoms become more severe.'" Choua continued.

"Are we finished with the letter?" I wanted to end the conversation.

"How often do you use steroids to treat allergy?" Choua asked.

"Almost never. But ..."

"How do steroids work for allergy?" Choua didn't let me complete my sentence.

"They suppress symptoms."

"And what else do they suppress?"

"Choua, why do you keep asking me these questions? You know steroids suppress the entire range of immune responses," I protested.

"What do steroids do for the underlying problems in allergy?" he pressed on.

"Nothing!"

"Nothing. Good! I was hoping you would say that," Choua tilted his neck.

"Steroids do save lives in acute, life-threatening conditions," I said lamely.

"How many life-threatening conditions does little David suffer from?" Choua asked belligerently.

"You miss the point. When someone is very uncomfortable with allergy symptoms, steroids help. You know real treatment for allergy works slowly. Sometimes it takes months." I put forth the usual defense of steroids used by mainstream physicians.

"So why don't you use it more often?" Choua was unrelenting.

"Because I do nutritional medicine. That's why! I don't find that necessary. If I did, I would use them," I answered, exasperated.

I walked out to my car in the parking lot, opened the car, threw my briefcase on the back seat. As I bent to slide into the driver's seat, I saw Choua leaning on the railing by the door out of the corner of my eye. He was looking at me. I knew he wasn't through with his thing about little David. I hesitated for a minute before walking back toward him.

*Your gurus of the body-mind-spirit business are so obsessed with the "inner" children that they don't see how our "outer" children are mauled by toxic drugs, toxins in food and stress.*

"Are you staying here tonight?" I forced a smile as I approached Choua.

"Suppose someone is a lawn freak," Choua spoke, seemingly oblivious to the hesitation in my steps. "He waters his lawn twice a week. He hand-pulls the weeds every week. He feeds the lawn every two weeks. Now suppose his lawn is like a rug — deeply rooted, freshly cut and neatly trimmed. His neighbor is annoyed at the way his unkempt lawn looks next to this man's manicured grounds. Now ..."

"Are we talking about David or are we talking about somebody's lawn?" I interrupted Choua.

"Now suppose the lawn freak goes away with his family for a three-week vacation." Choua again ignored my question. "The neighbor, out of sheer spite, decides to wreck the lawn. He sprays a potent herbicide over the lawn and kills all the deep-rooted grass. Then the rain pours down and is followed by bright sunshine and then the rains come again. So the cycles of heavy rain and warm sunshine continue until the man returns. What do you think he will find when he returns?" Choua asked me.

"The killed grass cannot come back in just three weeks," I ventured a guess.

"Right! Right!" Choua became animated. "What will the lawn look like when he returns?"

"I guess when the grass is gone, weeds will grow," I guessed again.

"Yeah! Yeah! And what next?" Choua pressed me.

"What next? I guess the weeds will flourish and overgrow everything."

"Why? Why would the weeds overgrow everything?"

"Because the weeds are hardier than grass?" I gave a tentative answer.

"Exactly! That's it. Exactly right," Choua gloated with excitement. "The delicate grass will be no more. Instead, the hardy weeds will raise their heads and will crowd out everything else."

"I suppose that will happen. But tell me, Choua, what does the lawn have to do with David?" I protested again.

"You don't get it. Do you?" Choua's eyes narrowed.

"I think I'll understand if you would speak plainly. Your *Chouese* is sometimes hard on me," I complained.

"Oh! Is that so? Really! You have trouble deciphering my bits of Chouese. How do you think your patients cope with heavy barrages of your *medicalese*?" Choua retorted.

"Okay, so you're saying David's gut is like the man's lawn. Is that it? And every time an antibiotic is prescribed ..."

"Some part of the lawn in David's bowel dies." Choua completed my sentence.

"So what do you propose, Choua? Infections in children should be allowed to go unchecked without antibiotics? Do you want to return to the pre-antibiotic era? Do you have any idea how many children died of infections in those days? Do you have any idea how many of them might die today if physicians were to become your disciples and withhold antibiotics?" Choua had made a silly statement and I let him have it.

"How is David's *bowel ecosystem* different from that of his grandfather when he was a toddler?" Choua again sidestepped my question. He often does that. When he cannot win an argument directly, he tries to throw my own words back at me.

"I don't know what his grandfather's bowel ecology was like when he was a toddler," I tried to brush aside the question.

"Oh yes, you do! You wrote the wolf book. You do know! When David's grandfather was born, his mother planted the virgin field of his bowel with seeds of love through her breast milk — bifidobacteria and acidophilus and all. But David's gut was planted with a formula, rich in salt because the formula companies want to make it agreeable to the mothers' palates. How much that salt hurt the babies is not their concern. When David's grandfather was some months old, he was given little bits of foods that were fresh in season. David was given foods *preserved* with killer molecules that money-making moguls of your food industry call preservatives. When David's grandfather looked out, he saw trees and brush and hills and moving clouds. When David looks at something, it is usually TV with whirlpools of images — images of animated things beating up on each other, sprinkled with images of commercials for sugary cereals. That's in the mornings. In the evenings and nights, what gets killed are real people and what is sold are more toxic foods. When David's grandfather breathed, he took in clear, fresh, pristine air. When David inhales, his lungs are inundated by pollutants. When David's grandfather took his first steps, he walked out to play with chicken and baby goats. When David walks out, he is engulfed in 57,000 chemicals — or is it 67,000 different chemicals that we Americans breathe in with every breath?"

Choua was on a roll again. I didn't see any point in

fighting back. It was late and I hoped his tirade would soon end.

"When David's grandfather didn't seem well, someone found a herb or two for him. When David sneezes, his pediatrician is awfully fast with his prescription pad. David's bowel ecosystem is violated with each dose of antibiotic. Each teaspoonful of the designer killer batters some part of that delicate ecologic balance. Each course of antibiotic annihilates the healthy bowel flora and makes room for yeasts to grow. And when little girls get vaginal irritation and rashes, the pediatrician gives them vaginal creams. Do they ever think that the vaginal problem is really a spill-over problem from the gut? Treating vaginitis with creams and suppositories is like building dams downstream and hoping the water might flow upstream. How many of your pediatricians really understand the bowel ecosystem and how it is battered with antibiotics? They just keep prescribing more and more antibiotics. And so it goes on and on and on."

Choua stopped. As he spoke the last few lines, he had slowly turned his face away from me and to the wild bush by Interstate 80 as it skirts by the side of our office building. We stood there in silence. As he gazed into the dark bush and the shadows it created, his eyes looking vacant, his delicate frame seemed to sway with the wind just as the bush did. I stood there in silence. It is not unusual for Choua to become passionately involved in his discourses, but he is never as passionate as when he talks about children. Sometimes I can't tell where his intellectual compassion ends and his visceral hurt begins.

"So, what do you advise?" I broke the silence. "What should pediatricians do when they see children with acute infections? Let the infections spread? Let some children risk death?" I offered what I thought was a realistic counterpoint.

"That's not the point!" Choua suddenly erupted, nearly startling me.

"What, then, is the point?" I recovered quickly.

"I'm sorry." Choua's chest heaved a little as he also recovered.

"What should the pediatricians do?" I repeated my question.

"It's not important what they do then! Not when the little ones come down with acute infections. It's what they *don't* do when the children recover. How long has David been with you?"

"Probably a little over a year," I replied.

"Was he allergic?"

"Of course! But you already know that."

"Any food sensitivities?"

"The usual — dairy, egg, chocolate, peanut, tomato and others."

"Did you treat his mold allergy?"

"Yes!"

"And his food sensitivities?"

"You know how I do it. Eliminate some, rotate others."

"How many infections did he get?"

"I don't remember offhand. Maybe once or twice. His mom said our throat protocol did the trick."

"How many courses of antibiotics has he gotten from you?"

"None! But I am not that lucky every time."

"What does his mom say about mood swings?"

"Dramatic improvement." I recalled the exact words she had used during a recent follow-up visit.

"How much sugary stuff is he eating?"

"Very little, if any. At least that's what his mom tells me."

"What was it that you wrote about in your butterfly

book? About the strategy that pediatrician had for keeping his kids busy in order to be left alone?"

Choua now referred to a small piece I had included in *The Butterfly and Life Span Nutrition.* A pediatrician in our hospital one day told us at lunch how he took his children to a public swimming pool during his vacation. The children were predictably very excited and difficult to manage until he came up with what he thought was an absolutely brilliant strategy. He gave them a dollar an hour for ice cream and they left him alone after that.

"How much do you think pediatricians know about *your* sugar and insulin and adrenaline roller coasters?"

"There are some pediatricians in the Academy of Environmental Medicine who are good, I mean really good — you know, Frank Waickman and Doris Rapp and others." I tried to mitigate Choua's hostility toward my fellow physicians.

"Don't! Don't bull sh ....'Choua restrained himself. "I ask you about thousands and thousands of pediatricians who dole out prescriptions for Amoxicillin and Ceclor and Augmentin syrups as if they were holy waters." Choua now shook visibly with disdain.

"Okay! Okay! I don't think the average pediatrician really understands how food choices hurt children," I conceded.

"And how much does your Dr. A. Average understand about mold exposure and chemical sensitivities?"

"Not much," I conceded.

"Do you agree with them when they talk about allergic children growing out of their allergies?"

"No, I don't, Choua. You know that."

"Why so?"

"Because every time I see a young woman or man who

has rheumatoid arthritis, or ulcerative colitis, or vasculitis, or asthma, or hives, he is allergic."

"They were allergic as children and they are allergic as adults!" Choua rubbed in.

"Yes! I don't think allergic genes simply go away as children grow older." I realized Choua was now chastising me for the very reasons I use to chastise others. "Why do you think, Choua, that pediatricians tell such things to their little patients' moms?" I asked.

"Because they never learned how to properly diagnose and treat allergies and food sensitivities. That's why!" Choua answered testily.

We were silent again for some time. Choua seemed lost in the bushes and the shadows they made on the ground as it bulged to meet the tar on the highway. I looked across the street. The parking lot of the A&P supermarket was now deserted.

"It's late, Choua," I tried one more time to disentangle myself from this after-midnight discourse about the prevailing dogma of what Choua calls $N^2D^2$ medicine.

"You asked how it all begin." Choua ignored my plea. "This is how chronic fatigue begins," Choua murmured as he visibly tried to be calm. "This is how it all begins." Choua's voice quivered again in the dim light of the parking lot.

"We will talk more about David some other day, Choua." I tried to break off the conversation.

"How many Davids are there," Choua resumed, "whose gut ecologies are being battered with antibiotics for throat and ear infections? How many Davids there are who continue to be assaulted in their teen years with tetracycline for acne? How many Davids are there whose immune systems are being suppressed with steroids? How many Davids are there whose food sensitivities and allergies go unrecognized and unmanaged? And how many of these Davids will go on to become chemically sensitive, and be referred to psychologists and psychiatrists? How many of them will grow up with damaged host defenses? How many of them will have their impaired defenses totally destroyed with Epstein-Barr and other viruses? And, then, how many of them will proceed to full-blown, paralyzing chronic fatigue? How many of them will see those fatigue experts who will run up lab bills for thousands and thousands of dollars, and then write prescriptions for Prozac and Elavil and God knows what other triumphs of synthetic chemistry?"

Choua stopped and looked at me with his intense eyes. I didn't try to answer any of his questions. I didn't think any of them needed to be.

"Do you know what your wizards of $N^2D^2$ medicine cannot see!" Choua resumed, still in an angry tone.
"What?" I asked with resignation. I had no answers for Choua.
"Antibiotics add up. And steroid pills add up. And *not* doing the right things month after month adds up. And feeding children foods that they react to adds up. And all *your* sugar and insulin and adrenaline roller coasters add up. And mold exposure adds up. And inhalant exposure adds up. And allergy sets them up for infections. And all those infections add up. And all those pesticides in their foods add up. And all those fumigants sprayed on their fruit add up. Everything adds up. Everything takes it toll. Each such insult weakens David's defenses — and the defenses of all the other Davids of this world. Each viral infection leaves them diminished. Each bacterial infection leaves them diminished. Each course of

antibiotics leaves them diminished. Diminished until they become the canaries. In the old days, canaries died quickly in mines because there was so little of them to be killed. The life enzymes of children are being poisoned slowly because there is so much of them to be poisoned."

Choua stopped and looked at me with his piercing eyes.

"You are preaching to the converted." I didn't know what else to say.

Choua stopped again and looked away at the bush by Interstate 80. I watched his gentle frame, heaving with each breath. There was nothing there for me to refute. No challenge to Choua's rumblings. Choua looked at me after a while. I made no attempt to respond.

"Do you know what's so ironic?" Choua spoke in a whisper.
"What?"
"It's ironic how the gurus in the body-mind-spirit business are so obsessed with their 'inner' children that they do not see how their 'outer' children are mauled."

Choua moved slowly away from me and then he vanished in the darkness of the wild bush by I-80.

***********

Choua stopped by me early the next morning. "Are you going to write about little David in your fatigue book?" he asked.

"I don't know," I answered, not wanting to engage him so soon after his late night tirade.

"Write about Dawn," Choua advised quickly.

"You don't want me to write about David. Is that it?" I asked with puzzlement.

"No, you write about David first and then about Lucia and then about Dawn. Some readers might understand the problem better that way."

"I'll think ..."

Choua walked out before I could finish my sentence.

## THIS YEAR I GET TIRED MORE EASILY

Lucia is a 14-year-old girl. Her mom asked me to see her for eye irritation, nasal allergy symptoms and sinus congestion. Her symptoms had progressively become more intense with passing years. Now she was concerned because on some mornings she experienced some wheezing and difficulty in breathing. She had received antibiotics "a few times" for bronchitis during the preceding few months. That was all the history that she and her mom thought was necessary. I reviewed the detailed history sheet. There was nothing else there. I started to question her on the subject of energy.

"How active are you?" I asked.

"Very! She is very active," her mom answered with evident pride. "She is always doing things, in the classroom and outside the classroom."

"How is your energy level?" I peered into Lucia's eyes.

"Great! It's great!" she answered enthusiastically.

"Do you react to perfumes?" I changed the subject.

"Yes," She replied.

"How?"

"I sneeze."

"What else?"

"Nothing!" She looked a little puzzled.

"Car exhaust?"

"No, that doesn't bother me."

"Bleach? Other cleaning solutions?"

"No. They don't do anything."

"Were you in a fabric store recently?"

"Yes."

"Anything happen?"

"Nothing," she answered quickly and then looked at her mother. Her mother looked back at her blankly.

"Remember, Mom, I developed an eye rash when I went to a fabric store and the rash cleared up right after we left the store."

"Do you sometimes wake up tired?" I continued.

"Yes!" her mom intervened again. "But that is because she studies until very late."

"Okay! Now tell me, do you have as much energy this year as you did last year?" I persisted.

"Yes!" She looked at her mom and thought for a moment.

"Yes?" I pressed her.

"Well ... No! Yes, there is a difference."

"What's the difference?"

"This year I get tired much more easily than I did last year."

"This is where chronic fatigue begins," Choua spoke after Lucia and her mother left my consultation room for the examination room. "This is what your pediatricians do not know. This is what your chronic fatigue experts who spend thousands of dollars doing laboratory tests and then prescribe antidepressants do not understand."

"Many pediatricians do understand these things," I protested.

"Yeah! Yeah!" Choua taunted. "Allergy leads to chemical sensitivity. Parents and children don't see the link between the two, but what excuse do your pediatricians and allergists have for that?"

"It's changing," I asserted.

"Allergy and chemical sensitivity cause undue tiredness. Allergy sets children up for frequent viral and bacterial infections that add to the problem of undue tiredness."

"Yes! That it does," I consented.

"Antibiotics prescribed for infections disrupt the normal bowel ecology, and add to the problems of adverse food reactions and digestive-absorptive problems in the bowel, and cause fatigue."

"Yes! But, Choua, I thought we have covered this stuff many times," I provoked him.

"And that leads to yeast overgrowth and infections." Choua ignored my remark. "And that further feeds the problem of undue tiredness and delayed recovery from the state of being tired. This is the beginning of chronic fatigue. While you celebrate your *blessed* double-blind, cross-over, the poor children are getting sicker and sicker." Choua breathed hard.

"You can be brutal, Choua." I tried to appease him.

"This is how fatigue begins. This is where fatigue is so easy to reverse. This is also where the minor problems assume

major significance while most of your colleagues innocently —
and many of them arrogantly — dismiss the problem as
supratentorial." Choua surmised.

"Supratentorial! I haven't heard that in so long."

"Your beloved and *blessed* all-in-the-head syndrome,"
Choua blurted and walked out.

## DAWN: A REFUGEE FROM A TOXIC CITY

January evenings are very quiet in the woods by our
house in Blairstown. The ground is usually covered with snow.
The woods are still. The wild life is deep in slumber, hidden
from view. One can hear one's own breath.

It was quite warm one winter some years ago in New
Jersey. One evening I finished a follow-up telephone visit with
Dawn, one of my patients who had been totally disabled by
chronic fatigue and severe environmental sensitivity. I stepped
out for a walk in the woods and I saw a family of squirrels
frolicking on a bed of dried leaves. They seemed to celebrate
the renewal of life that one sees in springtime. My thoughts
drifted to the phenomenon of hibernation in squirrels, and
returned back to Dawn's plight. Dawn was very sick that day.
She had cried repeatedly during the telephone visit. I felt
helpless.

Dawn lives by herself outside a small village in Upstate
New York. She cannot live in her house in New York City
where she grew up and which she loves dearly, because "It is

too toxic for me."

## DAWN IS A UNIVERSAL REACTOR

Dawn is a universal reactor. During the first visit she said, "I react to everything."

I know many of my colleagues in drug medicine will scoff at the term universal reactor, and I understand. I myself used to scoff at many things patients would say. Then I learned the hard way. Some of the things I scoffed at came back to haunt me. When a physician doesn't understand what his patient is saying, and instead chooses to scoff at him, two things happen: First, he misses an opportunity to learn and become enlightened about the true nature of his patient's suffering; and second, he robs his patient of an opportunity for relief of his suffering.

What is a universal reactor? Dawn's story unfortunately makes an illustrative case study. Universal reactors are individuals who begin to react to an increasing number of foods and environmental agents as their energetic-molecular defenses are shattered and their general condition deteriorates precipitously. Many clinical ecologists call this a spreading phenomenon — the sensitivities spread as the energetic-molecular events within their cells and tissues feed upon each other to create domino effects.

## REVERSE SPREADING PHENOMENON

Fortunately, this spreading phenomenon in most instances can be reversed with optimal use of nondrug therapies outlined in the chapters dealing with the management of chronic fatigue states. When my patients begin to "shed" their sensitivities — and begin to tolerate many foods that they previously couldn't and cease to react to common air pollutants such as formaldehyde and organic solvents — I tell them they are manifesting a "reverse spreading phenomenon." After relating Dawn's clinical history, I describe in depth the disruptions of the energy and detoxification enzyme pathways that cause the spreading phenomenon and lead to the universal reactor status, and then those reversals that restore health and provide for the energetic-molecular basis for the reverse spreading phenomenon.

Dawn had been an allergic child. She was given large doses of drugs for control of allergy symptoms. She suffered from frequent throat and sinus infections for which she was prescribed antibiotics. During her school years, she was given yet more broad-spectrum antibiotics for acne for a few years.

In her early college days, she developed recurrent episodes of yeast vaginitis, Trichomonas infections, symptoms of colitis, frequent headaches, menstrual irregularities, and chronic fatigue. She underwent an extensive diagnostic work-up including gastroscopy and colonoscopy which showed nonspecific inflammation. An anal mucus test showed the presence of

Giardia lamblia, a common intestinal parasite. Following these tests, she was treated by several physicians with various painkillers, multiple courses of antibiotics, Nystatin, Flagyl, caprylic acid, paramycocidin, Artemisia ennui, Lactobacillus, and finally Nizoral. After each treatment, she felt better for some time. Then she would relapse, feeling more debilitated with each episode.

During the two years before she consulted me, she had developed sensitivity to cooking gas, paint, formaldehyde, tetrachloroethylene (dry cleaning solution), common organic solvents, tobacco smoke and automobile exhaust. She developed joint pains, muscle stiffness, frequent mood swings, and mental confusion. Predictably, Dawn was under unrelenting stress and became very depressed. She began to wonder if her problems were psychiatric in nature. And so did most of the physicians she consulted during those years, including a psychiatrist who promptly prescribed an antidepressant.

A repeat diagnostic work-up some months later showed abnormal laboratory test results indicative of an autoimmune disorder.

Oral and intravenous vitamin supplements relieved some of her symptoms initially. Within months she became intolerant to nutrients, and all such therapies had to be discontinued. She was exquisitely sensitive to many environmental chemicals. Like most patients with severe chemical sensitivity, she was unable to tolerate any synthetic drugs. During some months before I saw her, she also developed intolerance to nutrient supplements.

## CAN'T LIFT MY HEAD OFF MY PILLOW

Dawn played varsity tennis in college. Now at the age of 33 years, she is incapacitated with chronic fatigue. She said, "On some mornings, I cannot lift my head off my pillow." She lives with severe, intractable and debilitating chronic fatigue, literally incarcerated in her one room apartment, away from her loving family.

Dawn's clinical ecologist referred her to me to see if I could try my luck at autoregulation to stabilize her condition enough so that he and I together could try to use our nondrug therapies for chronic fatigue states associated with severe chemical sensitivity — this time with utmost caution and in a carefully orchestrated, slow and sustained fashion.

I repeated the IgE micro-elisa tests for allergy for Dawn and confirmed that she was strongly positive to all of the 35 yeasts, pollen, and foods that I tested her for.

Self-regulation is not an easy road. It requires patient and persistent efforts. This is hardest for patients who need it most, those in the throes of relentless suffering. But it does work. For Dawn, this seemed to be the only way. My hope was that self-regulation would give her some grip on life. It would eventually allow me to slowly and very cautiously use my allergy and nutritional protocols to stabilize her immune system. This would be a long and a grueling effort for Dawn. Would she see all this as clearly as I did? Could I help her see beyond the usual diagnostic labels? Could I help her see the true energetic-molecular nature of her suffering? Could I sustain her for that long? I was offering her self-regulation when she knew "the best of modern medicine" had failed her completely. Would she understand all this? Many people still see self-regulation as a mystical phenomenon, a simple-minded pursuit of things that could not happen — or worse, plain deception. Would Dawn rise above all this despite all the failures of past therapies? By now Dawn was convinced that her illness could not be treated with any drugs. Would this knowledge help her to consider autoregulation a viable option?

## A LIMBIC WINTER OF RENEWAL

The ground squirrel comes close to a near absence of breathing during hibernation. Its respiration rate drops from 150 breaths/minute during summer to 1-2 breaths/minute during hibernation in winter. The heart rate slows down from about 350 beats/minute to 2-4 beats/minute. The metabolism is reduced to one to five percent of the rate during active months (Biochemica et Biophysica Acta, 988: 123; 1989.)

The physiologic changes in the ground squirrel during hibernation are accompanied by several changes in the function and structure of cell membranes in various tissues. Saturated fatty acids are reduced and unsaturated fatty acids increased in the cell membrane as part of the "homeoviscous adaptation" of Sinensky. My thoughts go to the cell membrane in discussions like this because it is the integrity of the human cell membrane that determines the integrity of the human frame. I discuss this subject at length in the preceding chapter.

Hibernation changes allow the tissues of the squirrel to conserve energy and return to life, renewed and without chronic fatigue. No squirrel ever told me this, but I donot recall seeing a squirrel with obvious signs of the so-called chronic fatigue syndrome. What would happen if the heart and breathing rates of squirrels stayed at their summer rates during hibernation ? Squirrels would not be expected to live their normal life-span of about three years.

*Each person is allotted a definite number of breaths. He can breathe fast and live less or breathe slow and live longer.*

This was the advice the ancient philosophers of healing arts often gave to their pupils. I do not know what might have led them to such advice. What I do know is that slow breathing with prolonged breathe-out periods — limbic breathing — is one of the most effective methods for self-regulation. I describe some methods of slow, sustained breathing that I have found very effective from personal experience as well as from the experience of my patients in *The Cortical Monkey and Healing*. I strongly urge the reader to read the chapter Lata and Limbic Breathing in that book.

Science eventually does catch up with the intuitive wisdom of the ancients — though it often moves painstakingly slow. Science is that part of the poet's world that has been measured. The researchers at the National Institutes of Health proved with their careful studies in the late 20th century what the ancients had learned several millennia earlier.

## OXIDATIVE RATES AND LIFE SPAN

Dawn's insufferable anguish — and my hope that autoregulation might help stabilize her situation just enough to undertake nutritional and environmental therapies — cannot be understood with the prevailing notions of diseases and their cures with drugs.

To trace events in Dawn's illness and the energetic-molecular events that led to it, I return one more time to the *core* theme of this book — that chronic fatigue states are states of accelerated oxidative molecular injury — for it is only with sound understanding of such events that rational management strategies can be formulated.

Spontaneity of oxidation — in my view — is the true nature of the aging process in man. I discuss this subject at length and furnish scientific evidence for my hypothesis in the preceding chapter. If we accept this hypothesis, then it follows that the oxidative rates in tissues of aerobic (oxygen-utilizing) living beings must be related to their life spans. This indeed has been shown to be true.

Studies at the National Institutes of Health have shown that there is an inverse relationship between mammalian life spans and the rates of tissue oxidation. In such studies, rates of auto-oxidation — spontaneous oxidation or natural decomposition of living matter in common language — in the tissues of different organs of over 70 mammals were determined. They measured the rates at which tissues undergo spontaneous oxidation. These rates of oxidation represent the innate capacity of tissues for self-destruction. They observed that the mammalian species that showed the highest rates of auto-oxidation had the shortest life spans, and those with the lowest rates of auto-oxidation had the longest life spans. There was almost a perfect inverse correlation between the rates of oxidation and the species life spans.

Selected data for various species, including man, are shown in the table given below.

### Rates of Auto-Oxidation
### and Life Spans of Mammalian Species

| Species | Oxidation Rate | Life Span (years) |
|---|---|---|
| Man | 25 | 90 |
| Orangutan | 24 | 50 |
| Baboon | 35 | 37 |
| Green monkey | 41 | 34 |
| Squirrel monkey | 74 | 18 |
| Rat | 104 | 4 |
| Mouse | 182 | 3.5 |

*Proc Nat Acad Sci* 77:2777;1981

The above table illustrates clearly the inverse relationship between life spans and auto-oxidative rates: Animal species that oxidize their tissues rapidly live the shortest life spans, while those that oxidize their tissues slowly live the longest life spans. Man with the lowest rate of tissue breakdown has the highest longevity, while the mouse which has the highest rate among the species listed in the table, has the lowest longevity.

---

SPONTANEITY OF OXIDATION
IS NATURE'S GRAND DESIGN TO ASSURE
THAT NO LIVING BEING LIVES FOREVER

Old life must be cleared away so new life can begin. This is the grand design of Nature. Nature made oxidation a spontaneous reaction; it requires no energy. Reduction, the flip side of the coin of oxidation, by contrast is a non-spontaneous process; it requires energy expenditure. Living matter decomposes spontaneously with time; decomposed matter cannot become undecomposed with time.

Life is energy. The language of biology is energy. We live, get sick and die as our tissues are progressively oxidized. The lipids in our cell membrane get oxidized just as butter turns rancid on our kitchen counters. The proteins in our bodies get oxidized, cross-linked and denatured just as animal hide turns into leather with tanning. The sugars and starches in our bodies get oxidized, their molecules turned and twisted and distorted so they cannot link up with fats and proteins to be useful in the body. The vitamins — the moderators in the molecular talk shows of our metabolism — get oxidized and robbed of their communication skills. The cell membranes get shot full of holes, and what is inside the cell hemorrhages out and what is outside floods the cell innards. The essential minerals leak out. The toxic metals are oxidized to organic forms that are much more dangerous than they are in their elemental forms. For instance, elemental mercury is toxic but nowhere near as toxic as its oxidized form, methyl mercury.

Oxidation in human tissues is the process of energy release from molecules; reduction the mechanism of storing it. Breathing provides the tissues oxygen, the essential spark for life. The animals that breathe rapidly live shorter lives. Those who breathe at slower rates do not burn their tissues as fast and live longer. Of all mammals, man has the slowest breathing rate and the longest life span.

Research in aging, accelerated aging, and the energetic-molecular basis of disease is of great interest to us in our understanding of the state of chronic fatigue. Studies designed to explore these areas show how, in the natural order of things, a balanced state of redox regulation preserves health, and how redox dysregulation — an unbridled, chaotic oxidative arm of this fundamental energy mechanism of life causes accelerated aging, and, of course, by clearly defensible implication, a state of chronic fatigue.

Oxygen is life-giving; tissues and cells need oxygen to sustain them. This we understand well in our study of basic science. Tissues and cells are also "aged" by oxygen in the process of "living."Of this we have but little understanding in the clinical practice of medicine. Oxidation is a spontaneous process; reduction requires expenditure of energy. Molecular duality of oxygen essentially represents the economy of nature at its best.

## DAWN'S STORY IS ONE OF
## SHATTERED HUMAN MOLECULAR DEFENSES

Sadly Dawn's story will be all too familiar to clinical ecologists. The Dawns (and the other human canaries) of this world face triple jeopardy:

### First,

their genetic makeup that renders them vulnerable to the growing oxidant stress on their internal and external environment in ways that are different from others.

### Second,

a system of health care that stubbornly refuses to acknowledge the essential chemistry of human biology, and refuses to accept the potential of nondrug therapies based on such understanding.

### Third,

the tools of Star Wars medicine that, while affording necessary symptom suppression on a short-term basis, do nothing to reverse those basic energetic-molecular mechanisms that cause chronic fatigue states (and other degenerative and immune disorders.)

Dawn's story is a telling indictment of $N^2D^2$ medicine and a sad comment on the utter failure of Star Wars medicine and of all its glorious tools.

## MOLECULAR DEFENSES

The true nature of chronic fatigue, I wrote earlier, cannot be understood without basic knowledge of human energy and detoxification enzymes. In chronic fatigue, such enzymes are oxidatively damaged. In the next several pages, I include a brief discussion of molecular defenses in health and chronic fatigue states.

*Chronic fatigue in many people is associated with the inability to concentrate. Thus, the material I cover in this segment may be difficult to understand for some chronic fatiguers. I suggest that such readers skip this discussion and return to it some other day when it is easier to concentrate.*

## FIRST LINE OF MOLECULAR DEFENSES: OXIDATIVE DETOXIFICATION

The *central* tragedy of the prevailing standards of care in the United States is this: Practitioners of drug medicine fail to understand the breakdown of molecular defenses that occurs in chronic fatiguers like Dawn. Instead, they attribute the complaints of such patients to all-in-the-head syndrome. This is where the real chance of recovery for Dawn (and other human canaries) exists, and this is where $N^2D^2$ medicine fails, totally and utterly. The plain reason for this is that $N^2D^2$ medicine has pronounced all nondrug and nonsurgical therapies useless and wasteful (and fraud), yet, one thing its wonder drugs cannot do is repair the injured energy and detoxification enzymes.

Oxidation is the loss of electrons by atoms and molecules. Electrons are the tiniest balls of energy that spin in their specific orbits within atoms. Simple oxidation is the first line of human molecular defenses and usually involves the breakdown of large, complex toxic molecules into simpler non-toxic molecules. To cite one example, many environmental pollutants are oxidized into inert substances by free oxidizing radicals in the air. This is the principal mechanism by which air on the mountains and beaches is purified and made "fresh and crisp."

This appears to be a contradiction. Here, I tout oxidation as the first line of molecular defense, while in the preceding chapter, I theoriz that chronic fatigue is caused by accelerated oxidative molecular injury. The best way for me to explain this apparent contradiction is to return to the example of how a mere matchstick can burn down a whole forest. Clearly, a matchstick does not have the energy to turn tree pulps into ashes. How does it occur? The matchstick acts like a spark plug in an automobile engine: It *triggers* the reaction — ignites the fire. The oxidizing chemistry of fire now feeds upon itself and perpetuates the "oxidant flame" that keeps turning massive trees into ashes. We know that most forest fires do not proceed to conflagrations that annihilate the whole forest ecosystem, even when human intervention does not exist. How does that happen? Because of the "antioxidant" effects of rain or surface water or of the water within the bodies of the trees.

The problem in many chronic fatigue states is that either the oxidative sparks do not work to begin with — the "metabolic matchsticks" are dead — or that, once ignited, the oxidative frenzy in the tissues feeds upon itself uninterrupted. It is as if the spark plugs of an automobile engine fail to ignite the fuel, and when they do, there is no carburetor to regulate the flow of the combustible mixture. The engine either does not start to begin with, or when it does, it explodes.

## FAILING OXIDATIVE SPARKS AND VIOLENT OXIDATIVE STORMS

What do failing oxidative sparks and oxidative storms have to do with Dawn's problems? Everything!

Clinically, damaged oxidative sparks — redox

dysregulations in scientific jargon — cause vague, shifting, hard-to-define symptoms such as weakness, frustration, malaise, confusion and memory lapses — symptoms that are attributable to multiple organ systems and that are usually dismissed by the practitioners of drug medicine as all-in-the-head problems. One chronic fatiguer expressed it eloquently: "I used to be a ball of fire, now I have no oomph!"

When the sparks do fire, they bring forth oxidative storms. Chronic fatiguers suffer anxiety, sweating, heart palpitations, tightness in the chest, labored breathing, nausea and abdominal cramps. The energetic-molecular events that trigger such oxidative disruptions include allergic reactions, sugar-insulin-adrenaline roller coasters, stress responses, neurotransmitter surges, abnormal bowel responses to foods and reactions to environmental pollutants. Most commonly performed laboratory tests in such states yield negative results. Clinicians unfamiliar with the basic energy dynamics rush to their favorite all-in-the-head label. In the uncommon circumstances that such symptoms are acknowledged as valid, they are treated with drugs. Such therapies, while suppressing symptoms and offering some temporary benefits, almost always exaggerate the problems. The reason for this again is simple: Drugs work by impairing, blocking or destroying the very enzymes that are needed to restore normal energy pathways.

## DETECTION OF OXIDATIVE INJURY

In reality, accelerated oxidative injury at this early stage is not difficult to document, provided laboratory tests are specifically designed to study initial oxidative injury. One of the best laboratory tests for this purpose — in my clinical experience — is the microscopic study of the cell membrane of red blood cells. I described in the preceding chapter the results of one of my own studies in which I observed oxidative damage to red cell membranes in up to 80% of all cells in patients with chronic fatigue. The absolute proof that the red cell membranes are being deformed by oxidative stress is the fact that these abnormalities are readily reversed with an intravenous infusion of vitamin C (probably the most powerful, water-phase antioxidant in human blood). This correction, I might add, usually lasts for a short time initially.

What can the Dawns of this world do when they experience initial, vague symptoms before they plunge into severe chronic fatigue states? This, of course, is the thrust of this book and the companion volumes *The Butterfly and Life Span Nutrition, The Ghoraa and Limbic Exercise, The Cortical Monkey and Healing* and *RDA: Rats, Drugs and Assumptions.* The answer is: read, read and read; learn, learn and learn; experiment, experiment and experiment; and finally, know, know and know. As long as the main body of physicians is utterly devoted to drug medicine, people like Dawn have no other choice. They need to seek out and find professionals who can offer the right advice and the right nondrug therapies. I return to this subject several times in this book because it is one of the *core* issues under discussion.

The toxic and fatigue-causing effects of excess oxidant molecules are normally prevented by a host of life span molecules. These include:

1.   Water-phase antioxidants such as vitamin C

2. Fat-phase antioxidants such as vitamins E and A
3. Life span enzymes such as:
   A. superoxide dismutase
   B. catalase
   C. glutathione peroxidase
4. Plasma proteins, thiols and certain other plasma antioxidants
5. Life span minerals such as magnesium, potassium, molybdenum and others that are essential co-factors for enzyme functions
6. Certain amino acids that are essential for the functional integrity of the above mechanisms such as taurine


Increased oxidant stress plays a central role in the failure of energy enzymes — the root of chronic fatigue. The oxidative mechanisms operating at this level include:

A. Aging-oxidant molecules in our internal and external environment
B. Metabolic acidotic stresses


## INCREASED ACIDOTIC STRESS IN CHRONIC FATIGUE


Accelerated oxidative stress increases total body acidity. Acid wastes are generated as a normal consequence of metabolism. The Fourth-of-July-chemistry — it is easy to see — enormously increases acid waste. In chronic fatigue, detoxification enzymes are impaired, and this substantially increases the total body acid burdens. Thus, most patients with chronic fatigue are acidotic unless, of course, they are under the care of a professional knowledgeable in essential aspects of nutritional and environmental medicine. The diagnosis of increased acidotic stress in chronic fatigue can be accurately and easily made and requires a simple blood test. Increased body acidity can also be diagnosed by sequential urine tests. From a practical standpoint, the two most effective strategies for reducing the total acid burden are: 1) life span food choices and 2) limbic breathing. I discuss these subjects at length in *The Butterfly and Life Span Nutrition* and *The Cortical Monkey and Healing*. I include a synopsis later in this volume.

Where does increased acidotic stress take us? This is largely determined by the impact of accelerated oxidative injury upon an individual's genetic makeup; the human canaries get hurt first. *The health of an individual cell depends on the integrity of its surface membrane.* Likewise, the health of the tiniest structures within the cells (organelles) depends upon the plasma membrane of these structures. Diseases begin when these early changes of oxidant cell membrane injury are not expediently reversed with effective clinical anti-oxidant strategies that include:

A.  Reduction — and elimination when possible — of all relevant allergic triggers (molds, grasses, trees, foods and chemicals)
B.  Nutritional antioxidant therapies
    1.  Nutrition in the kitchen
    2.  Oral anti-oxidant nutrient therapies
    3.  Whenever indicated, intravenous antioxidant nutrient drips
C.  Self-regulatory methods for reducing oxidant stress

D.  Slow, sustained (limbic) exercise

I discuss all four sets of antioxidant therapies in the chapters dealing with management of chronic fatigue.

---

## GLUTATHIONE: THE GLADIATOR IN THE MOLECULAR ARENA

---

Glutathione is an important player in the essential oxidation-reduction equation of life. Indeed, it may be regarded as the quarterback molecule of the redox reaction. Glutathione is a tripeptide, composed of three important amino acids: cystine, glycine and glutamic acid.

Like gladiators in the Roman era, each molecule of glutathione is sacrificed at the end of the battle it engages in. Sometimes the terrorist molecules — pollutant molecules that invade from outside and the toxins produced metabolically within the body — are so powerful that individual glutathione molecules cannot cope with them. In such instances, two or more glutathione molecules team up to corner and subdue the terrorist molecule, and are all wasted together along with the terrorist as it is expelled from the body. It is as if many cops get roped up along with the single terrorist that they apprehend, but when that terrorist is expelled from the country, the roped-up cops also get expelled because they cannot untangle themselves from the terrorist.

The essential protective role of glutathione has been documented by many studies conducted in man and experimental animals. I cite below several studies to illustrate the role of glutathione in health and disease.

Research studies in aging have shown the central role glutathione plays in the integrity of electron dynamics in the basic pattern of the flow of energy in the redox reaction and enzymatic pathways in human metabolism. In essence, it counters and neutralizes the acid molecules produced by tissue oxidation in health and tissue burnout in disease.

In human longevity research, the impact of glutathione dynamics on life span has been established with different studies. In women living long, healthful lives, blood and tissue glutathione levels are higher than those seen in control male populations. Glutathione levels decrease with age, but the rate of decrease is lower among women over sixty than in men of the same age.

## THE 3 M STUDIES

The "3 M" longevity studies — research studies of mosquito, mouse and man — are of considerable interest to us in our discussion of chronic fatigue.

In mouse longevity research, a similar role of glutathione in tissue metabolism has been documented in many studies.

In mosquito longevity research, prolongation of life span by increasing glutathione levels has been shown. Small doses of a chemical (thiozolidine carboxylic acid) were used for this purpose.

There is a large body of research studies demonstrating the central role of glutathione in antioxidant defenses against microbes and chemical toxins in man and experimental animals. I cite below two such studies to illustrate this role. In asymptomatic HIV-infected men, subnormal levels of glutathione were found in blood and bronchial secretions, indicating impaired antioxidant defenses (*AIDS Alert,* Jan. 1990,) Cocaine is toxic to liver cells. Alcohol potentiates the toxic effects of cocaine. Studies in mice have shown that cocaine and alcohol toxicity of liver cells is associated with diminished concentration of glutathione in these cells. (*Alcoholism: Clinical and Experimental Research* 14:28; 1990.)

## URINE TELLS THE FATIGUE STORY

Measurement of mercapturic acid in the urine is a simple test that tells us how rapidly glutathione is being sacrificed in chronic fatigue. Similarly, measurement of D-glucaric acid in urine tells us how hard our detoxification enzymes are driven in their fight to cope with environmental pollutants. Specifically, increased quantities of D-glucaric acid in the urine indicate induction of liver detoxification enzymes by xenobiotics (alien chemicals). Many oxidant chemicals that cannot be disposed of by the simple processes of oxidation, reduction or hydrolysis are detoxified by conjugation with molecules such as glutathione. Compounds formed when glutathione is conjugated with xenobiotics are called mercapturic acids (acetyl-cysteinyl-xenobiotic complexes). Increased amounts of mercapturic acids, thus, indicate excessive wastage of glutathione.

## SECOND LINE OF MOLECULAR DEFENSE: ENZYMATIC DETOXIFICATION PATHWAYS

The enzymatic detoxification pathways are the second line of molecular defense against those chemicals that the body cannot dispose simply by oxidizing them.

Star Wars medicine is as patently helpless in coping with oxidant damage to the second line of molecular defenses as it is in dealing with damage to the first line of molecular defense. Indeed, it pours yet more fuel on the oxidative fires. The tools of Star Wars medicine — miracles of its synthetic chemistry — further add to the injury of damaged energy and detoxification enzymes. In relating Mr. Latimer's story in the chapter Pasteur's Sheep and My canaries, I describe how commonly used ulcer drugs such as Tagamet can so damage some detoxification enzymes — such as cytochrome P-450 system — in vulnerable individuals that they set the stage for chronic fatigue states, progressive immune disorders and cancer.

Oxidative injury disturbs human energy and detoxification enzymes in two major ways:

*First,*

Enzyme function is impaired by:

1.   Enzyme destruction

2. Enzyme inactivation
3. Enzyme blockage
4. Enzyme consumption

*Second,*

Enzyme function is dysregulated by enzyme induction.

In medical schools, students are taught pharmacology (science of drugs) and are usually glibly told how drugs are either cleared by the liver or by the kidneys — the clearance of drugs with stools and with breathing are far less important mechanisms. What is rarely taught to medical students is the true "molecular cost" of these mechanisms. Many drugs work by fooling the enzymes — drugs are mistaken by the enzymes for the molecules they normally encounter during their energy-generating or detoxification mechanisms. Molecule for molecule, such drugs literally waste a molecule of essential life span enzymes. Many drugs such as ace-inhibitor drugs for hypertension work by directly inhibiting essential enzymes. Yet other drugs block or simply destroy enzymes.

In *The Ghoraa and Limbic Exercise,* I describe how vulnerable the endocrine trio of thyroid, pancreas and adrenal glands is to oxidant stress. Hypothyroidism (underactive thyroid gland) is an autoimmune disorder — and since all immune injury in my view begins with oxidant injury — it seemed certain to me many years ago that future research will show that this disorder results from oxidative injury to enzymes that play critical roles in thyroid metabolism. This, indeed, is beginning to happen. Recent studies show that de-iodinase enzymes — enzymes that convert inactive thyroid pro-hormone into active thyroid hormone — are functionally impaired. Although these studies have not yet clearly documented that de-iodinase enzymes are functionally impaired due to oxidant injury, I am certain it is simply a matter of time before this will be proven to be so.

Enzyme induction describes an excessive response triggered by persistent stimuli. While such a response is initially necessary and desirable for molecular defense against the stimulus, with time it becomes "autonomous" and destructive. All drugs that are metabolized in the liver are capable of causing such enzyme dysregulation. An example of this phenomenon is induction of liver enzymes in children given barbiturates.

Cytochrome P system is an essential system of detoxification processes. This enzyme system is almost always affected by chronic drug use, and often leads to chronic metabolic deficits — changes that we frequently dismiss as side-effects of drugs. (I sometimes wonder why some drug effects are considered effects and others as side-effects.)

I include below a list of some essential biochemical processes that the body uses to rid itself of drugs and environmental pollutants:

1. acetylation
2. methylation
3. conjugation
4. glucuronidation
5. carbon-oxidation
6. sulfur-oxidation

However, these mechanisms are often unable to cope with insoluble organic compounds with long half-lives. For instance, the half-lives of dioxin and chlordane have been estimated to be over 6 and 15 years respectively. Evidently, these second lines of molecular defense are, for practical purposes, totally ineffective against dioxins, chlordane and other families of related molecules. Enzyme systems frequently activated by xenobiotics include cytochrome P-450 systems and enzymes frequently inactivated by xenobiotics include choline esterases, sulfite oxidases and phenol sulftransferases.

The enzymatic efficiency of sulfite oxidases and enzyme systems involved with trans-sulfuration steps are of special importance to individuals with chronic fatigue associated with allergic disorders such as asthma, chemical sensitivity and chemical toxicity. These enzymatic functions can be assessed by measurements of urinary sulfites and sulfates.

I cite here one more example for the reader with a biology background. The general reader may wish to skip this paragraph in view of the technical language. Cysteine oxygenase catalyzes the first step in the oxidation of cysteine to inorganic sulfate. This enzyme plays a role in the formation of sulfoxides from S-carboxy-L-methylcysteine. This reaction varies widely among individuals. Impaired sulfur oxidation has been documented in many autoimmune disorders including primary biliary cirrhosis, rheumatoid arthritis, and systemic lupus erythematosus. These observations are clinically significant, since an inadequate supply of inorganic sulfate limits the rate of formation of non-toxic sulfates (conjugates of compounds such as steroids, drugs and environmental pollutants that can then be readily excreted).

## THIRD LINE OF MOLECULAR DEFENSE: TOXIN-GENE-ENZYME-IMMUNE DYNAMICS

The Dawns of this world do not fare any better with Star Wars medicine in this phase of their illness any more than they do when their first two lines of molecular defense are damaged. At this rather late phase in their illness, they are frequently prescribed large doses of multiple drugs. Whatever chance they had of recovering on their own, they lose it now.

I coined the term TGEI (toxin-gene-enzyme-immune) dynamics to refer to a host of interactions that occur between toxins, genes, enzymatic pathways and the various components of the immune system. Oxidant injury can injure each and every part of this continuum, singly or in combination. Oxidant injury to genes provides the missing link in several molecular mysteries. Injured genes can induce certain enzyme systems so that uncontrolled enzyme activity begins to chew out healthy molecules when it is finished with the alien molecules — very much like what one sees in science fiction movies where a genetically engineered microbe begins to destroy everything in its way. Oxidant injury to genes can also so damage the gene that it orders the production of abnormal enzymes or of no enzymes at all. In this, I only refer to abnormal enzyme responses that have been documented.

Gene-toxin-enzyme-immune dynamics are the third line of molecular defense against environmental injury. Evidence is rapidly accumulating that the mechanisms of chronic degenerative, immune and environmental disorders involve complex TGEI interrelationships. Genes provide the hitherto missing links between the toxin exposure and persistent clinical symptomatology. Although direct, clear evidence for such inter-relationships in chronic fatigue is not yet forthcoming, I am confident that future research will provide the missing links in this story as well.

Toxins can directly bend or otherwise so disfigure the DNA molecules that they become vulnerable to deletion or transcription by a host of proteins. In health, DNA is usually packed tightly within the nucleus — the central, well-defended compartment of the cell — and is quite hard to reach for alien toxic molecules. When bent or disfigured, DNA becomes more accessible to proteins in its vicinity. When the DNA so injured happens to encode specific enzyme systems, enzyme activation so caused may persist for long periods of time and eventually lead to clinical disorders. A good example to illustrate such dynamics is the case of DNA injury caused by a family of potent chemical poisons known as dioxins. The herbicide Agent Orange that the United States used in the Vietnam War belongs to this family.

## FOURTH LINE OF MOLECULAR DEFENSE: CLASSICAL IMMUNE REACTIONS

*This is the stage in which the practitioners of $N^2D^2$ medicine gear themselves for action* — their laboratory tests begin to show abnormal results. They now exult with their positive test findings — devastatingly *negative* for the patient, I might add —

such as immune cell counts, immunoglobulin levels, complement, immune complexes, ANA and anti-DNA antibodies, lymphokines (messenger molecules of immune cells), interleukins such as IL-2, and a host of other enzyme markers of advanced stages of damage to the immune system. The practitioners of drug medicine now pull out their prescription pads and — with their customary authority — dole out prescriptions for steroids and other immunosuppressant drugs. The Dawns of this world have no chance now. Whatever parts of the immune system are still working prior to this point will be totally suppressed by such drugs.

I have seen a fairly large number of patients who consulted me for symptoms attributable to multiple organ systems and who showed positive ANA, anti-DNA antibodies and rheumatoid tests. We can look at such positive test results as evidence that this or that "immune disorder" exists or we can regard them as evidence that there are oxidative stresses on the energetic-molecular defenses. The first interpretation leads one to use one or more drugs — usually steroids and other immunosuppressant drugs — to suppress the immune system. The second interpretation leads one to nondrug therapies designed to enhance the energetic-molecular defenses. This is an essential point.

*The Dawns of this world need to know this.*

The study of several classical immune functions is undertaken all too often at a prohibitive cost to chronic fatiguers who can ill-afford lavish spending to satisfy the intellectual curiosity of the chronic fatigue "authorities." Such tests are generally of little, if any, value in the clinical management of this problem. I included a list of such tests in the chapter What Is Chronic fatigue? Some of the tests especially favored by some fatigue experts — I am at a loss as to why this is so — are expensive T and B lymphocyte counts, helper-suppressor cell ratios, immune complexes, complement components and interleukins. Such testing is of little value because it tells us about immune injury that we already know exists in chronic fatigue.

Gell and Coombs classification of immune disorders, while of enormous value for students of immunology, looks at the tail-end of immune injury. It is of limited value for patients with chronic fatigue except for IgE antibodies that, in my judgment, provide essential diagnostic information of immense clinical value as far as management is concerned.

## FIFTH LINE OF MOLECULAR DEFENSE: STRUCTURAL TISSUE RESPONSES

Structural tissue responses — or diseases that we diagnose with the microscopic study of biopsy materials — are the inescapable consequences of damaged and neglected first, second, third and fourth lines of energetic-molecular defenses.

Drugs often become necessary for suppression of symptoms. Cellular, tissue and organ damage are late events, and their treatment with drugs, in my judgment, represent tail-end medicine. The majority of patients with unreversed chronic fatigue unfortunately will proceed to develop what will then be labeled as "specific immune diseases." This is a dire yet inescapable prediction. Human canaries — Dawns of this world

— need to know this.

---

| SCIENCE AND PSEUDOSCIENCE |
| IN CHRONIC FATIGUE RESEARCH |

In chronic fatigue, muscles ache and feel tired even when the person is lying in bed. Any and all muscular activities become herculean tasks. Previously active, athletic individuals cannot perform simple tasks. Yet, many fatigue "researchers" continue to proclaim it to be a mere all-in-the-head phenomenon. Pseudoscience continues to thrive. Consider the following:

*The results from both intermittent and sustained leg exercise protocols indicate that the patients did not demonstrate excessive muscle fatigue relative to controls, which is consistent with previous reports. Similarly, the changes in phosphate metabolism, pH, and EC coupling were not different from controls. In fact, there was a trend toward both greater fatigue and a more marked metabolic response in the controls.*

*Neurology* 43:125-31;1993

Translation: Muscles in chronic fatigue are really not

tired. Chronic fatiguers are liars. The problems in chronic fatigue are all in the head — "suggesting a central component of muscle fatigue in CFS (chronic fatigue syndrome)." Indeed, the study claimed, that the muscles of chronic fatiguers were less tired than the muscles among healthy people used as controls — the study showed "a trend toward both greater fatigue and a more marked metabolic response." So much for the high priests of "scientific research" in chronic fatigue. *Long live the all-in-the-head dogma!*

When I read such reports, I cannot always recognize the methodological errors that might have led the experimenters to such conclusions. Nonetheless, I dismiss such studies for a simple reason: The conclusions drawn about chronic fatigue are utterly inconsistent with what chronic fatiguers say chronic fatigue is. True science is self-correcting. I have no doubt that the results of such "scientific" studies will be proven totally erroneous with future studies. For now, the problem of separating true science from pseudoscience in chronic fatigue remains difficult.

## IMPAIRED OXIDATIVE METABOLISM IN MUSCLES IN CHRONIC FATIGUE

What is truly remarkable about the article cited above is that it appeared after clear evidence of disturbed energy dynamics, including the changes in "phosphate metabolism" had already been documented with sensitive methods using radioactive phosphorus nuclear magnetic resonance spectroscopy.

Studies with radioactive phosphorus show that drastically reduced capacity for activity occurs in the absence of any reduction in the cardiac performance or neuromuscular dysfunction in most cases that have been studied (*Chest* 102:1716;1992.). It is my strong sense, however, that further research will reveal that oxidant injury that causes failure of energy enzymes in skeletal muscle — the type of muscle that is under our voluntary control — also damages energy enzymes in the heart and at the neuromuscular junctions.

The immediate source of mechanical energy in the muscle is provided by chemical bond energy. Energy is released when the premium energy molecule in the body called ATP (adenosine triphosphate) splits into a molecule of adenosine diphosphate and one molecule of inorganic phosphate. In health, such loss in ATP is quickly followed by resynthesis of ATP in the muscle, thus restoring muscle ATP stores for further activity. This essential step in human energy dynamics appears to be blocked to varying degrees in chronic fatigue.

Virtually all muscle ATP is resynthesized by one or more of the following four mechanisms:

        A.   oxidative phosphorylation
        B.   glycolysis
        C.   creatine kinase reaction
        D.   adenylate kinase reaction

Of these, the first pathway — the oxidative phosphorylation — is clearly the major mechanism of ATP generation (source of energy) during both rest and sustained activity. At first blush, diminished oxidative metabolism in chronic fatigue may seem to contradict my theory that the state of chronic fatigue is a state of accelerated oxidative molecular injury. On deeper reflection, it provides further evidence for my viewpoint: Specifically, oxidant injury to energy enzyme pathways — by any of the several mechanisms I described earlier — would logically interfere with and diminish oxidative metabolism.

The second energy pathway listed above — glycolytic metabolism — refers to the release of chemical bond energy from the breakdown of glycogen in the muscle. It plays only a limited role in energy generation. The remaining two mechanisms are even less important. To-date, these mechanisms have not been well studied in chronic fatigue.

**\*\*\*\*\*\*\*\*\*\***

*What will become of me?*
*Will I ever live a normal life again?*
*Will I ever have any children?*

Those are some of the many questions Dawn asked me. I often wonder if the high priests of American medicine who sit on the editorial boards of our prestigious medical journals and who pride themselves on their standards of *scientific rigor* ever hear such questions. If so, I wonder if they ever reflect on the principles and practice of nutritional medicine, environmental they are fortunate enough to live in clean, nontoxic environment and make optimal food choices in the kitchen. Living near a beach where air is usually clean allows many such persons to, slowly and painstakingly, hold to a bare minimum their exposure to chemical triggers. Spiritual work is also easier to do for them in such areas rather than in crowded, polluted environment.

Dawn, of course, is not alone in her vulnerability to environmental chemicals.

*No man is an island,*
*entire of itself,*
*Any man's death diminishes me,*
*Because I am involved in mankind;*
*and therefore never send to know*
*for whom the bell tolls;*
*It tolls for thee. "*

John Donne

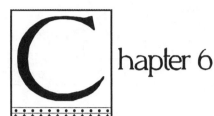

# Chapter 6

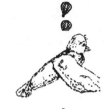

# On Reviving
# Injured
# Enzymes

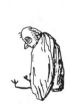
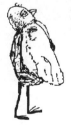

The management philosophy for chronic fatigue states I describe in this book is based on five central elements:

## First,

chronic fatiguers are genetically predisposed to oxidative injury, the root of chronic fatigue states.

## Second,

the frequency and degree of exposure to oxidative agents determines whether such a genetic predisposition remains dormant or initiates oxidative injury.

## Third,

the sum total of *all* burdens on an individual's biology determines whether such oxidative injury is efficiently repaired or leads to chronic, disabling fatigue.

## Fourth,

each chronic fatigue sufferer is unique and requires an individualized enzyme revival program tailored — figuratively and literally — to his needs.

## Fifth,

each chronic fatigue sufferer requires a comprehensive, holistic program that integrates all the necessary elements of nutritional and environmental medicines, self-regulation and slow, sustained (limbic) exercise.

The main importance of a genetic predisposition is to recognize that a risk exists, and that this information can be used to make choices that diminish the frequency and degree of oxidant agents. I often hear enthusiasts of gene therapy exclaim — with voices pregnant with anticipation — that they are on the verge of breakthroughs in genetic rearrangements with which they will achieve *any and all* goals. While I laud their determination and respect their technical skills in gene manipulation, they have to date no record of any achievements in reversing oxidative, degenerative or immune disorders. There is no reasonable hope that gene therapy enthusiasts will be able to offer any clinical benefits to chronic fatiguers in the foreseeable future.

The second element calls for well thought out strategies to reduce to a bare minimum all environmental exposures that lead to enzyme injury. These include mold and pollen allergy, chemical triggers, viral, bacterial and parasitic infections, stress-related factors and issues of physical fitness.

The emphasis of the third element is on *host* defenses — how human energetic-molecular defenses can be enhanced. This is where all the miracles of synthetic chemistry completely fail. And this is where the true preventive potential for holistic-molecular medicine lies.

The fourth and fifth elements point to the fact that holistic physicians are harshly criticized by disease doctors of drug medicine for their alleged inability to distinguish between specific lesions and what specific drugs or surgical treatments to use for them. Such criticism shows how little these champions of drug medicine understand the philosophy and practice of holistic molecular medicine. In reality, holistic-molecular medicine, as described in this volume, addresses health issues of individual patients in a highly specific fashion. The difference is that disease doctors focus on names of diseases and drugs, while holistic physicians focus on the underlying energetic-molecular derangements.

## SPECTRUM OF CHRONIC FATIGUE STATES

In the chapter Seven Canaries, I illustrate the spectrum of chronic fatigue states with true-to-life case histories. The case histories of Little Joe, Father Thomas and Zena represent the early, benign and easily reversible states of chronic fatigue. Molecular defenses of such people have not yet been badly violated by the tools of Star Wars technology. I usually start my nutritional and environmental therapies all at once, and proceed to give them training in autoregulation and limbic exercise without any detail. With such nondrug management protocols of holistic-molecular medicine, they snap back — usually within a few weeks — and regain their normal energy patterns.

Recurrences of chronic fatigue can be easily prevented in such individuals. They quickly learn what works and what does not. They do not fall for the false promises of $N^2D^2$ medicine.

The case histories of Bruce, John and Mr. Latimer represent the other end of the spectrum of chronic fatigue states. They require carefully thought out management plans that must be executed cautiously. Such individuals cannot afford many missteps on the part of the professional caring for them.

Certainly, they cannot tolerate the interventions of Star Wars medicine.

Before I describe my clinical approaches and give details of my nondrug therapies for chronic fatigue sufferers, I want to make three essential points:

I use three analogies to describe the principles and practice of the management strategy I apply to my human canaries, those patients literally incarcerated in their homes with chronic fatigue: a popcorn machine, a chessboard and quicksand.

## THE OXIDATIVE PLATE

In one aspect, human biology works the way a popcorn machine does. When a popcorn machine is not plugged in and its heating plate is cold, nothing happens to the kernels that are placed upon it. If the machine is defective and the heating plate heats only halfway, kernels put upon it roast but do not pop. If the machine is working well, the heating plate heats up all the way and every kernel put upon it readily pops.

Human canaries need to understand that. As long as the "oxidative plates" of their energetic-molecular dynamics are red hot, they will react and adversely respond to every trigger that comes along. Every allergic trigger causes debilitating fatigue. Every chemical exposure feeds the oxidative fire. Every sugar-insulin-adrenaline roller coaster fuels the oxidative pump. Every angry thought fans the oxidative flame. On and on, it feeds upon itself — just as the flames of a forest fire spread the fire once a carelessly hurled lighted matchstick sets the dry brush on fire. The essential element is this: The super-heated oxidative plate must be cooled down before the healing processes of the body can resume their normal functions.

## THE OXIDATIVE BOARD

In the game of chess, the queen is the most powerful piece, with the ability to strike out in all directions. By contrast, a pawn is a lowly piece that can move only one step at a time, essentially in only one direction. Chess players know that this is only part of the story. The essence of a good game of chess is not in simply knowing what the pieces are and how they can move on the board, but what the pieces can and cannot do within the context of a given board. A good chess player is able to position himself in such a way that the weakest piece can tower over the strongest. Thus, the all-powerful queen of one player succumbs to the lowly pawn of his opponent. Likewise, in human biology there are some very powerful and some weak enzyme systems. In disease states, sometimes the powerful enzyme systems become less important and some weak systems grow in importance.

There is much in common between a good chess player and a good holistic physician: The chess player *reads* his board and the physician his patient. The success of the chess player depends on how good his judgment calls are, and so it is with the physician — how he *reads* the oxidative board and how he plans to cool the oxidative plate.

I consider caring for chronic fatiguers in the same light. The skill of the physician is not merely in knowing what individual nutrients and herbs can and cannot do. Rather, it is in *reading* the total clinical picture of a chronic fatiguer and making the right judgment call.

I commonly see patients with overheated oxidative plates and maddeningly mangled oxidative boards. Attempts to relieve their severe allergy symptoms with immunotherapy injections only make them sicker. Efforts to treat their yeast overgrowth and infections further intensify their miseries. They may strongly react to IV infusions. Even small doses of oral nutrients may be poorly tolerated. Indeed, I have seen such patients respond negatively even to simple methods of self-regulation. So how does one begin one's work for cooling off their heated oxidative plates and rearranging their oxidative boards? With hope and with spiritual work! Some of the drug doctors may ridicule me for this statement. But if they do, it will only tell me how far removed they are from their severely fatigued patients, and how uninformed they are about the devastating reality of severe chronic fatigue. I discuss this subject further in the chapter On Hope, Spirituality and Chronic Fatigue.

## OXIDATIVE QUICKSAND

Persistent chronic fatigue is oxidative molecular quicksand. Thrashing around in this quicksand with quick-fix therapies such as antidepressants, anxiolytics, antibiotics, antiviral drugs and antiglobulins may give some temporary benefits. The underlying oxidative frenzy persists. Steroid therapy creates a false sense of well-being while suppressing the already weakened immune defenses. The drug doctors usually prescribe a host of other symptom-suppressing drugs — therapies that seek to silence whatever body organ happens to serve as the spokesorgan for the whole body at the time. Such therapies only make the real problems worse. The oxidative quicksand grows wider and deeper.

Antiyeast drugs such as Nystatin, Diflucan and others fare no better — they also create the illusion of success for short periods of time. With prolonged use, these antiyeast drugs kill off the sensitive strains of yeast and allow the resistent strains to take over. The result: Easily correctable patterns of yeast overgrowth are turned into indolent, difficult-to-eradicate yeast overgrowth and infections.

Chronic fatigue does not spare fitness trainers, dancers and models. Some of these individuals often try to pull themselves out of the oxidative quicksand with sheer willpower. Other chronic fatiguers are prescribed ill-advised exercise programs with Star Wars exercise technology. The results are usually disastrous. Such exercise adds fuel to the fire — oxidative storms gather strength and turn into oxidative hurricanes.

The use of antiyeast herbs, yeast diets and antioxidant formulations are steps in the right direction but are rarely sufficient by themselves.

The mind-over-body approach — my patients have taught me — does not work. It is nothing more than a cruel joke. I discuss this popular misconception in *The Ghoraa and Limbic Exercise*. Affirmations usually are of limited benefit unless they lead one to deeper spirituality.

Persons with severe, disabling chronic fatigue need a hand that can reach out to them in the quicksand and help them to slowly—often maddeningly slowly—pull themselves out of the quicksand. They need physicians who understand the essential oxidative equation of life — professionals who know something about the impact of environment on human biology, something about human nutrition. They need companions with whom they can do some true spiritual work.

Sometimes, for very ill patients, I begin my restorative program with simple choices in the kitchen. Such patients are so sensitive that they cannot tolerate common nutrients until the blazing hot oxidative plate is cooled off. I discuss this subject in the chapter Choices in the Kitchen. I recommend *The Butterfly and Life Span Nutrition* as a source of useful information on this subject.

My next area of focus for severely fatigued patients is self-regulation. I offer three two-hour training periods to each of my patients for this. My purpose here is to address the difficult problem of Fourth-of-July chemistry. Such chemistry — in my clinical experience — can rarely be brought down to a steady, even state by mere talk therapy. The mind-over-body approach does not work for such patients. Most of my patients have learned this the hard way by the time I see them. Energy over mind is the only viable option. This, they quickly learn by true-to-life experience, *does* work. I recommend *The Cortical Monkey and Healing* for useful information about slow, sustained breathing for this purpose.

Once the oxidative storms have cleared — or at least have subsided — I begin oral nutrient and herbal therapies. I discuss this subject in the chapter Oral Nutrient and Herbal Protocols.

I find intravenous nutrient therapy necessary in less than half of all chronic fatiguers who consult me. Usually a set of five or fewer infusions is all that is necessary to "jump start" the energy and detoxification enzymes. I describe intravenous nutrient therapy in detail, and give clinical outcome data for such therapy in the chapter Intravenous Nutrient Protocols. For further information, I refer the professional reader to my monograph *Intravenous Nutrient Protocols in Molecular Medicine.*

Chronic fatiguers almost always suffer from allergic and autoimmune disorders. Immunotherapy for allergy often needs to be postponed in severely fatigued persons, but is absolutely essential for preventing recurrence of chronic fatigue states after initial success. I address some essential issues later in this chapter and refer the professional reader to my monograph *Allergy: Diagnosis and Management* for further information.

## "CAP" AND "ENERGY" PHILOSOPHIES FOR CHRONIC FATIGUE SUFFERERS

The letters in the word *cap* stand for the three essentials of my core philosophy of caring for chronic fatiguers, and the letters in *energy* for the core elements in my clinical strategy. Thus:

**C**atch in early stages

**A**void drugs

**P**revent relapses

**C**atching chronic fatigue in early stages is clearly the best strategy. I have cared for hundreds of Little Joes, Father Thomas' and Zenas, and chronic fatigue in such patients can be relieved in *all* cases and in an entirely *predictable* fashion. Energy enzyme systems have an enormous capacity for regeneration. All we really need to do is address two issues: Reduce, and when possible, eliminate altogether the oxidative exposures that injure them, and provide optimal nutritional support for the regenerative processes.

**A**voiding drugs is imperative both for the chronic fatiguer and for the individual who cares for them. It is simply a matter of understanding the true oxidative nature of the problem and the true interruptive nature of drug mechanisms. Interruptive strategies cannot revive energy enzymes that were damaged by interruptions caused by oxidative injury in the first place. *It's that simple.*

**P**reventing recurrence of chronic fatigue after initial success is the third core element. Two common causes of recurrence in my experience are discontinuance of restorative measures and severe viral and bacterial infections. *Both elements are self-explanatory.* I strongly advise my patients with chronic fatigue to aggressively manage common infections early on and to avoid antibiotics unless such therapy is *truly* necessary. Now, what is truly necessary? If such a patient consults a drug doctor, antibiotics will be deemed truly necessary for every infection because he really has no tools for managing such infections except antibiotics. If he consults a knowledgeable holistic physician, he will likely be managed without antibiotics. *I cannot too strongly recommend intravenous nutrient therapy for common infections.* The risk of ignoring common infections is simply too great for chronic fatiguers. I describe such therapies in the chapter Intravenous Nutrient Protocols. In over 95% of my patients with chronic fatigue who contract common viral and bacterial infections, I do not find the use of antibiotics necessary.

The six letters in the word *energy* stand for:

**E**nvironment

**N**utrition

**E**xercise

**R**estoration    (of energy enzyme pathways)

**G**od

**Y**ou

**E**nvironment, in the context of chronic fatigue states, requires focus on the following:

Chemical sensitivity and chemical toxicity
Mold and other types of inhalant allergy
Body burden of toxic metals

Indoor air for most Americans today is far more polluted than outdoor air. I often think about it when I take the New Jersey Turnpike and pass the refineries near Newark Airport. On many days, the air is thick with pungent odors. And yet, study after study of environmental pollutants document how indoor air has a much higher content of pollutants than outdoor air. There are four issues here:

## First,

toxicity of pollutants is not a function of their odor. Indoor pollutants may not be as pungent and odorous as outdoor pollutants, but that does not mean they are less toxic.

## Second,

chemical toxicity is dose-dependent, and, hence, its effects are measurable with the established scientific methods for studying chemical toxicity. By contrast, chemical sensitivity is dose-independent. This cause of ill-being cannot be measured with the narrow-focused methods of prevailing drug medicine.

## Third,

our sensory perceptions are numbed by prolonged exposure to pollutants. Thus, we become "acclimatized" to toxins in indoor air, and so become insensitive to the magnitude of the threat. Chronic exposure to indoor pollutants causes slow-onset, vague symptoms attributable to multiple organ systems — the stuff that supports the old all-in-the-head theory. Such symptoms are simply dismissed by drug doctors as they dole out prescriptions for antidepressants. (The *New York Times* on

October 31, 1993, ranked *Listening to Prozac* number seven on its best-seller list. The book by the Prozac guru, psychiatrist Peter Kramer, extols the virtue of Prozac, subtly suggesting that perhaps we all should drink from this chemical fountain of enlightenment. I wonder how many prescription pads Dr. Kramer has used up practicing what he preaches.)

## *Fourth,*

air pollutants, by and large, are lipophilic — fat-loving with special affinity for the fats in brain tissue. That means that these molecules tenaciously stick to the brain and other types of neural tissues in the body — such as cells and fibers in the autonomic nervous system that controls blood circulation and regulates body temperature. Indeed, this is an important cause of undue cold sensitivity from which chronic fatiguers almost always suffer. There is no easy, quick-fix method for ridding the body of these aging-oxidant molecules.

## *Fifth,*

I have a strong sense that the cumulative burden of air, water and food pollutants is compounding the problems caused by the classical hay-fever type (IgE-mediated) of allergy. Recently, I reduced my dose schedule for immunotherapy I prescribe for allergy sufferers. As late as 10 years ago, I did not see the problems with dose tolerance that I see now. What is making the problem of allergy so much more difficult?

It is not commonly recognized that allergic reactions are triggered by oxidant injury to the cell membranes of mast cells — the tiny bombs in the tissues that are primed to explode —

and release into tissues their payload of chemicals — when triggered by allergic agents. The oxidant effects of allergic triggers and pollutants combine to compound the problems of allergic persons.

## SOME PRACTICAL SUGGESTIONS FOR MINIMIZING INDOOR POLLUTION

Chronic fatigue sufferers can take several short-term measures and some long-term measures to reduce their body burden of indoor air pollutants.

### *Short-Term Measures*

1.  Drinking liberally good waters and fluids (See Choices in the Kitchen)
2.  Eating foods that sustain energy enzymes and avoiding foods that deplete energy enzymes (See Choices in the Kitchen)
3.  Eating organically grown foods whenever possible
4.  Using natural and organic household cleaners
5.  Using air filters in the living rooms and bedrooms
6.  Using water filters
7.  Eliminating all cosmetic chemicals from bedrooms
8.  Reducing — and eliminating when possible — all synthetic chemicals from the home environment
9.  Wearing common surgical masks to reduce exposure to chemicals during household cleaning and other activities
10. Completely avoiding exposure to pesticide, fungicide and

other chemical sprays. I cannot overemphasize this point. (I have seen many tragic case histories similar to that of Mr. Latimer's given in the chapter Seven Canaries.)
11.  Carefully avoiding freshly painted rooms

## *Long-Term Measures*

1.  Using cotton area rugs (dhurries) rather than wall-to-wall carpeting
2.  Using electrical cooking ranges rather than gas cookers. (Natural gas ranks high among the agents that cause and exaggerate chemical sensitivity.)
3.  Using nonmercury paints rather than wallpapers
4.  Living in less polluted geographic areas (Oceanside locations are ideal. Cities like Denver and Phoenix are actually very high-pollution areas.)
5.  Residing in areas away from major industrial complexes (Information about wind currents from such areas is extremely useful when buying homes. I know of people for whom wrong home locations turned out to be very expensive mistakes.)

## BODY BURDEN OF TOXIC METALS

I test every adult patient who consults me for chronic fatigue for total body burden of toxic metals. In about one-fourth of all such patients, the total toxic metal burden is high. Fortunately, this problem is not difficult to manage. Six to 10 EDTA chelation infusions significantly lower the metabolically active toxic metal burden. Metals bound down in some tissues such as bone are not easily chelated out. However, "fixed" toxic metals sequestered in these tissues do not seem to carry the same threat to energy and detoxification enzymes.

Toxic metals such as aluminum, mercury, lead, cadmium, nickel and arsenic are known enzyme poisons. Evidently, this risk is far greater for chronic fatiguers than it is for the general population — fatigue sufferers have damaged enzymes to begin with. For instance, a 24-hour urinary excretion of mercury of 18 micrograms in a woman in good health indicates a significant body burden of mercury. It poses a clear hazard to her enzymes though she may not suffer from any visible adverse effects for 20 years. By contrast, a 24-hour mercury excretion of 10 micrograms in her husband who suffers fatigue may be enough to impede his recovery from fatigue.

I sometimes wonder why physicians practicing drug medicine do not recognize this threat. Health hazards posed by lead have been the subject of scrutiny by the media, and pediatricians frequently test for lead in children. It must be a rare pediatrician or internist who routinely tests his patients for mercury, aluminum and other toxic metals. There are three possible reasons for it. First, disease doctors generally do not understand the cumulative risks of environmental toxicants. Second, no drug company is promoting such testing since there is no drug to be sold when the test comes back positive — EDTA is an orphan chelating agent, and without patent protection, no drug company wants to throw its money behind it. Third, the only effective therapy for toxic metal overload is chelation — and that, the main physician body has been told, is quackery.

Aluminum overload — in my view — is a far more important threat to human biology than are lead or mercury. One reason for this is that I encounter increased body burden of aluminum in chronic fatiguers much more frequently than that I see of lead or mercury. Second, Americans are far more frequently exposed to aluminum in their general environment than they are to other toxic metals.

The body burden of toxic metals can be assessed with random urine and blood tests. Blood tests, in my experience, do not nearly yield diagnostic information as valuable as the urine tests. The ideal way to test for increased body burden of toxic metals is to do a three-phase urine test as follows:

1.   A pre-challenge 24-hour urine sample for toxic metals
2.   DMPS or EDTA chelation challenge dose
3.   A post-challenge 24-hour urine test for toxic metals

DMPS and EDTA are chelating agents that bind to metabolically active toxic metals in soft tissues — and to a lesser degree to heavy metals embedded deep in the meshwork of bone — and bring the metals out in the urine. The difference between the pre-challenge and the post-challenge amounts of toxic metals excreted in the urine is a good indicator of total body burden of toxic metals.

## EDTA: THE ENZYME SAVER

Apart from reducing the increased body burden of toxic

metals, EDTA infusion therapy offers several other important advantages. For example, it has been known that EDTA slows down the aging process of the mitochondrial energy enzymes under experimental conditions (*J Mol Cell Cardiol* 9:897; 1977.) Furthermore, EDTA can directly *revive* injured enzymes quite apart of its indirect beneficial effects on enzyme function brought about by removing excess calcium from within the cells (*Nature* 187:162; 1960.)

When EDTA chelation therapy becomes necessary to reduce body burden of toxic metals, such therapy brings unexpected dividends in terms of saved and rehabilitated enzymes. Toxic metals, I wrote earlier, are enzyme poisons, and EDTA revives enzymes by dissociating them from toxic metals.

## INHALANT ALLERGY

Treatment of mold and other types of inhalant allergy that exists in almost all chronic fatiguers is essential to a good long-term clinical outcome. *The case for such therapy cannot be overstated.* I discuss the subject of food sensitivity in *The Butterfly and Life Span Nutrition.* I refer the professional reader to my monograph *Allergy: Diagnosis and Management* for detailed information about immunotherapy I administer to my patients for IgE-mediated allergy. In this chapter, I limit myself in this chapter to making some essential points for the general reader.

## *First,*

allergy must be considered in a much broader context for chronic fatiguers — as a large burden on energy and detoxification systems of the body and a profound pathophysiologic derangement, not merely a matter of running nose or itchy eyes. The traditional ideas of diagnosing and managing nasal and sinus allergy with the RAST test have very little relevance to chronic fatigue states. Chronic fatigue sufferers should seek out physicians who understand this essential issue.

## *Second,*

allergy exists in almost *all* persons who suffer from chronic fatigue. I see many chronic fatiguers who insist they do not have any allergies. A careful review of the past medical history going back to infancy almost always brings out the existence of allergic symptoms. (Colicky babies are always allergic babies. Eczema of infancy is often forgotten. Tonsillectomies are almost always done for undiagnosed and unmanaged allergy. Fatigue after eating is rarely recognized as caused by food sensitivity.)

## *Third,*

commonly used RAST tests are inadequate for allergy diagnosis. Specifically, such tests fail to detect up to one half of mold sensitivities. My colleague, Madhava Ramanarayanan, Ph.D., and I observed this phenomenon in the early 1980s and published extensive data defining the magnitude of this problem.

## Fourth,

issues of mold and food allergy, and its impact upon
bowel ecology and the ecosystem in other body organs —
in my view — are much more significant for chronic
fatiguers than the commonly recognized nasal, eye and
sinus allergy.

## Fifth,

immunotherapy for allergy in chronic fatigue should be
broad-based, and should include all relevant allergens.
Again, narrowly defined concepts of allergy that pervade
our medical schools are of limited value.

## Sixth,

immunotherapy should not be expected to produce early
clinical benefits. Rather, it should be considered as an
essential therapy for long-term support of energetic-
molecular defenses.

Immunotherapy with allergens — allergy shots in common
language — enhances the immune response. One of the changes
observed is an increase in the production of blocking antibodies
(allergen-specific IgG antibodies that literally block allergic
reactions.) On the following page, I use two case histories to
illustrate the difference in the immune responsiveness of
individuals with intact molecular defenses and those with badly
battered defenses. The first patient is a 15-year-old boy who
wrestled for his school team but had experienced progressive
fatigue for about six months. The second patient is his mother

who had suffered from persistent fatigue for about three years before she consulted me. The table below compares the data for specific IgG antibodies assayed in the pre- and post-treatment samples.

For the professional reader, the numbers in the columns represent milliunits of Absorbance obtained with a micro-elisa assay for allergen-specific IgG antibodies. Both the pre- and post-treatment samples were assayed within the same assay run.

| SPECIFIC IgG RESPONSE TO IMMUNOTHERAPY | | | | |
|---|---|---|---|---|
| Antigen | Son Nov. 18, 92 | Son Aug. 9, 93 | Mother Feb. 5, 93 | Mother Sep. 18, 93 |
| Bermuda | 83 | 783 | 84 | 71 |
| June | 128 | 708 | 66 | 33 |
| Ragweed | 186 | 1093 | 155 | 59 |
| Plantain | 1,454 | 1,958 | 359 | 915 |
| Maple | 660 | 1,194 | 340 | 245 |
| Sycamore | 324 | 403 | 188 | 87 |
| Alternaria | 2,041 | 2,046 | 609 | 697 |
| Penicillium | 2,362 | 2,542 | 610 | 1,041 |
| Candida | 2,554 | 2,596 | 2,602 | 2,644 |
| Cat | 1,098 | 1,524 | 822 | 885 |

The clinical response in both the mother and the son was

satisfactory. The son regained his normal level of energy and
was able to return to school athletics within months of nondrug
therapies and immunotherapy. The mother responded well to
the management plan but still suffered from fatigue on some
days.

Comparison of specific IgG response to immunotherapy
injections in this mother-son twosome illustrates some important
points.

### First,

the immune response of an individual to various
antigens included in the treatment varies over a wide
range.

### Second,

the immune response to antigen immunotherapy
varies among different individuals over a wide range.

### Third,

the immune response to immunotherapy in children
suffering from chronic fatigue is usually brisk — their
molecular defenses have not been damaged yet by
antibiotics, other drugs, viruses, and environmental and
nutritional factors.

### Fourth,

the immune response to immunotherapy is markedly

impaired in adult chronic fatigue sufferers.

Chronic fatiguers do eventually respond to immunotherapy. I have observed this phenomenon in most adult chronic fatigue sufferers who continued immunotherapy for two to three years — although the IgG response in such patients is rarely as strong as seen in children who suffer from chronic fatigue.

Antigen immunotherapy for chronic fatigue sufferers should be an integral part of long-term strategy for restoring damaged energy enzymes. In one of my series of 200 consecutive patients, every single patient showed clear, unequivocal evidence of IgE-mediated allergy.

Nutrition is what we are, to paraphrase the ancients. Nutrition for chronic fatiguers has three core aspects:

1. Optimal choices in the kitchen
2. Oral nutrient and herbal protocols
3. Intravenous nutrient protocols when deemed necessary.

I devote the following three chapters to these three aspects. Here, I make the following three points:

*First,*

the nutrition science of practitioners of drug medicine is utterly irrelevant to chronic fatigue sufferers. Regrettably, so is that of nutritionists who are limited in their work to narrow limits defined by such physicians.

## *Second,*

the prevailing concepts of nutritional deficiencies are equally irrelevant to human canaries. The chemistry of life in chronic fatiguers is often in the Fourth-of-July mode. Such individuals require large doses of nutrients to put out the oxidative fires. To cite one example, one of my patients had blood levels of various vitamins measured about 36 hours after she received 15 grams (15,000 mg) of vitamin C for a viral infection. Her blood vitamin C level turned out to be 0.15 mg/dl — below the range of 0.2 to 2 mg/dl reported among health subjects not taking any supplemental vitamin C.

## *Third,*

the prevailing notions of balanced diet (including large quantities of highly reactive foods such as dairy and eggs) are also utterly irrelevant to the nutritional needs of chronic fatigue sufferers.

Exercise for chronic fatiguers must be slow, sustained and non goal-oriented. Demand exercise fuels the oxidative storms of chronic fatiguers. It's easy to understand why: Exercise requires tissues to generate more energy, and energy generation is an oxidative function. I return to this subject in the chapter Limbic Exercise for Chronic Fatigue.

Restoration   of energy and detoxification enzymes calls for integrated, holistic-molecular, nondrug therapies. For emphasis, I reproduce the list of essential areas from the chapter Seven Canaries.

1.   Restoration  to normal states of bowel ecology
2.   Restoration  of even, steady-state  molecular  dynamics  of health (eliminating sugar, insulin, adrenaline and neurotransmitter   roller coasters)
3.   Restoration  of normal body temperature (through self-regulation and normalization of thyroid gland function)
4.   Restoration  of cell membrane  structure  and function (through food choices in the kitchen, oral and, when necessary, intravenous  nutrient  protocols)
5.   Restoration  of normal energy dynamics by reducing, and eventually eliminating, stress-related molecular events
6.   Restoration  of energy systems that have been blocked or impaired by toxic metal overload such as aluminum, mercury, lead and others

In a global sense, these restorations can be achieved by nondrug therapies that prevent oxidative injury to energy enzymes and allow these enzymes to regenerate by the natural order of things. To this purpose, I make a large number of specific recommendations  both for the chronic fatiguer and the professional who cares for him in the following six chapters. Here I want to address two special issues: the matter of the troubled trio and temperature  dysregulation.

---

| THE TROUBLED TRIO |
|---|

*Chronic fatiguers almost always suffer from excessive cold sensitivity and low body temperatures.*
*Chronic fatiguers almost always suffer from sugar-insulin-adrenaline roller coasters.*
*Chronic fatiguers almost always suffer from severe stress states.*

The thyroid, pancreas and adrenal glands are a troubled trio in chronic fatigue states. Regardless of the initial events that set the stage for chronic fatigue, the accelerated oxidative molecular injury to human enzyme pathways will *always* lead to oxidative damage to enzymes and receptors that preserve the functional integrity of these three body organs.

The thyroid gland is the primary gland that regulates the body temperature — and through it the metabolic functions of *all* energy and detoxification enzyme systems of the body. Thus, undue sensitivity to cold temperatures and lack of energy are two of the major clinical symptoms of chronic fatiguers.

The pancreas regulates the blood sugar level. Beyond that, through its insulin secretion, it profoundly affects a host of other molecular dynamics and cardiovascular functions. Injury to the pancreas causes the sugar roller coasters that are well known to chronic fatiguers. Sugar roller coasters evoke insulin roller coasters that, in turn, bring on adrenaline roller coasters. Adrenaline roller coasters, of course, cause the symptoms that are commonly believed to be due to hypoglycemia — sudden mood swings, weakness, sweating, nausea, lightheadedness and palpitations. Almost all chronic fatiguers suffer from such symptoms at one time or the other.

The adrenal gland is the primary stress organ of the body. It produces several essential hormones including:

1. 'Fight or flight' hormones — adrenaline and its cousin molecules, catecholamines — that help us gear our energetic-molecular defenses for coping with life-threatening events

2. Cortisone and its cousin molecules that energize many receptors — including those for adrenaline — for various body functions.

3. Aldosterone hormone that regulates kidney function, and through that water and salt balance of the body

4. DHEA (the "mother" hormone that prevents accelerated aging), androgen (male) and estrogen (female) hormones that provide a counterbalance to such hormones produced in other organs of the body.

The adrenal gland is, in many of its functions, regulated by ACTH hormone of the pituitary gland, which in turn is regulated by the hypothalamus. It was entirely predictable that the adrenal-pituitary-hypothalamus axis would draw much attention from chronic fatigue researchers. That indeed has happened. Below I include some research findings:

1. Low blood cortisone levels in chronic fatigue

2.   High blood levels of ACTH — not unexpected, because the pituitary senses the low adrenal activity and tries to drive it harder

3.   Low prevalence of dexamethasone nonsuppression

4.   Increased sensitivity (and reduced maximal response) of adrenal gland to ACTH and reduced maximal response of the adrenal glands

5.   Reduced ability of CRF (corticotrophin releasing factor) to stimulate ACTH release
                              (*J Clin Endocrinol Metab* 73:1224;1991)

## TEMPERATURE DYSREGULATION IN CHRONIC FATIGUE

Most chronic fatiguers have a significant problem with cold hands and feet by the time they consult me. Eventually all chronic fatiguers develop temperature dysregulation and low body temperature — and with that lose the efficiency of their enzymes much like a defect in the furnace reduces the efficiency of a home heating system. There are five core points in this discussion:

*First,*

the oxidative injury that damages energy enzymes also damages the autonomic nerve receptors, which regulate regional blood flow and the temperature of that part of the body. This is not mere speculation on my part. Every Wednesday evening, I spend two and half hours in my autoregulation laboratory teaching my patients how to flush their cold hands and feet with warm blood by allowing their arteries to open up by shutting out the thinking mind. I do not recall a single laboratory session in which one or more patients did not see their skin temperature shoot up from below 80 degrees to 90 degrees or over. Clearly, this is an autonomic function. (The term autoregulation actually derives from my early work in this area when I used to call it autonomic regulation. My patients shortened it to autoregulation and then autoreg.) Equally clearly, such a rise in skin temperature cannot be deemed a consequence of thyroid manipulation because no thyroid hormone is used in such work. Furthermore, temperature regulation through thyroid hormone therapy takes several days to some weeks, while I observe changes in the skin temperature in minutes.

## Second,

the accelerated oxidative injury in chronic fatigue states that damages energy enzymes also damages the enzymes that are involved in the synthesis of thyroid hormones such as de-iodinases.

## Third,

all energy and detoxification enzymes are highly sensitive to temperature. Even a small drop in body temperature, such as three-quarters to one degree, can be expected to significantly impair the efficiency of enzymes. In laboratory conditions, such changes can sometimes cause as much as a 50% drop in enzyme efficiency. This question within the context of human total body metabolism has not been well investigated. I am confident when it is, it will reveal a large drop in metabolic enzyme efficiency. In common language, this turns into a major physiologic handicap for those who run low body temperature.

### *Fourth,*

the combined effect of the above three factors is that cold hands and feet become increasingly colder as the body metabolism lumbers on to cope with the intensified demands of the Fourth-of-July chemistry in chronic fatigue states.

---

## TEMPERATURE  UP-REGULATION WITH $T_4$ AND $T_3$ THERAPIES

---

This subject is generally considered very complex. It need not be. In the chapter What Is Chronic Fatigue? and in the section dealing with the troubled trio in this chapter, I describe how thyroid dysfunction occurs in chronic fatigue states. Seven mistakes are commonly made in this area:

### *First,*

the impact of persistently low body temperature  on energy and detoxification enzymes is not recognized, both by the patient and the physician. The fundamental difference between living beings and nonliving things, I wrote earlier in this volume, is that living beings are enzymes beings. *All* enzymes are temperature-dependent.   Lowering of the body temperature  by one-half to one degree has the same effect on human metabolism as lowering the thermal efficiency of a home heating system — the fuel burns inefficiently with waste of valuable energy. *The firm proof for this phenomenon is the common observation that chronic fatiguers feel better and more energetic on days when their temperature is normal and do poorly on days when their temperature is low.*

## Second,

the enzymes that convert inactive and weakly active thyroid hormone precursors to active hormones are damaged by oxidative injury. I am certain of this, though this has not been proven yet with actual studies. This leads to diminished production of active $T_3$ hormone and persistently low body temperature. The proof of this is in the common observation that daily temperature  cannot be normalized in many patients even with large doses of natural thyroid extract or synthetic $T_4$ preparations  such as synthyroid. Yet, the temperature  rises within days when optimal doses of $T_3$ are used. Furthermore, oxidative injury damages the thyroid hormone receptors. I discuss this subject further, later in this section.

## Third,

in the prevailing dogma of endocrinology, thyroid function is frequently assumed to be normal if the commonly performed $T_4$, $T_3$ uptake, quantitative $T_3$, and TSH tests show negative results. Rather large drops in the blood hormone levels are ignored simply because the test value falls within the "normal" range. The frequency with which otherwise knowledgeable physicians make this mistake amazes me. For example, the normal range for $T_4$ in most laboratories is 4.5 to 12 mcg/ml. However, a fatigue sufferer with a normal hormone level of 12 mcg/ml might drop it by 50% down to 6 mcg/ml. According to the prevailing dogma, this would be considered a negative result, while in reality it represents a significant degree of hypothyroidism (underactive thyroid gland).

## *Fourth,*

hypothyroidism is assumed to exist when the body temperature is below normal, and no attempts are made to investigate dysfunction of the autonomic nervous system. Predictably, when low body temperature is due to autonomic dysfunction, thyroid replacement fails to restore the body temperature to the normal range.

## *Fifth,*

the dose of thyroid hormone is continually increased even when such therapy neither affords clinical benefits nor raises the body temperature. I have seen cases where the dose of $T_4$ or $T_3$ was pushed to a very high value with resulting rapid heart rate, palpitations, and in some cases, cardiac arrythmia.

## *Sixth,*

sufficient attention is not paid to impaired function of the adrenal gland and other hormonal dysfunctions that frequently coexist with underactive thyroid status. The oxidative injury that slows down enzymes involved with thyroid hormone synthesis can also be fully expected to slow down the enzymes that are essential for production of adrenal hormone. This indeed does happen. The blood levels of DHEA, an adrenal hormone, are almost always low, often markedly, in patients with persistent chronic fatigue.

## *Seventh,*

little, if any, attempts are made in clinical endocrinology to consider the nutritional basis of hormonal dysregulations. This is remarkable because even a cursory look at the biochemistry charts outlining enzyme pathways will shows how multiple nutrients are essential for each enzymatic step in hormone synthesis. My thoughts go to Clinton's campaign. His aides came up with the campaign slogan, *It's economy, stupid!* After his election, they changed the slogan to, *It's taxes, stupid!*. For clinical endocrinology, I suggest the slogan, *It's nutrition, stupid!*

I carefully study temperature dysregulation in every single chronic fatiguer by ordering appropriate blood tests as well as by asking the patient to take oral as well as axillary (underarm) temperature readings immediately after waking up and before leaving the bed. The oral and axillary temperature readings are again taken three and six hours after the morning reading. In addition, I ask the patient to record her/his pulse in the morning. These steps are repeated on three consecutive days.

The oral temperature should range from 98.2 to 98.6 degrees. Axillary temperature should range from 97.5 to 98 degrees. If the temperature is more than a half degree lower on average, I focus on the functional integrity of both the autonomic nervous system and the thyroid gland.

For thyroid hypofunction, I usually prescribe a small dose of one grain of natural thyroid extract (Armour brand). Four weeks later, I do a clinical evaluation and repeat body temperature readings — oral, axillary or both, depending on the pattern of temperatures observed during the initial readings. If the small dose of thyroid extract fails to raise the body temperature to the desired level, I increase the dose by small increments such as one-half to one grain at a time. *It is essential to monitor pulse rate during all types of thyroid therapy.* I clearly instruct the patient not to increase the thyroid dose if the pulse rate begins to rise by more than 10 beats per minute above the initial reading or when the pulse rate climbs above 90 per minute.

## $T_3$ TEMPERATURE   UP-REGULATION

At times, thyroid extract therapy fails to give any clinical benefits and low body temperatures persist. After careful re-evaluation, if I still think the thyroid gland is not functioning properly, I move on to the use of small doses (7.5 to 30 mcg daily in two divided doses) of slow-acting $T_3$ preparations, and increase the dose in small increments of 7.5 mcg (as suggested by my friend, Dennis Wilson, M.D.), carefully watching the pulse rate and body temperature and looking for clinical signs of improvement.

In my office, I use temperature and pulse sheets for recording daily temperatures, pulse rates and symptom scores. I designed these worksheets specifically to assist and guide the patient in following my instructions. I cannot overemphasize the *absolute* need for careful monitoring of both the body temperature and the pulse rate so that both the thyroid gland and the heart are not needlessly overdriven.

## DHEA, PROGESTERONE AND RELATED HORMONAL DYSREGULATIONS

It should be evident from my discussion of thyroid dysfunction that accelerated oxidant injury in chronic fatigue states should be expected to also cause dysfunctions of other hormonal systems in the body. This indeed happens. I see clinical evidence of this in almost all patients with severe chronic fatigue. As for the laboratory abnormalities, clear evidence of dysfunction is easily established for some hormone systems — such as DHEA for the adrenal gland — while it is not readily forthcoming for some other systems such as estrogens and progesterone in women and androsterone in men. I believe such evidence will be forthcoming as highly sensitive laboratory methods are developed.

## DHEA-DEHYDROEPIANDROSTERONE

DHEA is a primary adrenal hormone that has been called the "mother hormone" by some investigators. There are excellent reasons why this hormone should be of considerable clinical value in chronic fatigue states. Indeed, most physicians practicing nutritional and environmental medicines report good results with DHEA in their fatigue patients.

I frequently use DHEA in doses of 50 mg on alternate days for periods of some months for my canaries. In most cases, such therapy can be discontinued within some months when the normal enzyme functions — and energy levels — are restored.

DHEA has many established beneficial effects on several arms of the immune system.

It is involved in regulation of lymphokine production.

It depresses production of interleukin 4 and 5 and gamma interferon but not IL-2 in activated murine T cells.

DHEA enhances IL-2 production in cytotoxic effector function of human T cells.

It protects against acute lethal viral infections (Coxsackie and viral encephalitis).

DHEA is a predictor of progression of AIDS in HIV positive individuals and in men with CD4 counts between 200 and 499.

Stress states are associated with suppression of lymphocyte proliferation.

Steroids such as dexamethasone depress the immune system (blastogenic responses), DHEA prevents such depression.

DHEA levels are usually reduced in chronic fatigue states, and replacement therapy with DHEA improves the overall energy level and reduces many associated symptoms.

A role of DHEA in the cause of systemic lupus — autoimmune disorder — has been suggested.

DHEA opposes the physiological effects of cortisone in several animal models.

## PROGESTERONE AND ESTROGEN THERAPIES

Biology adapts to the environment slowly. Natural selection of favorable genes to support adaptation to adverse changes in the environment is a very slow process — and often requires several millennia if not longer. By contrast, oxidant injury can damage genes quickly — perhaps in some hours.

Menstrual periods are Nature's design to ensure the perpetuation of humankind. To this purpose, the endometrium — the inner lining of the uterus — prepares itself for conception every month. That is the natural order of things, and was established to preserve homo sapiens in an era when the principal threat to the survival of humankind was extinction by a shrinking population. Predators and accidents were the principal threats. Human genes needed to be preserved, and the simplest and most efficient mechanism for that was more babies.

Times have changed — and so have the demands for survival. Now the twin principal threats to humankind are progressive oxidant stress and overpopulation, each feeding upon the other. Families today cannot afford pregnancy at the rate planned in nature. Natural monthly demands of the endometrium for pregnancy cannot be met, and hence are foiled every month.

How does the endometrium prepare itself every month for its evolutionary role? By putting out bursts of estrogen. How does the body cope with such bursts of estrogen in the natural order of things (when pregnancy does occur)? By providing a counterbalance with bursts of progesterone from the corpus luteum of the ovary as the fertilized egg settles into the pregnant endometrium. What happens when the endometrium prepares but the fertilized ovum does not make the scene?

Disillusioned — and frustrated — the endometrium strikes back. This is the natural order of things. And this is where female hormonal problems begin. Unbridled estrogen is the villain for women today — and not the commonly perceived estrogen deficiency. The hot flashes of menopause are confused responses of the body — estrogen withdrawal symptoms akin to the misery of a cocaine addict when his fix is not forthcoming. (Most of my patients respond well to rather large doses of folic acid — 10 to 30 mg in two divided daily doses — and natural progesterone therapy.)

Accelerated oxidative injury can be expected to injure the enzyme system involved in the synthesis of estrogen and progesterone as well as the hormone receptor molecules. This indeed does happen. It is very common for women with severe fatigue to suffer from menstrual irregularities, severe PMS symptoms, and, in persistent cases, absence of menstruation. *The return to normal menstruation is utterly predictable when chronic fatigue is managed well and enzyme functions are restored.*

Should synthetic estrogen be used for prevention of osteoporosis? No, except as a last resort. The best prevention of osteoporosis is with a reduction in the total oxidative stress — with optimal choices in the kitchen and self-regulation — and direct vertical stress on the axial skeleton with rebounding exercises such as jumping with a rope or on a trampoline. I recommend *The Ghoraa and Limbic Exercise* for a discussion of exercise for osteoporosis. Osteoporosis is caused by oxidant injury to hormone receptors and enzymes involved with laying down of new bone. I discuss this subject at length in *What Do Woodpeckers Know About Osteoporosis?*

If hormonal treatment is deemed necessary, I prefer to use natural progesterone rather than estrogen. I try to avoid the use of synthetic estrogen preparations unless all other alternatives have been exhausted. It is a rare woman who does not respond to integrated, holistic nondrug therapies as described in this book to such a degree that the use of synthetic estrogens becomes necessary. I do not oppose short-term use of very small doses of synthetic estrogens in refractory cases.

I use natural progesterone products — such as those derived from wild yam — liberally for my female patients with chronic fatigue. The favorable results include improvement in general energy level, mood swings, PMS symptoms and skin texture. I recommend one or two daily skin applications of natural progesterone creams or oils for 15 to 20 days in each month. It is advisable to rotate the skin areas for application of creams and oils between face, neck, chest, abdomen and thighs. Again, the use of natural progesterone products can be discontinued when normal energy patterns are restored. *In general, the best strategies for prevention of chronic fatigue are right choices in the kitchen, oral nutrient supplementation, immunotherapy for IgE-mediated allergy, intravenous nutrient infusions for managing common infections, self-regulation, and slow, sustained, nongoal-oriented (limbic) exercise.* I do not recommend long-term hormonal therapies as preventive measures.

In closing this section, I wish to emphasize that hormonal therapies for chronic fatigues states should not be undertaken without the supervision of a knowledgeable physician.

## THE TYRANNY OF THE 17-YEAR LAW

I expect my women readers to ask me the predictable question at this time: If my viewpoint about hormonal dysregulation described above is true, why don't all the women physicians in the country who prescribe synthetic estrogens by the ton pay attention? They *do* care for their women patients. Of this, there is no doubt. Then why don't they try simpler, natural — and clearly safer — therapies first? (No one yet knows the increased risk of cancer of the uterus and the breast from synthetic estrogens and increased oxidative stress among women fatigue sufferers.)

The simple answer is this: The tyranny of the "17-Year Law" prevails in synthetic estrogen and progesterone therapies just as it does in other drug therapies. The use of natural hormones cannot be patented — and hence made richly profitable for 17 years — by the drug companies. No drug company is foolish enough to fly its "experts" around the country lecturing about — and extolling the virtues of — natural hormone therapies. So synthetic hormone therapies prevail at considerable peril to the safety of their recipients.

No funds are made available for researching the clinical efficacy of nutrients and natural substances. Indeed, when physicians conduct such research with their personal funds, they are actively harassed by their peers, the state medical licensing boards and government regulators. This goes on while billions of dollars flow freely to develop synthetic — and toxic — analogues of effective natural substances with the sole purpose of profitability under the protection of the 17-year law. I cite one example: The amino acids tryptophane and tyrosine were used by nutritionists successfully for depression throughout the country until tryptophane was banned a few years ago. How many Americans might have been hurt by tryptophane? A dozen? Two dozen? And why did tryptophane, an essential amino acid, suddenly become toxic after decades of safe, nationwide use?

The year tryptophane was banned, the sales of Prozac skyrocketed and its makers rang in a billion dollar in sales. (Now the figure must be much larger.) Some strange events occurred at that time. I am told three Japanese companies used to manufacture tryptophane. Two of these companies stopped manufacturing tryptophane, while the third mysteriously changed its manufacturing process. Mere coincidences? Then came an onslaught of magazine articles and books extolling the virtues of Prozac. How many people were injured by amino acids? How many will be injured by Prozac? And by other antidepressants? How many will be given chronic fatigue by such drugs? How many human canaries will stay incarcerated in fatigue with the false promise of antidepressants?

Such is the tyranny of the 17-year law.

## MISCELLANEOUS THERAPIES

Some other therapies have been reported to give good clinical responses in chronic fatigue. Kutapressin is an injectable preparation of crude liver extract. I have observed only limited clinical benefits with this therapy.

Nitroglycerine in patch form has been recommended for chronic fatigue. This drug may be of some value in patients with severe muscle pains and tender myofascial points located within the muscles. Again, I have not observed significant clinical benefits in my limited experience with it.

Malic acid used in conjunction with magnesium has also been reported to be of value. Malic acid is a safe, natural product derived from apples and is used widely in the food industry. It plays a role in ATP energy pathways, and, at least, on a theoretical basis seems worthy of larger trials. The initial recommended dose is 300 mg of malic acid and 1,200 mg of magnesium.

I do want to make one point forcefully here. Some patients consulted me for persistent fatigue and told me they had been treated with kutapressin injections with or without vitamin $B_{12}$ injections as the only therapy for months. Some patients had been given nitroglycerine as the only therapy. Such approaches are doomed to failure even if they offer some initial benefits. I think such therapies are a disservice to those who can ill-afford the cost — in prolonged suffering and expense — of such frivolous thinking.

Severely fatigued patients often suffer depression, anxiety, sleep disorders, abdominal bloating and a variety of other symptoms. The use of appropriate drugs for relief of symptoms often becomes necessary and should be considered. The essential point is this: *Drugs must never be considered as agents for restoring normal energy patterns.*

## BRUCELLA REMEDY FOR CHRONIC FATIGUE

I am unable to comment on the relative efficacy of homeopathic remedies for chronic fatigue because I do not have adequate experience with these remedies. I do have some reservations about the possible long-term benefits of such therapies. My view is based on the clinical outcome with such therapies related to me by my patients who received care from homeopathic physicians before they consulted me.

I relate my experience with one homeopathic remedy to make an important point. In a meeting of the Academy of Environmental Medicine a few years ago, I heard a colleague describe the use of Brucella homeopathic remedy for chronic fatigue. I wondered how anyone thought of using this remedy.

I asked my colleague if he knew how it might work. He shrugged his shoulders and told me he had learned about it from another physician who, in turn, had heard about it from a 91-year-old physician. Next, I tried to reach that old gentleman only to find that he cannot take any phone calls due to a hearing disability.

I recognized why anyone would propose Brucella remedy for chronic fatigue — chronic Brucella infection was supposed to cause chronic fatigue in sporadic cases at the turn of the century, and, indeed, chronic brucellosis was the diagnostic label used for it. I didn't think it would work for most chronic fatiguers now because Brucella infection is clearly not the cause of chronic fatigue in the majority of patients today.

Still, this possibility intrigued me and I decided to test it with ten patients. I soon confirmed my suspicions that Brucella remedy was not useful. I kept my reservation to myself until recently when I saw Dr. Hanna Chaim who I remembered was present at the meeting where I first learned about the Brucella remedy. I told her about my experience and asked if her experience had been any different. She grinned broadly and replied, "It doesn't work!"

I write these few lines about the Brucella remedy to answer a criticism that disease doctors in drug medicine often level at holistic physicians who use multiple therapies simultaneously: that holistic physicians do not follow scientific methods and use double-blind, cross-over studies with single agents at a time. *There is nothing more scientific than asking the patient whether a therapy works or not.* Astute clinicians have no difficulty figuring out what works and what doesn't. This is an essential issue and I discuss it at length in the chapter

Intravenous Nutrient Protocols.

## HERBAL REMEDIES FOR CHRONIC FATIGUE

I use herbal products liberally to restore altered states of bowel ecology (that almost always exist in chronic fatigue states) and to reduce detoxification overload in the liver. I give details of such therapies in the chapters Oral Nutrient Protocols and Battered Bowel Ecology.

## DRUGS FOR CHRONIC FATIGUE

The use of drugs sometimes becomes necessary for relief of a host of troublesome symptoms associated with chronic fatigue states. *Drugs, however, cannot revive injured energy enzymes — the root cause of chronic fatigue.*

Natural nutrients and herbs, in general, are not as potent as synthetic agents. Still, physicians who have never used natural therapies such as those described in this book are in for a pleasant surprise: Drug use can frequently be avoided altogether with nondrug therapies, and, when deemed necessary, drugs can be used in substantially lower doses when combined with natural therapies than would be case if drugs were to be used without nutrients and herbs.

I strongly oppose the use of drugs that are often

promoted to "treat" chronic fatigue. I rank antiviral drugs high among the drugs that carry serious potential for long-term injury to the energy mechanisms of the body, even though they may offer temporary benefits. Antiviral drugs essentially work by interfering with the synthesis of viral DNA or RNA. We must recognize that drugs that interfere with viral DNA and RNA eventually *will* interfere with the synthesis of human DNA and RNA.

A case can be made for short-term use of antiviral drugs in patients with severe fatigue and evidence of active replication of viruses in their bodies. My friend, Dr. Robert Bradford of San Diego, has reported good results with deoxychlor infusions in such cases. Deoxychlor has not been available to me, and I have not been able to evaluate its efficacy. Notwithstanding such reports, it is essential to regard short-term use of agents such as deoxychlor or live cell therapies as temporary measures in a global plan for restoration of damaged energy enzymes.

Several of my patients went to Mexican clinics that offer a variety of international therapies not permitted in the United States. They report some good initial results. Long-term results of such therapies are invariably poor unless they can be followed with holistic and integrated programs that address all the essential issues.

I strongly urge chronic fatigue sufferers to shun drug research trials that offer free treatment in chronic fatigue clinics at our medical schools and that are funded by the pharmaceutical companies. Such drug trials often lead to the publications of "landmark" papers and prestige for the fatigue "researchers" but leave the targets of their research — the fatigue sufferer — weaker, sicker and dispirited when the researchers are through with them.

## AFTERMATH OF DRUG RESEARCH

Fatigue drug researchers know little, if anything, about the aftermath of their studies. (When was the last time you read about a research study of people damaged during drug trails years after the researchers were through with their human subjects?) My clinical files contain a large number of charts of chronic fatigue sufferers who were the targets of drug research before they understood the real long-term dangers.

No research studies are ever done to document the slow, insidious enzyme injury — the type suffered by Mr. Latimer — years after the drug research is over. Why would any drug company throw good money after the bad? When astute clinical ecologists do recognize patterns of slow, insidious injury to energy and detoxification enzymes by drugs, the drug dollars fly disease doctors of $N^2D^2$ medicine all over the country to proclaim ecologists quacks. Many of them bring charges against ecologists before the state licensing boards.

## MENSTRUAL IRREGULAITIES, HAIR LOSS AND IMPOTENCE

The uterus often serves female chronic fatigue sufferers as the spokes-organ for other body organs — and their femininity. Thus, menstrual irregularities almost always develop, with infrequent or short periods being the common symptom. Not infrequently, such symptoms lead to total loss of menstruation. Another symptom that often troubles female chronic fatiguers is excessive loss of hair. All I need to do for these symptoms is to reassure the patient. Menstruation normalizes and hair return with successful revival of energy enzymes without exceptions.

Male chronic fatiguers often develop loss of sexual drive that sometimes leads to impotence. Again, normal sex drive is restored with successful management in most cases and no special therapies are necessary. Infrequently, injections of prostaglandin into the penile tissues are advisable to normalize the circulatory patterns. I obtain excellent results with two to four monthly injections of 60 mcg of prostaglandin in one ml of diluent.

***********

G<sub>od</sub> and Y<sub>ou</sub> are the subjects closest to my heart when it comes to caring for people paralyzed with devastating fatigue that persists for long periods of time even with the best possible management. I return to this subject in the chapter Hope, Spirituality and Chronic Fatigue.

## RETURNING TO WORK

Whether the person is a teenager returning to school after an absence of some months or a young man going back to his work in a T.V. production, there is a clear risk for overshooting the physical limits. As much as I try to caution chronic fatiguers against ambitious undertakings soon after returning to their vocations, I continue to see early relapses. A teenager may find the discipline of limiting classes to two to four hours a day initially difficult, and so may an adult as he begins to recapture his lost energy patterns. The main reason for this is the inability of the chronic fatigue sufferer to correctly estimate his reserve for energy and work. It is hard to know the mind of regenerating enzymes.

A second point worth making in closing this chapter is the need for chronic fatigue sufferers to continue the restorative programs well past the time of their near-complete recovery. Oxidative simmering coals have a way of rekindling themselves into open blazes.

*I slept and dreamt that life was joy.*
*I awoke and saw that life was service.*
*I acted and behold! Service was joy.*

Tagore

The most pleasant task I perform in my clinical work with chronic fatigue sufferers is to sign the physician's note for them to return to school or work. It is at such times that I see coming alive all the abstract theories of oxidatively injured enzymes, vague concepts of battered bowel ecology, the images of sugar-insulin-adrenaline roller coasters, inconspicuous food sensitivities, and the exhortations of persistent restorative work, and the language of silence and hope during long months when nothing seems to work.

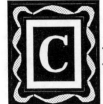 **Chapter 7**

# Choices
# In The
# Kitchen

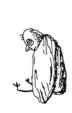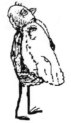

I establish five principles and make 18 practical recommendations at the outset regarding the subject of food choices:

## *First,*

I consider optimal choices in the kitchen the first and foremost strategy for initial stabilization of individuals who suffer from severe chronic fatigue and chemical sensitivity. Such persons often tolerate poorly nondrug therapies during the early periods of treatment.

## *Second,*

I consider optimal choices in the kitchen the first and foremost priority for preventing recurrence of chronic fatigue after initial recovery.

## *Third,*

from a global clinical standpoint, I divide foods into two broad groups for chronic fatiguers: high-compatibility foods, which sustain energy enzymes and low-compatibility foods, which deplete energy enzymes. Later in this chapter, I give my criteria for dividing foods into these two categories and include food lists.

## *Fourth,*

martyrdom in the kitchen is not the way to success. Nor is it necessary for chronic fatiguers to forever play a skunk at other people's garden parties. What is required for long-term success is a visceral-intuitive change that makes the things we *need* to eat the same as what we *like* to eat. This may appear to be wishful thinking to chronic fatiguers with multiple food sensitivities, but I see this in my clinical practice every working day.

After an initial period of recovery from severe fatigue, most chronic fatiguers can eat almost all foods on special occasions — such as family dinners or business meetings — as long as they primarily eat high-compatibility foods at home most of the time. Absolute abstinence from low-compatibility foods is neither feasible nor necessary.

## *Fifth,*

food sensitivities, abnormal bowel responses to foods, sugar-insulin-adrenaline roller coasters, acidotic stressors, sugar and salt cravings, and battered bowel ecosystems are essential issues. These issues are best addressed through a philosophy of nutrition — an abiding respect for the way foods affect the human condition — rather than through narrow-focused dieting plans.

## HIGH-COMPATIBILITY AND LOW-COMPATIBILITY FOODS

The concept of dividing foods into high-compatibility and low-compatibility foods evolved slowly in my mind as I closely studied the effects of food choices on the clinical status of chronic fatiguers. I use these two terms to consider the issue of compatibility of foods with an individual's energy patterns. The prevailing notions of a balanced diet are utterly irrelevant to the problems of chronic fatiguers. Furthermore, the traditional ideas of food allergy are inadequate for such persons.

## FIVE ESSENTIAL CRITERIA FOR HIGH- AND LOW-COMPATIBILITY FOODS

### *First,*

high-compatibility foods must not trigger allergic reactions. Evidently, foods that trigger the classical allergic reactions mediated by IgE type of antibodies and other incompatibility reactions caused by other mechanisms increase oxidant stress. Abnormal bowel responses caused by digestive-absorptive problems also add to such burdens. Food incompatibility is a paradox: It is a complex subject full of inconsistencies for physicians who lack training necessary for the diagnosis and management of food allergy, yet it is a patently simple matter for physicians who make the effort necessary to become familiar with the diversity of clinical symptoms caused by it. There are no perfect laboratory tests for the diagnosis of food sensitivity. Clinically useful information, however, can be obtained with electrodermal conductance, micro-elisa blood assays for IgE antibodies and diagnostic skin tests.

### *Second,*

high-compatibility foods must be able to prevent or suppress molecular roller coasters that generate bursts of oxyradicals, rapid acidotic shifts, sharp hypoglycemic-hyperglycemic shifts, quick releases of catecholamine surges (adrenaline and its cousin molecules), large cholinergic pulses, and sudden fluctuations in neurotransmitter levels.

## *Third,*

high-compatibility foods must fully support the normal bowel ecosystem. These foods must facilitate the digestive and absorptive processes in the bowel, not interfere with the normal motility (transit time) and blood supply of the bowel, sustain the normal bowel flora, and prevent parasitic infestation of the bowel.

## *Fourth,*

high-compatibility foods must provide for enjoyable meals and satiety.

## *Fifth,*

high-compatibility foods must provide all the essential nutrients as well as the total caloric requirements.

> *I advise my chronic fatigue patients to eat only high-compatibility foods for six to eight weeks, depending on the severity of symptoms and response to changes in food choices. Additionally, I ask them to refrain from eating any meat during this period. After that, I allow one selection from the low-compatibility foods one day a week.*

To help my patients make the right choices, I organize high- and low-compatibility fluids and foods in separate columns in tables devoted to different food types. These tables appear after the following 18 practical suggestions.

## NINETEENS PRACTICAL FOOD-CHOICE GUIDELINES FOR CHRONIC FATIGUERS

The 19 recommendations that I make to my human canaries are discussed at length in *The Canary and Chronic Fatigue.* I cannot overstate the case for a sound philosophy of nutrition. Martyrdom in food choices does not work. Good nutrition is neither denial of dieting nor euphoria of eating. One cannot eat well for a full life span except through a deep visceral-intuitive sense about how various foods affect his general level of energy and well-bing. This cannot come from cortical obsessions about studying foods charts and calorie tables.

1.  Seek steady-state energy metabolism.

Avoid starving-gorging-starving cycles.
Avoid sugar-insulin-adrenaline roller coasters

2. Maintain an optimal state of hydration.
Drink 50 to 70 ounces of high-compatibility fluids
every day.
Drink fluids even when you are not thirsty.

3. Know your food reactivities.
Avoid foods that cause allergic reactions.
Avoid foods that deplete energy.
Avoid foods that cause abnormal bowel
responses.

5. Focus on what you can eat
De-focus foods that should be avoided.
Try new foods, observe their effects.
Think high-compatibility foods when food-
shopping.

6. Never miss breakfast.
Body tissues need to be energized in the morning.
Missing breakfast is fasting for 15 to 18 hours and
sets us up for nutritional roller coasters.
Missing breakfast increases the need for
undesirable stimulants such as coffee and tea.

7. Get the most out of vegetables.
Develop a taste for uncooked vegetables. (Taste
is changeable.)
Develop a taste for steamed or stir-fried
vegetables.
Reduce acidotic stress on metabolism. (Vegetables

are alkaline-ash foods.)

8.  Cut back on fruits.
    Avoid allergenic fruits such as oranges.
    Avoid very sweet fruits.
    Avoid overripe fruits.

9.  Increase proteins in food choices.
    Proteins are time-release energy sources.
    Proteins are building blocks for tissues and for
    energy and detoxification enzymes.
    Minimize meat intake; increase lentils and beans.

10. Favor alkaline-ash foods.
    Favor vegetables on the top of the vegetable table
    (Chronic fatigue states are states of acidotic
    overload. All biologic stressors increase acidotic
    stress. SAD [standard American diet] increases
    the body acid burden.)

11. Minimize acid-ash foods.
    Reduce intake of all meats.
    (Grains are, in general, acid-ash foods, but are
    needed to balance the alkalinity of vegetables and
    fruits.)

12. Understand food cravings.
    Food craving is the other side of the coin of
        food addiction.
    Reduce salt intake.
    Reduce sugar intake.
    Reduce intake of artificial sweeteners.
    (Salt, sugar and sweeteners increase sugar

cravings.)

13. Have free access to ideal snacks.
    The ideal snacks: uncooked or steamed vegetables.
    Eat low-fructose fruits — those that are not very sweet.
    Soynuts, pumpkin, sunflower and other seeds are also recommended.
    Avoid walnuts and other tree nuts. (Tree nuts are among the most allergenic foods.)

14. Rotate foods.
    High-compatibility foods may be eaten on three or less days a week.
    Low-compatibility foods should not be eaten more often than once a week.

15. Ensure a healthy gut ecosystem.
    Seed the bowel with healthful lactic-acid-producing microbes.
    Feed the lactic-acid producers with nutrients such as pantothenic acid, vitamin $B_{12}$, fructose oligosaccharides and others.
    Weed out the toxin-producing microbes such as yeasts, bacteria and parasites. (See the chapter Battered Bowel Ecology.)

16. Eat limbically.
    Follow visceral-intuitive impulses.
    With time, one *likes* to eat what one *needs* to eat.
    Dieting plans are cortical traps.
    (Reading food labels becomes unnecessary after

some time.)

17.  Do not omit nutrient supplements.
         Take morning supplements with breakfast.
         Take evening supplements with dinner.
         Split daily supplements into three, four or more
             portions if problems of tolerance exist.
         (Pollutants in the air can only be neutralized by
             nutrients.
         Contaminants in food can only be neutralized by
             nutrients.
         Toxins in water can only be neutralized by
             nutrients.)

18.  Don't be a skunk in someone's garden party.
         It is not necessary.
         It is not desirable.
         Enzyme detoxification systems can cope with an
             occasional workout —but only occasionally.

19.  Bring some spiritual dimensions to your day.
         (Martyrdom doesn't work in nutrition. Good
         nutrition is neither denial of dieting nor euphoria
         of eating.)

| High-Compatibility Fluids | Low-Compatibility Fluids |
|---|---|
| Well water | Cow's milk |
| Spring water | Milk shakes |
| Ginger root water | Malt drinks |
| Vegetable juices | Coffee |
| Bancha and mu teas | Black (common) tea |
| Grain coffees | Regular cola drinks |
| Seltzer | Orange juice |
| Bottled waters | Sweetened fruit juices |
| Herbal teas | Alcohol |

The ideal drinking water is a fresh, natural, non-chlorinated spring or deep well water obtained from natural, noncommercial sources. (Problem: Where are we to find such water?) Bottled spring waters generally go through a packaging process: Some are good; others are not.

Ginger root water: This is the cheapest and best water. Boil one and a half inches of fresh ginger root with one gallon of water, let it cool, transfer it into a glass bottle discarding the last one inch of water, and refrigerate. Ginger alkaloids bind to water pollutants and precipitate them.

Lemon and lime water, taken hot as substitutes for other hot morning drinks and cold in the evening as substitutes for other cold drinks, is strongly recommended. However, I do not recommend that such waters should be taken every single day of the week — persons with allergy become allergic to the things to which they are most often exposed.

Herbal teas should be rotated as beverages as well as for their healthful effects. These teas are not recommended as treatment of specific active diseases except under the direct supervision of a physician.

Diet drinks that contain aspartame (NutraSweet) are acceptable on occasions, except for people with aspartame sensitivity (molecular individuality).

Grain teas (barley, brown rice, millet, corn-silk) are neutral-to-alkaline, caffeine-free life span teas. These teas restore gastric and bowel ecology, and have several known mild medicinal effects. Mu tea is a popular blend that contains ginseng and several other herbs. It is an alkaline, caffeine-free life span tea.

Bancha tea is highly recommended as a substitute for morning coffee and tea until such time that substitutes are not necessary. Bancha tea is alkaline and nearly caffeine-free. It protects the stomach lining from acidotic stress, preserves normal gastric ecology, promotes digestion, and hence is a life span tea. Common coffee (from coffee beans) is acidic and caffeine-rich (up to 80 mg of caffeine per cup). Decaffeinated coffee has much lower levels of caffeine (3-10 mg per cup) but is acidic and often contains residual methylene chloride and ethyl acetate, chemicals that many companies use to decaffeinate their coffee. Black tea (common tea) is an aging-oxidant tea. It is acidic, caffeine-rich and favors the aging-oxidant molecules. It decreases tissue levels of some life span enzymes such as transketolase, lactic dehydrogenase and thiamin diphosphatase. Green tea is milder than black tea, but is acidic, favors aging-oxidant molecules, and hence is an aging-oxidant tea.

As for the low-compatibility fluids, it is desirable to avoid them altogether except for special occasions.

A large glass of orange juice may contain as many as 6-8 teaspoons of fructose which causes a sugar overload even though it is metabolized somewhat slower than glucose.

Regular colas and other sodas should be avoided. (A can of coke may contain as much as 6-8 teaspoons of sugar.)

Alcohol is an aging-oxidant drink. However, when taken in modest amounts on special family and other occasions, it has some redeeming desirable effects on mood.

## HERBAL TEAS

Specific individual herbal teas listed below have several established biochemical medicinal effects and their regular use for specific health disorders should be physician-supervised.

Chamomile flower: Egyptians used it to slow the aging process.
Golden seal root: general life span tea. Biblical Rx, American Indian Rx.
Echinacea root: general life span tea.

Astragalus: general life span.
Linden flower: general life span tea.
Ginseng root: general life span tea.
Pau D'Arco inner bark: for altered bowel ecology states.
Flax seeds tea: for lung and bowel ecology.
Caraway seeds: for stomach and bowel ecology.
Thyme leaves: for stomach and bowel ecology.
Cascara sagrada: for bowel ecology.
Peppermint: for stomach ecology.
Alfalfa leaves and seeds: for stomach ecology.
Clover blossoms: for liver disorders.
Juniper berry: for bladder ecology.
Horsetail: for hair, skin and nail ecology.
Valerian root: for nervous system disorders (Latin *valere*=well-being).
Huckleberry: for hypoglycemia and hyperglycemia.
Hawthorn flower and berries: for hypertension and heart disease.
Rose petal tea: for eyestrain.
Black oats (with whiskers) tea: for anxiety.
Marigold petal tea: for anxiety.
Sage tea: for flu-like symptoms.
Ginger root: gastric and bowel ecology; for motion sickness.
Feverfew leaves: for chronic headache (also freeze dried in tablets).
Aloe vera gel: for bowel ecology. Taken as syrup or gel.

Herbal teas are excellent choices but must be taken in rotation and under the supervision of a knowledgeable professional. One or two teaspoons of food-grade glycerine may be added to herbal teas as a sweetener. Alcohol in small amounts has some good physiological effects and other positive effects on mood and spirits. These effects, as I wrote earlier, may indeed counterbalance the essential aging-oxidant effects of alcohol. Thus, complete abstinence, except in the case of persons with past or present dependence on it, is not necessary.

The bowel ecosystem is delicate and easily damaged by antibiotics, drugs, toxic foods, environmental pollutants and stress. Damaged bowel ecosystems can only be restored with nutrient and herbal therapies — and, categorically and unequivocally, not with any drugs. I discuss gut ecosystem at length in the companion volume *Battered Bowel Ecology — Waving Away a Wandering Wolf.*

## VEGETABLE JUICES

I cannot overstate the case for investing in a juicer for chronic fatiguers. Also, I cannot overstate the case for investing a few minutes in preparing fresh vegetable juice. Chlorophyll is what turns solar energy into chemical energy for the food chain in nature. Vegetables are the best sources of chlorophyll. Vegetables are the best source of minerals. And, of course, fresh vegetables are the best source of life span enzymes. Fresh vegetable juices are most desirable. Preferred choices of vegetables are given in the vegetable table. Carrot juice is very rich in its sugar content. The best vegetable juices are fresh unsalted juices. Cans of most commercially available vegetable juices contain as much as 500-600 mg of sodium (a "life span mineral" turned into an "aging-oxidant mineral" by the American food industry). Unsalted canned vegetable juices are acceptable compromises when circumstances do not allow fresh juices.

It is advisable that fresh vegetable juice be prepared with two or three vegetables at a time to improve the taste and enhance the nutritional value of the juice. Furthermore, vegetables for this purpose should be chosen in rotation from a long list that follows. A common mistake in this context is to use carrots for preparing the juice every single time. A patient once told me she notices slight yellow tinge to her skin and eyes, and consulted her doctor who ordered tests for jaundice. All tests were negative. She found out much later that her slight skin discoloration was due to carrot juice that she drank twice a day for six consecutive months. Her case of "carrot jaundice" was cured when she eliminated carrots from her juices altogether for two months.

| VEGETABLES OF SPECIAL VALUE | |
| --- | --- |
| Ginger | Broccoli |
| Garlic | Mushrooms |
| Burdock | Chinese cabbage |
| Radish | Brussels sprouts |
| Turnips | Cauliflower |
| Daikon | Lettuce substitutes* |
| Squashes** | Others*** |
| SEA AND WILD VEGETABLES | |
| Kombu | Wild burdock |
| Nori | Dandelion |
| Dulse | Lamb's Quarters |
| Wakame | Mugwort |
| Hiziki | Milkweed |
| Mekabu | Ferns |

\* Lettuce substitutes: green tops of beets, carrot, collard, daikon, kale, mustard, red radish, spinach and turnip.

\*\* Squashes: acorn, buttercup, butternut, hokaido, hubbard, spaghetti, star, yellow summer, zucchini.

\*\*\* Artichoke, asparagus, beets, Brussels sprouts, broccoli, bok choy, cabbage, cauliflower, celery, cucumber, escarole, garlic, ginger, parsnip, peas, plantain, rutabagas, sauerkraut, scallions, shiitake mushrooms, water chestnuts.

Lettuce is in the same family as ragweed, which is among the most allergenic weeds in the United States. There is a high degree of cross reactivity between lettuce and ragweed. For this reason I recommend that people with food and hay-fever type allergy cut down on lettuce and use lettuce substitutes given above.

## SNACKS

In general, snacks are best avoided. The best strategy for the life span is to eat regular meals at regular times. It is ironic that we offer children snacks for the slimmest of excuses while we adults struggle so hard to unlearn this awful habit. For chronic fatiguers, however, high-compatibility snacks sometimes serve as therapeutic items for the management of troublesome sugar-insulin-adrenaline roller coasters.

| High-Compatibility Snacks | Low-Compatibility Snacks |
|---|---|
| Fresh vegetables | Cookies, candy, chocolate |
| Stir-fried and steamed vegetables | Cakes, creams |
| Soynuts | Pies and other desserts |
| Sprouted grains | Doughnuts |
| Fruits with low fructose | Peanuts |
| Pumpkin seeds | Popcorn |
| Sunflower seeds | Fruits rich in fructose |
| Puffed millet | Walnuts and other tree nuts |
| Puffed amaranth | Dried fruits rich in fructose |

| High-Compatibility Fats | Low-Compatibility Fats |
|---|---|
| Ghee* | Margarine |
| Olive oil, cold pressed | "Cholesterol-free" foods |
| Avocado oil, cold pressed | Animal shortening |
| Flaxseed, cold pressed | Vegetable shortening |
| Sesame oil | Corn, palm and peanut oil |
| Evening primrose and borage oils | Fats used for deep-frying foods |

*Ghee (clarified butter) can be prepared by gently warming the butter and skimming off and discarding the top layer of "white fat" rich in saturated and polyunsaturated fats and milk proteins; the latter seems to improve the tolerance of ghee for many individuals who are sensitive to milk proteins.

Flaxseed oil is an excellent source of omega-3 and omega-6 oils. Cold pressed flaxseed oil should be purchased in dark bottles and should be kept refrigerated with the cap tightly closed. Three 200 iu capsules of vitamin E added to the bottle of flaxseed oil are very effective in preventing undesirable oxidation of flaxseed oil.

Margarine contains up to 35% trans fatty acids that cannot be utilized by human tissues. Trans fatty acids raise the blood levels of LDL ("bad") cholesterol and lower blood levels of HDL ("good") cholesterol.

Cholesterol-free fats are rendered "cholesterol-free" through chemical processes that introduce trans fatty acids and toxic cyclic compounds into these fats. Trans fatty acids and toxic cyclic fatty compounds cannot be metabolized by the body and, quite literally, clog up the molecular wheels of fat metabolism in the body. The immune system resents this onslaught of toxic molecules and mounts an immune response by making antibodies specifically directed against these toxic compounds. These antibodies try to capture these toxic compounds by making complexes with them and clear them, but have a limited capacity to do this. With passing years, denatured and toxic fats in supermarket foods prove to be too large a burden for the immune system to bear. I discuss this important subject in depth in *Choua, Cholesterol Cats and Chelation*.

| High-Compatibility Proteins | Low-Compatibility Proteins |
|---|---|
| Lentils | Beef |
| Beans | Veal |
| Hunted fish* | Pork, bacon |
| Proteins drink (sugar-free) | Cultured fish |
| Spirulina plankton | Egg (fried, broken yolks) |
| Venison and game | Salami |
| Duck, pheasant | Hamburgers |
| Goat, buffalo | Frankfurter |
| Chicken, turkey | Deep fried chicken |
| Egg (not fried, unbroken yolks) | Highly salted deli meats |

*Sea bass, red snapper, Atlantic paddock and rock fish are excellent low-fat fish. (A three and half ounce portion of each of sea bass and chinook salmon contains 595 and 1,355 mg of Omega-3; the respective numbers for total fat are 3 and 10 grams.) Other good choices are catfish, cod, grouper, halibut, haddock, herring, mackerel, mahi mahi, and pike. Cultured fish are increasingly raised in fisheries that use large amounts of fungicides and antibiotics to increase the fish yield. Beef and egg rank high among the causes of food allergy.

Beans, such as grains, can be budded (sprouted) to

enhance their nutritional value. Budding increases the vitamin B complex levels by many fold and also has the effect of predigesting these foods. Zuki and Mung beans are especially good for this purpose.

Egg is an excellent source of high-grade proteins and lecithin (the "good" fat that facilitates metabolism of fat and prevents fat buildup in the liver and other body tissues). However, as I indicated earlier, the frequency of egg allergy in the general population is quite high.

We need proteins for amino acids. We need amino acids as building blocks for tissue proteins, hormones and neurotransmitters. As a source of energy, I regard them as "time-release energy molecules." Amino acids are also the premium intelligence molecules of the body. Properly formulated amino acid and peptide products prepared from natural proteins by partial hydrolysis (predigestion) are excellent sources of these nutrients. Many of the name brand protein drinks carry 50% to 90% of their calories as carbohydrates. I do not recommend such products. Good amino acid, peptide and protein formulas should have as much as 90% of their calories calories as these nutrients.

Proteins are composed of amino acids. The life span advantages of amino acids are too numerous to list here. Unlike sugar, amino acids are time-release energy molecules. Sugar is a much bigger culprit than fat in the cause of degenerative and immune disorders. In this context, well-formulated amino acid, peptide (small chains of amino acids) and protein products, when taken with vegetable and fruity juices or with dilute soy or rice milk, make an excellent breakfast. Indeed, my own breakfast three to four days a week is composed of an amino acid and protein formula mixed with one of the above fluids. I do not need any coffee nor tea. It sustains me till my lunch. I use three formulas made from different sources of protein to balance the intake of the various amino acids contained in them. I recommend such well-formulated products to my patients, especially those who suffer from molecular roller coasters or experience rapid hypoglycemic-hyperglycemic shifts. *It is imperative, however, that amino acid, peptide and protein drinks be used under the general supervision of a knowledgeable professional.*

| High-Compatibility Carbohydrates | Low-Compatibility Carbohydrates |
|---|---|
| Wild and brown rice | Wheat |
| Amaranth | Barley |
| Spelt, kamut, teff | Oat |
| Tofu and other soy products | Rye |
| Quinoa, buckwheat | Corn |
| Beans | Potato, yam |
| Millet, artichoke | White rice |
| Seeds | Peanuts and tree nuts |

Gluten-sensitive persons need to avoid or restrict wheat, rye, oat and barley — grains that contain "free gluten"; other grains such as amaranth, buckwheat, quinoa, milo, teff, rice and corn contain small amounts of "bound gluten" that, in general, do not cause food incompatibility reactions in gluten-sensitive persons. Spelt and kamut are two types of ancient wheats that appear to be distinct enough from common wheat to be tolerated well by individuals who suffer from wheat incompatibility. These are usually grown without pesticides. Spelt has a strong hull that protects its kernel. Teff, an Ethiopian staple, is a highly nutritious grain that contains more than 10 times as much calcium as wheat and barley.

Sunflower seeds, sesame seeds, pumpkin seeds, melon seeds, watermelon seeds, soy nuts (actually a grain) are good choices. Almonds, cashew nuts, macadamia nuts, pine nuts, brazil nuts, chestnut, pecans, and litchi nuts should be eaten infrequently. *Peanuts and walnuts are common causes of allergic reactions and should be eaten infrequently.* Malanga, yuca, sesame meal, sunflower meal, breadfruit, lotus root, agar. Beans: black beans, pink beans, white beans, hokaido beans and others.

| High-Compatibility Fruits | Low-Compatibility Fruits |
| --- | --- |
| Organic apples | Orange |
| Berries (except strawberry) | Pineapple |
| Papaya | Coconut |
| Avocado | Strawberries |
| Plums, peaches, persimmon | Banana |
| Lemon and lime (with water) | Very sweet fruit |
| Grapefruit | Polished fruit |
| Fruits with low fructose content | Canned fruit |

The fruits in the low-compatibility category are included there for reasons of their high fructose content, acidity and the potential to cause allergy. Fruits should be eaten fresh in season. Avoid canned fruit completely. Depleted of their life-sustaining enzymes and laced with sugar, canned fruits in reality are canned candy. I refer the reader to *The Butterfly and Life Span Nutrition* for further details.

The issue of pesticide and fungicide residues on fruits and vegetables is important. All fruits and vegetables should be thoroughly washed to eliminate, or at least reduce, such residues. Polished fruits present a more complex problem. Organically grown unpolished apples are among the first choice group for their long-established empirical nutritional value. I list apples treated with pesticides and polished to improve their looks in the low-compatibility group   for equally obvious reasons.

## HIGH-COMPATIBILITY   DESSERTS

The critical issues in desserts for fatiguers are:

* Use of fruit juices versus sugar as sweeteners
* Use of natural food sweeteners such as licorice, carob, cinnamon, molasses, pilon cillo and honey.
* Use of other sweeteners such as food grain glycerine and herbs like Stevia and Tree Sweet.
* Occasional use of artificial sweeteners such as aspartame and saccharine except for people with a chemical sensitivity to these items.

## SUGAR: A NUTRITIONAL VILLAIN

Sugar is an antinutrient, and is a killer molecule for human canaries. I recommend that fatigue patients avoid all sugar items for six to eight weeks initially and whenever fatigue recurs. As a clinical situation improves, I do allow desserts on special occasions. Ideally, all desserts should be prepared with fruit juices or natural sweeteners such as honey and stevia. Fruits contain fructose, which is metabolized at a slower rate than glucose. More importantly, fruit juices are very rich sources of mineral cofactors and some digestive enzymes. Sugar, of course, is totally devoid of any nutritional merit and is one of the principal nutritional villains.

Preparing desserts with natural sweeteners within reason is an acceptable practice for those who can be comfortable with restraints implicit in this practice. Some good choices include rice syrup, maple syrup, persimmon, honey, almond syrup, and carob. For others, such desserts may be combined at times with those prepared with aspartame and saccharine. Similarly, diet sodas with aspartame are allowed within reason.

## FOOD COMPATIBILITY AND ALLERGY

In drug medicine, the subjects of food incompatibility and allergy and abnormal bowel responses to foods are considered subjects for fringe physicians. Scientists in medicine, I often hear, must steer clear of such hucksterism. I sometimes wonder if there is another area in medicine in which more irresponsible statements are made by otherwise responsible physicians. A great enigma for me is this: How can any physician engage in any healing art without making nutrition the centerpiece of his practice? After all, we are made of food, are sustained by food, fall ill when we eat the wrong foods, and die if food is withheld from us.

One man's food is another man's poison, observed Hippocrates almost 2,500 years ago. Hippocrates, it seems, learned his lesson from the Man from the Rift Valley who realized that some foods were healing while others made him sick. We physicians are the intellectual progeny of this Man from Africa, even though many of us are now infatuated with drugs and despise the word empiricism.

What is the most common cause of fatigue after eating? Milk allergy. Is egg an excellent food? Yes. Should everyone eat eggs? No. Egg is a very allergenic food. People with allergic genes are very likely to be allergic to eggs. Which is a better food for some one with allergic nasal and sinus symptoms, wheat or wild rice? Wild rice, because allergy to wild rice is very uncommon while wheat is one of the major allergens.

Dealing with food allergy and abnormal bowel responses is necessary for chronic fatiguers as well as for the professionals who care for them. It is also a subject full of apparent inconsistencies. Food allergy often causes chronic headaches; arthritis; colitis; asthma; disorders of mood, memory and mentation; and hyperactivity in children. In the prevailing mode of drug medicine, these afflictions are usually treated with drugs.

Food allergy as the true cause remains undiagnosed. Clinically useful diagnoses of food sensitivities and adverse bowel responses may be established with electrodermal conductance tests, micro-elisa blood tests or skin tests. None of these tests is perfect. In my view, electrodermal methods in the hands of an experienced professional gives a far superior total profile of food tolerance and intolerance than blood tests. As the benefits of this technology become better known to the physician community, it will likely become widely accepted for this purpose.

## SPECIAL FOODS FOR FATIGUERS

**Broccoli** restores bowel ecology, strengthens the immune system, contains organic sulfur compounds such as indole carbinol (which breaks down estrogen) and beta carotene which is an important antioxidant.

**Burdock** has long established empirical values in improving digestive and absorptive functions in the stomach and bowel. It speeds up the bowel transit time and so facilitates restoration of the bowel ecosystem.

**Celery** contains muscle-friendly phthalate and is helpful in normalizing fat metabolism. Celery is also beneficial for joint symptoms and for related disorders such as bursitis and fibrositis.

**Daikon** has a long-established empirical value in maintaining a healthy bowel ecology.

**Flaxseed** contains linolenic acid, an essential fatty acid that reduces the formation of hormone-like substances called prostaglandins of PG-2 series. These prostaglandins induce inflammatory responses in the lungs (asthma), the joints (arthritis), the skin (psoriasis) and other body organs. Prostaglandins may also contribute to the development of tumors. Flaxseed is a cereal grain that Europeans and Canadians consume in large quantities in their cereals and breads.

**Garlic** contains allicin and some other sulfur compounds that restore bowel ecology, prevent yeast overgrowth, thin blood, and prevents platelet clumping. It appears to act as an anti-inflammatory agent and antibacterial agent, and reduce the risk of cancer.

**Ginger** contains natural alkaloids that precipitate out (and render harmless) most environmental pollutants in drinking water. (See note about ginger root water in the beverage section of this chapter.) It has a long established empirical value in restoring altered bowel ecology. Ginger also reduces inflammation in arthritis.

**Grapefruit** contains pectin, the gelling agent present in the peel and membrane, which lowers cholesterol and facilitates blood flow in arteries. Pectin also appears to prevent blood clotting in arteries.

**Klongi** (onion seeds) are well known in Pakistan as immune-enhancing spices.

**Soybean** is an excellent source of minerals such as magnesium, calcium, molybdenum and others. It is rich in essential life span oils and high-quality proteins. Predigestion of food is an old discovery of man. Perhaps no food had intrigued man in his pursuit of predigested food than has soybean. Tofu, tofu p'i, tofu kan, tempeh, toya, natto and kabitofu are some of the soy-derived staple foods in the Far East. I have observed extraordinary benefits of some positively-charged components of soybean in restoring damaged bowel ecosystems, as I suspect the ancients did when I look at their inventiveness with this grain.

**Squashes** have a long established empirical role in improving digestive and absorptive functions. These vegetables are useful in restoring bowel ecology and decreasing bowel transit time (prevention of constipation and toxic effects of prolonged bowel transit time).

**Turmeric** has been used in Pakistan, India and the Far East since ancient times as a spice that prevents food from spoiling. Curcumin, the major yellow pigment in tumeric and mustard, is an antioxidant and anti-inflammatory agent that has recently been shown to have anti-neoplastic properties.

## WHAT IS A BALANCED DIET?

In the preceding chapter, I write that drug doctors' concepts of a balanced diet are utterly irrelevant to chronic fatiguers. Indeed, dairy products and red meats, two groups among the cherished foods of the enthusiasts of "balanced" diets, are actually among the most reactive foods for human canaries.

I have been a student of human biology for about 35 years and of human nutrition for about 15 years. I must admit I do not know what a balanced diet is. Next time you meet a nutrition expert, ask him what he considers a balanced diet. His answer is likely to be this: It is a diet composed of all four major food groups — of dairy, meat, cereal, and fruits and vegetables; it has 50% to 60% of its calories in carbohydrates, 20% to 25% in proteins, and 20% to 25% in fats; and it contains 60 mg of vitamin C, 1 mg of thiamine and RDA amounts of other vitamins and minerals. If he is very knowledgeable, he might add that the fats should be one part saturated, one part monosaturated, and one part polyunsaturated.

A sad, sad state of affairs. These nutrition experts are blissfully ignorant of almost all critical nutritional issues we face today. They know nothing (or act as if they don't) about the issues of molecular roller coasters caused by supermarket foods, food incompatibilities, abnormal bowel responses to foods, allergy to molds included in food items, toxic fats, denatured proteins, agricultural fumigants that coat our vegetables, pesticides and fungicides that cover our fruits, the toxic heavy metals that poison our foods, environmental pollutants that contaminate our water, and the industrial toxins that poison our air. Our nutrition experts do not seem to understand much about the health consequences of battered bowel ecology and disrupted ecosystems of other body organs.

Here is a simple test to distinguish between the experts of worthless knowledge of nutrition and the practitioners of nutritional medicine: If a physician, a nutritionist, or some other health professional talks about RDA values, you know that he cannot help you much. He is not even close to the real problems in nutrition. Here is a second simple test: Ask the professional if he has ever reversed any chronic diseases with nutritional protocols. If his answer is no, he is obviously not your man.

## LIFE SPAN NUTRITION

*Life span nutrition is a philosophy of food and its relationship to the human condition.*

Life span nutrition means respecting food so it can respect us.

Life span nutrition is not a "diet." It is *knowing* what we eat. It is knowing how food affects us after we eat it — after some minutes, after some hours, after some days, after some months and after some years. It is knowing how the food we eat affects our *life span.*

Life span nutrition is neither euphoria of eating nor denial of dieting.

Life span nutrition is not about martyrdom before we eat or guilt after it. It is not about calorie counting. It is not about dieting. It is not about starving-gorging-starving cycles.

Life span nutrition is not about "low sugar," "high protein," "low fat" or "megavitamin" regimens.

Life span nutrition is not about losing weight, though loss of excess weight occurs as a natural consequence of knowing the relationship between food and life.

Life span nutrition is a lifelong interest. It is about feeling better, looking better, and living better. It is about a slow and sustained change in the way we think about food, feel about it, and are nourished by it.

My philosophy of life span nutrition evolved over several years of clinical work with persons with severe immune and degenerative disorders. It represents a blending of the enormous intuitive wisdom of the ancients in matters of food and my concept that spontaneity of oxidation in nature is the essential cause of the aging process, and by natural extension of pre-mature aging, dis-ease, disease and death. In the preface of this volume, I defined the term life span foods as foods that promote optimal health for the full life span of an individual. I define aging-oxidant foods as foods that cause accelerated (premature) aging.

***********

I close this chapter by reiterating criteria that separate life span from aging-oxidant foods.

* High-compatibility foods are fresh and un-oxidized foods.
* High-compatibility foods are free of toxic residues of chemical food processing.
* High-compatibility foods do not cause adverse reactions. High-compatibility foods do not cause sugar-insulin-adrenaline roller coasters.

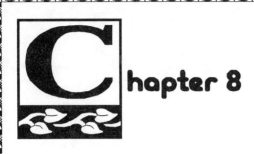

# Chapter 8

# Oral
# Nutrient
# and
# Herbal
# Protocols

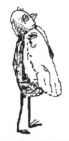

*I do not recommend that chronic fatigue sufferers consider the oral nutrient protocols that I describe in this chapter as recipes for treating chronic fatigue on a self-help basis. Such an approach would be fraught with many dangers. I strongly urge the reader with persistent chronic fatigue to seek out a physician knowledgeable and experienced in the use of nutritional therapies.*

In this chapter, I outline the oral nutrient therapies I use for reviving damaged energy and detoxification enzymes — the fundamental energetic-molecular derangement in chronic fatigue states. It is not my purpose to provide specific treatment measures for individual chronic fatigue sufferers. That must be done by the professional. Rather, my purpose is to give both chronic fatiguers and their physicians some general sense of the various nutrients and the required doses that I have found to be effective for my own patients.

In the chapters What Is Chronic Fatigue? and How Does It All Begin?, I describe at length the molecular events that cause oxidative injury to enzymes. I use oral nutrient protocols to restore damaged enzymes, and not to correct any putative nutrient deficiencies as narrowly defined in the prevailing practice of drug medicine. I address this critical issue in greater detail in the next chapter.

> ## IN BIOLOGY, IF WE CHANGE SOMETHING IN ONE WAY, WE CHANGE EVERYTHING IN SOME WAY

This is a central issue in nutritional medicine. There must be very few, if any, true indications for mononutrient therapies. It is my firm practice never to use *single* agents — any nutrient, any herb or any other natural product — to treat any specific disorder. Indeed, this would violate my core management philosophy of molecular medicine. I do not know of any molecule that functions in a vacuum in the human frame. In the cellular soup of life, every molecule is intricately involved with every other molecule, though such relationships may not always be apparent. The essential clinical implication of holistic molecular relatedness in human biology is this: A broad coverage of vitamin, minerals, and essential amino acids and fatty acids must be assured before prescribing nutrient therapies for specific metabolic roles for individual patients.

> ## GENERAL NUTRIENT SUPPORT

In the general support category, I prescribe the following nutrient protocols in varying combinations for every patient who consults me for chronic fatigue.

1.   Vitamin C protocol

2. TPM protocol (taurine, potassium and magnesium)
3. Antioxidant protocol
4. Antistress protocol
5. Mineral protocol
6. Pantothenic protocol
7. Cal-Mag protocol (calcium and magnesium)
8. Peptide and protein protocols (partially digested protein formula for amino acid support)
9. Bowel and gastric ecology protocols
10. Oxidative liver stress protocols

I give the formulations and the dose schedule for the above nutrient protocols later in this chapter. Some other protocols that I frequently use for chronic fatigue sufferers include neurotransmitter protocol, taurine protocol, omega-3 and omega-6 protocols, allergy protocol, fatigue-stress protocol and OMS (oxidative molecular stress) protocol. I prescribe these protocols on an empirical clinical basis, according to the individual needs of the patient.

Initially, I prescribe my nutrient protocols for a period of three months. During the follow-up visits, I specifically ask the patient to guide me. (In the prevailing drug medicine, we are cautioned not to let the patient influence our judgment as to the choice of drugs and drug dosage. In nutritional medicine, the rules are different. We *want* to be guided by the patient.)

*No two chronic fatigue sufferers are exactly the same; hence, nutrient prescriptions for no two patients can be exactly the same.*

The  content,  quality,  absorption  characteristics  and
bioavailability of nutrients  are critically important  in nutritional
medicine.  My studies  have revealed  wide — and  frightening —
disparities  between  what is on  the label  and  what is inside  the
nutrient  package.  It is the  physician's  responsibility  to monitor
the consistency  and characteristics  of the nutrient protocols that
he uses  on an ongoing  basis.

Several  years  ago,  a patient  brought  me  a tablet  of one
of my protocols  that she had  passed  in her stool.  In response,
I  asked  the  president  of  the  company  that  prepares  my
formulations  to join me  for lunch  and discussed  the matter  with
him  in  great  detail.  He  assured  me  he  would  personally
investigate  the incident  and report  back.  Of course,  I didn't stop
there.  I asked  my staff to specifically  ask every patient  if he had
ever encountered  the same situation.  We found three  other  such
incidents.  Next,  I carefully  studied  the  charts  of these  four
patients.  My finding:  All four patients  suffered  from  serious,
persistent  types  of colitis.  My conclusion:  The nutrient  tablets
that emerged  with stools  more  or less unchanged  were telling
me something  important  about  the patient's  bowel ecology, and
not about  the tablet dissolution  characteristics.  I might add here
that  I  do  not  allow  any  additions  to  the  nutrient  protocols;
hence,  they have their natural  aromas.  I do not recommend  the
glassy, polished  vitamin pills that may be aesthetically  pleasing
but often  carry  unwanted  contaminants.

## SLOW  AND  SUSTAINED  NUTRIENT  BUILDUP

It  is  not  uncommon  for  chronic  fatiguers  to  tolerate nutrients poorly in the initial stages of their management with nondrug therapies. These are almost always temporary problems that can be effectively managed with an incremental supplementation approach: Nutrients are prescribed in gradually increasing numbers and doses. It is my usual approach to begin with only two nutrient protocols that are least likely to provoke any reactions, and then add one or two protocols at one- or two-day intervals until all prescribed nutrient protocols can be tolerated without difficulty. This step-wise approach has three clear advantages:

## *First,*

it allows a slow and steady buildup of nutrients and prevents shocking the enzyme pathways that can occur with a rapid buildup.

## *Second,*

it significantly reduces the incidence of temporary abdominal symptoms that such therapies can produce.

## *Third,*

it identifies any nutrient protocols that may cause untoward responses, thus permitting necessary changes in nutrient selection in order to eliminate or minimize such responses.

## MANAGEMENT OF UNWANTED RESPONSES

Nutrient therapies as outlined here are remarkably safe therapies. To date, I have not encountered any serious side effects of such therapies. Patients with severe fatigue and chemical sensitivities commonly react to nutrients when administered intravenously, but rarely do so when nutrients are taken orally. The symptoms sometimes caused by oral nutrients include abdominal bloating (sometimes with cramps), loose, frequent bowel movements and diarrhea.

When nutrient formulations are prepared without the commonly used binders, excipients and asthetic coating materials, sensitivity reactions to nutrient formulations are extremely rare — probably occurring in fewer than one patient in a hundred. Some of my patients were convinced that they developed skin reactions — such as rashes or dryness in response to specific protocols — mostly an antistress formulation that contains vitamin B complex members. Almost always, such individuals were able to tolerate the incriminated protocol when their general condition was stabilized with self-regulation, optimal food choices and management of allergy. It has been my strong sense that their symptoms were caused by a multitude of factors rather than by the nutrient protocol in question, although the protocol may have contributed to the problem initially.

The nutrient protocols that contain magnesium and vitamin C, as well as the bowel ecology protocols, have been commonly linked to bowel discomfort such as flatulence, abdominal bloating, cramps and excessive mucus. Unfortunately, this represents a catch-22 situation as these are the protocols most needed. I simply advise the patient to reduce by 50% all protocols in these categories for two weeks and then slowly build up to the prescribed dose schedule. Sometimes I recommend that the dose be further reduced — to 25% of the original dose. On rare occasions, I discontinue all such protocols for two to three weeks and then start all over again. With such a flexible approach, *all chronic fatiguers can eventually tolerate nutrient protocols.* When my patients recover their normal energy patterns — or nearly so — I do reduce the total number of nutrient protocols I prescribe for them. The maintenance doses, in general, represent 50% to 75% of the starting doses.

## WHEN SHOULD NUTRIENTS BE DISCONTINUED?

When should a person stop breathing? This is the question I often pose when chronic fatiguers ask me about discontinuing nutrient supplements. I am only half joking in my response. The oxidizing capacity of planet Earth is rapidly rising. Human antioxidant defenses are under an unrelenting siege. Almost every advance in technology is increasing oxidant stress on human biology. The few exceptions are the technologies for restoring the geographic ecosystems that surround us and the ecosystems within our body organs. Drugs, while they can play powerful indirect antioxidant roles in acute, life-threatening disorders, are not indicated within a long-term, life span perspective. How can one provide an antioxidant counterbalance to the oxidant avalanches we face every day? By self-regulation, optimal choices in the kitchen, nongoal-oriented exercise and antioxidant nutrients.

## STATE OF OPTIMAL HYDRATION

My patients frequently complain in the initial stages of nutrient therapies that they must drink large quantities of fluids to take their nutrient supplements. I tell them that is good news. Nutrient protocols force them to increase their water intake. So much the better!

The simplest and most effective practical measure for reducing the excessive acidotic — and oxidative — stress on biology in chronic fatigue is to dilute and eliminate the acidotic — and oxidative — molecules with increased fluid intake. Parenthetically, one of the fundamental changes of the general aging process is cellular aging. Aged cells are shrunken and dehydrated. Chronic fatigue is clearly a state of accelerated molecular and cellular aging. A state of overhydration is not only desirable but necessary.

One-third of kidney diseases in the United States are considered to be iatrogenic — caused by prescription drugs. Three major culprits are nonsteroidal anti-inflammatory pain-killers, antibiotics such as aminoglycosides and contrast media used for X-ray and scan studies. The simplest safeguard against such kidney damage when taking drugs is optimal hydration.

I recommend a glass (six ounces) of suitable fluid every three hours. Frequent trips to the bathroom are a very small price to pay for up-regulated energy enzymes. I include some useful information about fluid selection in the section dealing with life span and aging-oxidant fluids in the chapter Food Choices for Chronic Fatigue.

## COMPOSITION OF NUTRIENT PROTOCOLS

Following are the composition and dose schedules of nutrient protocols I use in my practice. I discuss, in considerable detail, the life span functions of vitamin C, magnesium and taurine — three nutrients that stand out in their metabolic roles in *The Butterfly and Life Span Nutrition.* I recommend that volume to the reader for that discussion as well as for many other essential nutritional issues relevant to chronic fatigue.

| VITAMIN C PROTOCOL | |
|---|---|
| Vitamin C (niascorbate) | 750 mg |
| Vitamin C (calcium ascorbate) | 250 mg |
| Bioflavinoids (citrus) | 50 mg |

Vitamin C is the premium life span molecule in my view. First, it is the *principal* aqueous-phase (water-soluble) antioxidant in human redox (oxidative-reductive) dynamics. Second, it is a small molecule that is handled well by redox pathways — this vitamin is, in reality, a close cousin molecule of glucose. Animals turn glucose into vitamin C with an enzyme called gulunolactone oxidase. Goats make 13 grams of vitamin C every day for their antioxidant defenses — humans cannot make any because they lost their enzyme a long time ago (due to oxidative injury to the gene that encodes for it — I venture a guess, though I have no proof.) Vitamin C plays both sides of the field: In the rare instances where the oxidative arm of redox is weakened, it reverses its role and turns into an oxidant molecule. It is a weak chelating agent and helps lower the body burden of toxic metals. It speeds up the bowel transit time and so facilitates elimination of toxins in human waste. I am not aware of any long-term toxic effects of this vitamin, even though practitioners of drug medicine who do not use it are deathly afraid of it. (Why? Perhaps because the benefits of vitamins tarnish our wonder drugs.) Finally — and fortunately for us in molecular medicine — it is fairly inexpensive. I suggest that the reader be careful about commercial vitamin C products that sell for 99¢ a bottle and clearly are of low quality.

The subject of vitamin C is very close to my heart, and I devote a large part of the companion volume *RDA: Rats, Drugs and Assumptions* to it.

**Dose Schedule:** The usual starting dose I recommend for adult chronic fatigue sufferers is six to eight grams of vitamin C. For brief periods of time, I encourage some of my patients to take larger amounts until they have three to four loose bowel movements a day. Uncommonly, I use this vitamin for what I call C-Catharsis — using 15 or more grams of it to induce a state of watery diarrhea. Once I have achieved good clinical results in terms of restoring normal energy pathways, I usually drop the dose to four to six grams — a dose that I myself take for long-term health preservation.

| TPM PROTOCOL | |
|---|---|
| Magnesium (carbonate, sulfate | 150 mg |
| Potassium (citrate) | 50 mg |
| Taurine | 250 mg |

TPM is one of my key nutrient protocols for chronic fatiguers.

I discuss at length the occurrence and consequences of cell membrane injury caused by accelerated oxidative molecular stress in the chapters What Is Chronic Fatigue? and How Does It Begin?. Indeed, my core clinical strategy for reversing such injury and preventing further damage is based upon my focus on oxidant cell membrane injury. Oxidant injury pokes holes in the cell membrane — and for that matter, in the plasma membranes of cellular organelles — and causes "leaky cell membrane syndrome." (I coin this term to humor my colleagues who thrive on inventing lamppost labels.) The SAD (standard American diet) is in a sad state indeed. It makes us potassium-poor, magnesium-deficient and taurine-depleted.

Taurine — an antioxidant amino acid, and my favorite — is present in all cells, and has been ascribed many protective roles in brain, heart and kidney cells. On one of the walls of my office, I have hung a large, complex chart that shows innumerable metabolic pathways and interrelationships among various amino acids with uni-directional, bi-directional and multi-directional arrows. Sometime ago, my eyes wandered around over that chart before settling on taurine. I noticed something that I never had before: The taurine box showed arrows coming in from different directions — cysteine, cysteic acid and hypotaurine — but no arrow going out. Why would that be? I wondered. Why would nature design those pathways like that if not to ensure that other amino acids were to be used to produce taurine but taurine was to be reserved for some higher function?

In *The Butterfly and Life Span Nutrition,* I discuss at length the many essential roles of magnesium in enzymatic functions involved in the human energy pathways as well as in the metabolism of carbohydrates, proteins and fats. Potassium is the principal intracellular ion (electrically charged atom) and is intricately involved in the maintenance of the electro-magnetic charge (negative potential) at the cell membrane surface. When the cell is oxidatively damaged, potassium leaks out and sodium floods the cell innards. The cell vigorously defends such loss of potassium by pumping up the activity of $Na^+K^+$ ATPase — the enzyme that brings potassium back into the cell and expels unwanted sodium. The cell membrane, however, has a limit to its capacity for pulling back potassium and pushing out sodium — and this, indeed, is what happens in chronic fatigue. In addition to the cell loss of potassium and magnesium as a direct consequence of oxidant cell membrane injury, these two minerals are also lost indirectly due to molecular events caused by chronic fatigue such as unremitting stress. Chronic stress results in wasting of potassium, magnesium, taurine and other life span molecules such as zinc.

TPM protocol is my favorite because it gives me some of

the best clinical results in chronic fatigue states. In closing, I might add that I have learned from many patients with long histories of chronic constipation that this protocol helped more than any other to speed bowel transit time.

**Dose Schedule:** I usually begin my therapy with two tablets of TPM protocol in the morning with breakfast and two tablets with the evening meal. In cases of severe, chronic constipation, I increase the dose to two tablets three times a day. Can still larger doses be given? My answer is yes, though one should assess the total clinical picture again before simply pushing any one single protocol. I might add that it would be impossible to hurt anyone by giving too much TPM. The worst that might happen is that the patient would develop diarrhea and lose the extra TPM. Patients with chronic kidney diseases and those on dialysis treatment are obvious exceptions to it.

| TAURINE PROTOCOL | |
|---|---|
| Taurine | 500 mg |

**Dose Schedule:** I often presribe two tablets daily of this protocol to administer additional taurine as a cell membrane stabilizer by adding this protocol to my prescription for TPM protocol.

| ANTIOXIDANT PROTOCOL | |
|---|---|
| Vitamin A (acetate) | 2,500 units |
| Beta carotene | 2,500 units |
| Vitamin C (calcium salt) | 200 mg |
| Vitamin E | 100 units |
| Bioflavonoids (citrus) | 100 mg |
| Choline bitartrate | 40 mg |
| Zinc (gluconate) | 5 mg |
| Selenium (sodium) | 50 mcg |
| Taurine | 100 mg |
| Methionine | 40 mg |
| L-Cysteine HCl | 270 mg |
| L-Glutathione (reduced) | 25 mg |
| N-Acetyl-L-Cysteine | 25 mg |

**Dose Schedule:** I recommend one tablet of antioxidant protocol twice daily. After satisfactory initial clinical response, I generally reduce the dose to one tablet daily.

| ANTISTRESS PROTOCOL | |
|---|---|
| Vitamin $B_1$ | 30 mg |
| Vitamin $B_2$ | 30 mg |
| Niacin | 150 mg |
| Pantothenic Acid | 30 mg |
| Pyridoxine | 220 mg |
| Folic Acid | 400 mcg |
| Vitamin $B_{12}$ | 200 mcg |
| Vitamin C | 100 mg |
| Vitamin E | 100 IU |
| Biotin | 100 mcg |
| Choline | 50 mg |
| Inositol | 50 mg |
| Magnesium (oxide) | 25 mg |
| Zinc (chelate) | 4 mg |
| Manganese | 10 mg |
| Potassium (citrate) | 2 mg |
| L-Phenylalanine | 100 mg |
| L-Tyrosine | 75 mg |

**Dose Schedule:** I recommend one tablet of antistress protocol daily. If I find it necessary to consider additional nutrient support to alleviate anxiety, stress, sleep difficulty and panic attacks, I usually use neurotransmitter protocol.

| MINERAL PROTOCOL | |
|---|---|
| Magnesium | 175 mg |
| Potassium | 35 mg |
| Zinc | 7.5 mg |
| Manganese | 5 mg |
| Calcium | 75 mg |
| Copper | 0.75 mg |
| Iodine | 50 mcg |
| Chromium | 100 mcg |
| Boron | 1 mg |
| Molybdenum | 50 mcg |
| Selenium | 3 mcg |
| Vanadium | 50 mcg |
| Phosphorus | 70 mg |
| Vitamin $D_3$ | 75 IU |

**Dose Schedule:** I recommend two tablets with the evening meal.

| PANTOTHENIC  PROTOCOL | |
|---|---|
| Pantothenic   Acid | 165 mg |
| Pantetheine | 100 mg |
| Folic  Acid | 50 mcg |
| PABA | 5 mg |
| Potassium   (citrate) | 2 mg |
| L-Arginine | 25 mg |
| L-Histidine | 25 mg |
| L-Ornithine | 5 mg |
| Aloe | 5 mg |
| Licorice   root  (GLGE) | 50 mg |
| Spirulina | 20 mg |
|  |  |

**Dose Schedule:** Like TPM protocol, this protocol is one of my staple nutrient protocols for two main reasons: 1) Pantothenic acid and pantetheine  play critical roles in energy enzyme pathways; and 2) these vitamin factors, along with vitamin $B_{12}$, are among the principal growth factors for the protective bowel flora.

| CAL-MAG PROTOCOL | |
|---|---|
| Calcium (carbonate, citrate) | 240 mg |
| Magnesium (carbonate, sulfate) | 240 mg |
| Vitamin D$_3$ | 50 units |

Calcium is a misunderstood mineral. It is essential for optimal function of cell membranes, and specifically for the muscle contractibility of heart and skeletal muscle.

There are several interesting paradoxes about this life span mineral. Men of money with unlimited access to TV commercials have chosen to ride the calcium money trail. Calcium, they hammer into us every day, must be obtained from dairy or from makers of calcium pills. They frighten us with pictures of bones thinned out with osteoporosis that collapse and fracture. Yet, the practitioners of drug medicine dole out prescriptions for calcium channel blockers as if they are afraid the fountains of calcium channel blockers will dry out. What is it that calcium does that must be blocked with blocker drugs?

Years ago, as a pathology resident, I was baffled by the coexistence of two lesions that I commonly observed in elderly women and men at autopsy: Their coronary arteries were clogged with densely calcified arterial plaques while their bones were mushy with osteoporosis. I often wondered about it. My professors didn't have any answers. Now I know what is creating such a paradox: Calcium is *maldistributed* so that too much of it in the vessel walls destroys them while not enough of it in the bones renders them osteoporotic. Why? The old oxidant injury again? Yes! Absolutely yes! I discuss this subject at length in *Chirri, Cholesterol Cats and Chelation.* Here, I make two brief comments: First, my focus is on calcium homeostasis — normalization of patterns of calcium deposits in the body through a broad, global clinical approach for reducing the accelerated oxidant stress. Second, to restore normal cell membrane function. I am not really interested in frivolous notions of calcium deficiency as proposed by practitioners of drug medicine.

**Dose Schedule:** I usually recommend one tablet of cal-mag protocol with breakfast and one with the evening meal. Rarely, I use the calcium protocol to provide additional calcium in doses of 250 to 500 mg daily. (This is usually a very intuitive response on my behalf. Again, I supplement calcium for *functional* considerations and not for any putative deficiency states.)

| PROTEIN PROTOCOL 1* | |
|---|---|
| Protein*** | 19.5 gm |
| Carbohydrates | 2.0 gm |
| Fats | 0.2 gm |
| Calories | 84 |

* Amounts for both protein protocols I and II represent a serving size of one and half tablespoons. Protocols I contains

partially hydrolyzed milk and egg proteins and protocol II hydrolyzed proteins of soybean (90% of calories from peptides and proteins)

| PROTEIN PROTOCOL II | |
|---|---|
| Proteins* | 8.7 gm |
| Carbohydrates | less than 0.1 gm |
| Fats | less than 0.1 gm |
| Calories | 53 |

**Dose Schedule:** I recommend that protein and peptide protocols I and II be taken on an alternate basis, each for two to three days a week. One- to one-half heaping tablespoons of either protocol powder may be mixed with eight ounces of water and eight ounces of vegetable juice and drunk over a suitable period of time at breakfast. Fresh vegetable juices are preferred; canned juices are acceptable as a compromise. Occasionally, fruit juices, rice milk or soy milk may be used as substitutes. If desired, fruit such as banana, apple or peach may be added to such drinks to enhance taste as well as nutritional value.

Other suitable sources of proteins for such protocols include rice and spirulina.

Chronic fatiguers who suffer from unremitting symptoms of hypoglycemia may use such protocols a second time in the afternoon. Other permissible food items may be added, if found necessary, to such a drink. Five days a week, my own breakfast consists of protein protocols 1 or 2 taken with vegetable juices.

Initially, I required additional food items. Now I do not. Most of my patients who found such a breakfast not sufficiently filling in the beginning reported satisfaction with it within weeks or months. Human metabolism adjusts well to food offered it — both upward and downward.

Sugar-insulin-adrenaline roller coasters occur in all chronic fatiguers. There are no exceptions. Sometimes, the clinician needs to probe the symptomatology more deeply to bring out the difficulties caused by such roller coasters. The symptoms of hypoglycemia — such as sudden-onset weakness, jitteryness, nausea, sweating and heart palpitations — in the majority of cases are caused by sugar-insulin-adrenaline roller coasters. Such roller coasters can be effectively managed with protein protocols such as those described above. I discuss this subject further in *The Butterfly and Life Span Nutrition.*

## GASTRIC AND BOWEL ECOLOGY PROTOCOLS

I discuss my use of 9 bowel ecology protocols and four gastric ecology protocols in the chapter Chronic Fatigue and Battered Bowel Ecology. For readers who suffer from irritable bowel syndrome, spastic colitis, ulcerative colitis, Crohn's colitis, microscopic colitis, collagenous colitis, celiac disease, gastritis, gastric ulcer and other stomach and bowel disorders, I recommend the companion volume *Battered Bowel Ecology — Waving Away A Wandering Wolf.*

## ENHANCEMENT OF LIVER ANTIOXIDANT DEFENSES

The liver is *the* detoxification organ of the human body. Not surprisingly, this organ has fascinated men and women in the healing professions since antiquity. Presently, the role of the liver in health preservation is being increasingly recognized in view of the growing pollutant body burden. However, my research and clinical work in battered bowel ecosystem has led me to conclude that the liver cannot function well except when it is shielded by the gut. Hence, the gut ecosystem — in my view — is the true interface between man and his environment, and must be recognized as the principal protective body organ in matters of environmental toxicants. Notwithstanding, I recognize that chronic fatiguers require extra support for their liver antioxidant and detoxification enzyme systems. To this purpose, I liberally use several herbs and some nutrients combined in the following two oxidative liver stress (OLS) protocols.

Other herbs that can play protective roles for the liver include *Artemesia, Astragalus, Bupleurum Chinese Root, Canna indica, Curcuma longa, Catechin, Cynara scolymus, Dong kwai, Eleutherococcus senticosus (Siberian ginseng), Gentiana root, Glycyrriza glabra, Lycium chinense, Schizandra chinensis, and Swertia pseudochinensise.* Herba that stimulate and support adrenal gland function include *Aconite, Atractylodes, Codonopsis, Coix, Ganoderma, Eleuthrococcus, Epimedium, Panax* and *Rehmannia.* I have not had sufficient experience with these herbs to formulate specific guidelines for their clinical application in the management of chronic fatigue.

| OXIDATIVE LIVER STRESS (OLS) PROTOCOL I | |
|---|---|
| Dandelion Root | 100 mg |
| Beet Root | 50 mg |
| Black Radish | 50 mg |
| Goldenseal | 50 mg |
| Catnip | 50 mg |
| Methionine | 400 mg |
| Choline | 200 mg |
| Inositol | 20 mg |
| OXIDATIVE LIVER STRESS (OLS) PROTOCOL II | |
| Tumeric | 100 mg |
| Milk thistle | 100 mg |
| Red clover | 100 mg |
| Ginger root | 100 mg |
| Goldenseal | 100 mg |
| Jerusulum Artichoke | 100 mg |
| Fennel seed | 100 mg |

I recommend two to three capsules daily of these two protocols in weekly rotation for periods of two or three months.

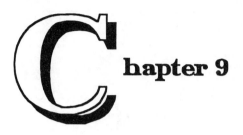

# Chapter 9

# Intravenous
# Nutrient
# Protocols

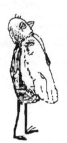

## *Intravenous Nutrient Infusions Can Jump Start Cellular Enzymes in Chronic Fatigue*

I begin my discussion of the clinical value of intravenous nutrient infusions (IV drips) by making four important points:

### *First,*

IV nutrient therapies are not essential for mild to moderate cases of chronic fatigue. In general, such cases can be managed successfully with nondrug therapies outlined in this volume without IV nutrient infusions — especially when the energy and detoxification enzymes have not been further damaged by prolonged drug therapies.

### *Second,*

IV therapies can greatly expedite recovery in moderate to severe cases of chronic fatigue. Thus, nondrug therapies, when administered with IV infusions, often produce the same clinical benefits in three to six weeks as they do in three to six months when IV infusions are withheld.

### *Third,*

IV therapies in severe to very severe cases are *essential*

for reviving badly damaged enzymes.

## *Fourth,*

IV therapies described in this chapter — and others described in my monograph *Intravenous Nutrient Therapies in Molecular Medicine* — are safe and effective when careful attention is paid to all the details. The uncommon untoward effects of such therapies are minor and self-limiting. In my extensive personal experience with such therapies, I have not had to institute any interventional medical or surgical measures to manage such untoward effects in a single patient to date.

Later in this chapter, I describe the composition of some intravenous nutrient protocols I use for my patients with chronic fatigue. For the professional reader — and the general reader with a biology or medical background — I recommend my monograph *Intravenous Nutrient Protocols in Molecular Medicine* published by Life Span, Inc., Denville, New Jersey; (800)-633-6226. In that monograph, I discuss several issues essential to safe and effective IV therapies, such as the composition of various protocols, preparation of protocols, solution osmolality, vein access, management of untoward reactions, proper informed consent and other related subjects.

## FREQUENCY OF IV INFUSIONS

A vast majority of chronic fatigue sufferers require only

a course of five IV nutrient infusions, administered twice weekly. Such patients often require some additional intramuscular injections of magnesium, potassium, calcium and vitamin $B_{12}$. Uncommonly — in less than 5% of patients — I find it necessary to administer a second course of five infusions. Patients with severe chemical sensitivity sometimes require prolonged IV therapy, as much as 20 or more infusions.

Following initial IV infusions, most chronic fatiguers can be managed with optimal food choices, oral nutrient protocols, immunotherapy for IgE-mediated allergies, environmental controls, self-regulation and special slow, sustained physical exercise. Still, I emphasize to my patients that if there is any recurrence — and most chronic fatiguers are prone to some recurrence — they should not delay IV therapy unnecessarily. Early recurrences can usually be managed expediently with just one or two IV infusions.

## IV THERAPY FOR VIRAL INFECTIONS

*Chronic fatiguers cannot afford a slow recovery from common viral infections.* Increasingly, I see patients who consult me for viral infections that do not clear for weeks and months and leave behind persistent cough, muscle weakness and aches, irritability or abdominal symptoms. I have seen many cases in which months of restorative work went down the drain when viral infections were aggressively treated with broad-spectrum antibiotics by physicians unfamiliar with the special problems of chronic fatiguers. Human canaries, I write earlier, have a peculiar vulnerability to broad-spectrum antibiotics. I strongly urge my patients to receive an IV infusion if there are no clear signs of clinical improvement of a viral infection in 48 to 72 hours. In such cases, I use infection control IV protocol described later in this chapter. Repeated empirical observations with IV nutrient infusions have convinced me of their significant value in preventing cases of delayed resolution when such infections lead to dry hacking cough, muscle aches and malaise for weeks after acute symptoms have subsided.

## SEEKING OUT THE RIGHT PHYSICIAN

This is a major problem facing chronic fatiguers at present. There is a severe dearth of physicians who are knowledgeable and experienced in management of several molecular and practical issues of IV nutrient therapies. On a positive note, a growing number of physicians are beginning to recognize that chronic fatigue is linked to nutrition, environment and stress, and that these problems will continue to have a significant impact on chronic fatigue. More important, none of these issues can be addressed with drug therapies. Such physicians are turning to nutrient therapies. I am comfortable predicting that within the next 20 years, intravenous nutrient therapies will become mainstream therapies.

For several years, I have conducted IV therapy courses for chronic fatigue and related disorders at the annual meetings of the American Academy of Otolaryngic Allergy and at the Institute of Preventive Medicine (Denville, New Jersey). During these years, I have also taught such therapies at the Instruction Courses of the American Academy of Environmental Medicine.

I use my monograph *Intravenous Nutrient Therapy in Molecular Medicine* as a comprehensive syllabus for teaching these courses. This monograph is published by Life Span, Inc., and may be obtained by physicians as well as the general reader by calling (800)-633-6226 or (201)-586-9191.

IV therapy for chronic fatigue states and related disorders is not an area where physicians who do not practice nutritional medicine can, on short notice, acquire the necessary depth of perspective. Fortunately, and judging from the calls my office gets for information about IV therapy, a growing number of physicians recognize this and are receiving training in such therapy.

It is my sense that it is not hard now for anyone to find a physician experienced in IV nutrient therapies in most parts of the United States. More important, a growing number of physicians are now willing to consider my IV protocols when their patients plead for such therapies. The number of calls our staff receives in this context is also increasing.

## INDICATIONS FOR IV THERAPY

In my clinical practice, I have observed good results with intravenous nutritional supplements for a host of clinical disorders commonly associated with chronic fatigue states. Similar clinical benefits have been obtained by many other physicians who are well-versed in the principles and practice of nutritional medicine.

Chronic fatiguers commonly suffer from various types of immune and degenerative disorders, bowel disorders and recurrent infections. Such disorders frequently require multiple drug therapies. Yet, they need to avoid drug therapies as much as possible. The judicious use of optimally formulated intravenous nutrient protocols is extremely valuable in this context. Following are some of the disorders for which I have observed satisfactory clinical benefits either without or with minimal reliance on drug therapies:

1. Acute viral infections where the commonly used antibiotics are of no significant value.

2. Altered states of bowel ecology. These states include a host of entities including, but not limited to, multiple food allergies, malabsorptive dysfunctions, recurrent episodes of Candida overgrowth or infection, C. difficile colitis, antibiotic-associated colitis, and bowel parasitic infestations such as Entamoeba, Giardia, Blastocystis, Endolimax and others. It also includes different variants of chronic bowel inflammatory disease such as ulcerative colitis and Crohn's colitis. I discuss this subject in detail in the companion volume *Battered Bowel Ecology — Waving Away A Wandering Wolf.*

3. Asthma and incapacitating bronchospasm associated with pulmonary emphysema.

4. Autoimmune and immunodeficiency syndromes.

5. Bacterial infections under treatment with appropriate antibiotics. The purpose here is to protect the tissues from drug toxicity.

6. Major surgery (before and after). The purpose here is to facilitate and expedite wound healing. It provides a counterbalance to the oxidative and other molecular stresses caused by the surgical procedures.

7.   Major chemical exposures.
8.   Major food and inhalant allergy reactions.
9.   Heavy metal toxicity and heavy metal overload without clinical evidence of enzymatic inactivation.

## GOALS OF IV THERAPIES

The goals of intravenous nutritional therapy are in essence the same as goals for oral nutritional therapy. The main difference, obviously, is the time frame, immediacy of the desired nutritional support and the intended clinical results. Following are the principal goals for such therapy:

1.   to bypass the bowel mucosal barrier, to circumvent absorptive dysfunctions, and to deliver the nutrients directly to the tissues.
2.   to deliver the necessary nutrients to the tissues in optimal proportions, concurrently and for maximal synergistic effects.
3.   to restore the functional integrity of enzymatic pathways in chronic disorders known to result in vitamin, mineral and amino acid deficiencies.
4.   to eliminate the need for drugs when feasible.
5.   to reduce the dose of needed drugs during the early period of caring for a patient.
6.   to protect tissues from injury caused by chemotherapy and radiotherapy.

7.  to expedite recovery from acute infections.
8.  to provide healing tissues extra supplies of nutrients before and after surgery (times of increased demands).

## NUTRIENT GRADIENT

I indicated earlier that the intravenous nutrient protocols described here are not intended to correct any *nutrient deficiencies*. Rather, these protocols are used to create a high gradient of nutrients across the cell membranes to deliver "nutrient boluses." In chronic fatigue states, there are often *large functional* differences between the intra- and extra-cellular compartments even though blood and cellular mineral levels mat not appear significantly different from each other. The demands of cells for such nutrients are high, and IV therapies are designed to meet such demands. My colleagues in nutritional medicine and I regularly see the clinical proof of such states when chronic fatiguers respond well to IV infusions.

There are two critical issues in transmembrane nutrient gradient:

### First,

flushing the tissues with a high gradient of various essential nutrients.

### Second,

concurrent availability of nutrients in optimal

proportions.

Vitamins, minerals, and amino acids administered intravenously are very effective for short-term nutritional support in acute exacerbations of chronic disorders. These protocols are also very effective in clinical situations where serious damage to the immune system is anticipated, i.e.,as with chemotherapy and radiotherapy for cancer and extensive surgery for various diseases.

The intravenous route of therapy, bypassing the bowel mucosal barrier, eliminates all problems of absorption. It allows expeditious delivery of these essential elements to all the tissues. Furthermore, IV therapy provides the tissues necessary nutrients, concurrently and in the proper proportions.

*Intravenous nutritional protocols must be chosen and administered according to the specific needs of the individual patient. Clinical benefits must be carefully assessed on an on going basis.*

## PHLEBITIS AND PHLEBOTHROMBOSIS

Phlebitis is a term used to indicate inflammation of veins. Phlebothrombosis is a term used to indicate formation of blood clots in the vein lumen. These two terms are often used interchangeably because blood clots within the vein invariably lead to some inflammatory response.

All patients requiring intravenous infusions face the risk of phlebitis, whether the infusions carry drugs for hospitalized patients or nutrients in the clinical practice of nutritional medicine. Who is likely to develop phlebothrombosis? It has been a very rare occurrence in my personal experience with chelation therapy for cardiovascular disease. This has not been the case for patients with severe chemical sensitivities and disabling chronic fatigue. Patients requiring chelation therapy almost always have easily accessible large veins; those with chronic fatigue sometimes do not. More important than the issue of large accessible veins is the vulnerability of vascular endothelium to trauma associated with intravenous infusions containing large quantities of ascorbic acid and other nutrients. Indeed, spontaneous bruising and vasculitis unassociated with intravenous infusions is a common occurrence in chemical sensitivity and chronic fatigue.

Unfortunately, human canaries are more vulnerable to this than other people. People with environmental sensitivity and indolent autoimmune disorders often have a tendency to easy bruising. The reason for this is simple: Toxins and immune complexes circulate in blood, and the vascular endothelium (the delicate inner lining of the blood vessels) gets the most exposure. When this delicate lining is further irritated with IV nutrient solutions, it leads to blood clotting.

In the list of intravenous nutrient protocols given in this volume, I include three primer protocols. I designed these protocols with the specific purpose of eliminating or reducing the potential for incompatibility reactions. I have not seen phlebothrombosis with primer I protocol, and I believe the risk of such an event is very small.

## MANAGEMENT OF PHLEBITIS

What are the true risks of phlebothrombosis — or phlebitis — that may result from intravenous nutrient therapy? I have not yet encountered a single case of embolism, symptomatic or otherwise, occurring as a complication of such phlebothrombosis. It must be conceded that this indeed may occur.

The phlebitis that I have encountered in my work has been a self-limiting problem. No surgical or medical drug intervention has been necessary. The blood clot has been firmly tethered to the vein wall, and the risk of the clot traveling within the vein has been extremely small. In rare cases, warm packs and elevation have been deemed necessary. The veins in such cases have nearly always opened again, though sometimes it has taken months. As undesirable as phlebitis is, it is a small price to pay for the many clinical benefits offered by IV therapies.

## A NOTE ABOUT VITAMIN C

It is my practice to measure the serum ferritin level for every patient requiring intravenous nutrient therapy. If the ferritin level is raised, I eliminate or reduce the amount of ascorbic acid added to the infusion to minimize the risk of oxyradical injury due to Fenton's reaction. It is also my practice to reduce the amount of ascorbic acid used in cases where access to large veins is limited and the patient experiences pain with intravenous infusion in spite of the use of rheologic agents included in the protocols.

Intravenous nutrient therapies are grossly misunderstood. Most practitioners of $N^2D^2$ medicine still cling to the silly notion that all anyone can achieve with intravenous nutrient therapies is expensive urine. This viewpoint holds that SAD — the standard American diet — provides all the required amounts of vitamins and minerals, and injected nutrients simply pass through the body.

## PRIMER INTRAVENOUS PROTOCOLS

Many chronically fatigued patients who benefit most from intravenous nutrient therapies initially do not tolerate well the full nutrient doses given in the fatigue protocol that follows. Such patients suffer from a variety of initial symptoms including headache, lightheadedness, lethargy, fatigue and abdominal symptoms. Indeed, full nutrient doses can exaggerate, albeit temporarily, any or all symptoms that the individual patient suffers as a result of multiple organ involvement in the accelerated molecular oxidative process that causes chronic fatigue. This is a point of considerable clinical importance. My staff and I are very careful in briefing IV therapy patients about this temporary phenomenon. Except for patients with devastating, chronic chemical sensitivities of several years duration, I have not seen chronically ill patients who cannot tolerate or who cannot benefit from intravenous nutrient therapies.

In order to limit to a bare minimum the initial unwanted reactions to intravenous nutrient therapies, I recommend the following primer I, II and III protocols that in my experience have not caused significant problems. These protocols include nutrients that are least likely to cause initial intolerance. In general, it is my practice to prescribe a single IV infusion of primer I, II and III protocols each for severe to very severe chronic fatigue cases before moving on to the full-strength fatigue protocol. Uncommonly, I have to move more slowly and repeat one or more of the primer protocols depending upon patient tolerance. Also, in general I prescribe IV infusions twice weekly during the initial period of therapy.

| PRIMER I PROTOCOL | |
|---|---|
| Vitamin C | 5 gm |
| Magnesium Sulfate | 1 gm |
| Heparin | 4,000 units |
| Sodium Bicarbonate | 2.5 ml |
| Dextrose 5% * | 500 ml |

* Other suitable carrying solutions for all three primer protocols are Ringer's lactate and 0.45% saline. These solutions are hyperosmolar; however, these are clinically better tolerated than those prepared with sterile water to lower the solution osmolality.
**Administration Time:** two to three hours for all three primer protocols

| PRIMER II PROTOCOL | |
|---|---|
| Vitamin C | 10 gm |
| Magnesium Sulfate | 1.5 gm |
| Pantothenic Acid | 250 mg |
| Heparin | 4,000 units |
| Sodium Bicarbonate | 2.5 mEq |
| Dextrose 5% * | 500 ml |
| PRIMER III PROTOCOL | |
| Vitamin C | 15 gm |
| Magnesium sulfate | 2 gm |
| Pantothenic Acid | 500 mg |
| Zinc | 10 mg |
| Multivitamin | 2.5 ml* |
| Heparin | 4,000 units |
| Sodium Bicarbonate | 2.5 mEq |
| Dextrose 5% * | 500 ml |

*Multivitamin formula contains: vitamin A, 3,300 IU; vitamin D, 200 IU; vitamin E, 10 mg; biotin, 60 mcg; folic acid, 400 mcg; niacin, 40 mg; thiamine, 3 mg; riboflavin, 3.6 mg; pantothenic acid, 15 mg; pyridoxine, 4; cyanocobalamine, 5 mcg; and vitamin C, 100 mg.

| FATIGUE PROTOCOL | |
|---|---|
| Thiamine | 15 gm |
| Riboflavin | 3.5 mg |
| Niacinamide | 40 mg |
| Biotin | 60 mg |
| Pantothenic acid | 515 mg |
| Pyridoxin | 154 mg |
| Folic acid | 400 mcg |
| Cobalamine | 2,500 mcg |
| Vitamin A | 3,300 IU |
| Vitamin C | 15 gm |
| Vitamin D | 200 IU |
| Vitamin E | 10 IU |
| Magnesium | 2,000 mg |
| Calcium | 125 mg |
| Zinc | 24 mg |
| Chromium | 100 mg |
| Selenium | 100 mg |
| Molybdenum | 150 mg |
| Manganese | 0.4 mg |
| Potassium chloride | 6 mEq |
| Taurine | 50 mg |
| Heparin/NaHCO/Lidocaine | * |
| Dextrose 5% ** | 500 ml |

\* Sodium bicarbonate 1.25 mEq; Xylocaine, 60 mg; heparin, 4,000 units. \*\* Ringer's lactate and 0.45% saline are other suitable fluids. Vitamin $B_{12}$ (1,500 mcg) is given separately with an IM injection.

**Administration Time:** two to three hours

## INFECTION IV PROTOCOL

This protocol is recommended for use with acute and chronic viral infections in patients with an impaired immune status. Following are some clinical examples:

1. History of frequent viral infections with delayed or prolonged resolution.
2. History of chronic sore throat with dry cough lasting for weeks or even months.
3. History of pulmonary infiltrates that develop after upper respiratory infections and fail to clear for weeks.
4. History of chronic persistent fatigue.
5. History of frequent upper respiratory infections in patients with severe mold and food allergy.
6. History of autoimmune disorders such as rheumatoid arthritis, vasculitis, SLE, autoimmune thyroiditis and others.
7. History of recurrent episodes of candida vaginitis and infections with herpes simplex virus, human papilloma virus and other viruses.
8. Some acute viral infections in otherwise healthy individuals such as acute infectious mononucleosis.

| COMPOSITION OF INFECTION PROTOCOL ||
|---|---|
| Vitamin C | 15 gm |
| Vitamin A | 3,300 IU |
| Vitamin D | 200 IU |
| Vitamin E | 10 IU |
| Biotin | 60 mcg |
| Folic acid | 400 mcg |
| Niacinamide | 40 mg |
| Riboflavin | 3.5 mg |
| Thiamine | 3 mg |
| Pantothenic acid | 515 mg |
| Pyridoxine | 154 mg |
| Cyanocobalamine | 2,500 mcg |
| Calcium glycero/lactate | 125 mg |
| Copper sulfate | 1.6 mg |
| Chromium | 16 mg |
| Magnasium | 2,000 mg |
| Managenese | 0.4 mg |
| Molybdenum | 150 mcg |
| Zinc sulfate | 24 mcg |
| Selenium | 100 mcg |
| Taurine/Potassium chloride | 50 mg/ 6 mEq |

Other fluids for the infusion that may be used on a selective basis are Ringer's lactate or 0.45% saline or distilled water. Volume 450-550 ml. Vitamin $B_{12}$ (1,000 mcg) is given separately with an IM injection.

**Administration Time:** two to three hours

## IV BOLUS THERAPIES

Many clinicians report good results with intravenous nutrient bolus therapy. In general, my own clear preference for intravenous therapy is with an intravenous drip. There are two main reasons for this. First, it is difficult to administer integrated vitamin and mineral formulations with simple intravenous injections due to the volumes of these solutions (often 50 to 75 ml). Second, slow intravenous drips of diluted solutions are generally much less likely to provoke adverse reactions than direct injections of highly concentrated solutions. Still, there are situations in which bolus IV therapies may be used expediently, i.e., IV Bolus I for severe headache, acute musculoskeletal strains and other acute pain syndromes, and IV Bolus II for acute viral infections. Extreme care must be used when administering one gram of magnesium in 20 minutes in view of the potential for cardiac arrhythmias induced by a rapid increase in the serum magnesium levels. On rare occasions, IV bolus therapies indeed may be necessary because of the poor status of peripheral veins (again, warming the hand or the arm with a heating pad or with a heater will usually make collapsed invisible veins quite visible and suitable for access for intravenous infusion therapy.

| IV BOLUS I PROTOCOL | |
|---|---|
| Magnesium   Sulfate | 750  mg |
| Zinc | 12  mg |
| Multimineral | 2  ml |
| Calcium   Glycero/lactate | 75  mg |
| Pantothenic   Acid | 375  mg |
| Pyridoxin | 100  mg |
| Vitamin   C | 5  gm |
| Vitamin   B Complex | 1  ml |
| Molybdenum | 125  mcg |
| Sterile   Water | 50  ml |
| IV BOLUS II PROTOCOL | |
| Vitamin   C | 20  gm |
| Magnesium | 750  mg |
| Molybdenum | 125  mcg |
| Pyridoxine | 100  mg |
| Zinc | 12  mg |
| Dextrose 5% | 50  ml |

**Administration Time:** IV bolus therapies should be administered slowly over a period of 15 to 20 minutes as minidrips. The vein should be flushed with five ml of saline after the infusion.

## INTRAMUSCULAR PROTOCOLS

The following two intramuscular (IM) protocols may be used expediently to provide nutrient support to patients who may not need the larger IV protocols described earlier, or when poor vein condition or personnel and time constraints make IV therapy impractical. Whether to use IM I protocol or IM II protocols depends on the clinical judgment of the clinican for the potential benefits of giving supplemental pantothenic acid, molybdenum, zinc and vitamin B complex to an individual patient.

| INTRAMUSCULAR I PROTOCOL | | |
|---|---|---|
| Magnesium Sulfate | 500 mg/ml | 1.5 ml |
| Calcium Glycerophos | 25 mg/ml | 1.5 ml |
| Vitamin $B_{12}$ | 1,000 mcg/ml | 1 ml |
| Vit B Complex | * | 1 ml |
| Pantothenic Acid | 250 mg/ml | 0.5 ml |
| Pyridoxin | 100 mg/ml | 0.5 ml |
| Zinc | 5 mg/ml | 0.6 ml |
| Molybdenum | 25 mcg/ml | 0.5 ml |
| Selenium | 40 mcg/ml | 0.4 ml |
| Multivitamin | ** | 0.5 ml |

* Vitamin B complex includes the following per ml: Thiamine, 100 mg, Riboflavin, 2 mg; Nicotinamide 100 mg; dexpanthenol, 2 mg; pyridoxine, 2 mg. ** Described in the section on primer protocols.

| INTRAMUSCULAR II PROTOCOL | | |
|---|---|---|
| Magnesium sulfate | 500 mg/ml | 2 ml |
| Calcium glyc/lac | 25 mg/ml | 104 ml |
| Vitamin B$_{12}$ | 1,000 mcg/ml | 1 ml |

**Dose Schedule:** I usually prescribe five doses of either of the two IM protocols to be administered twice weekly. Subsequent injections may be given once weekly according to the needs of the individual patient. It is desirable to inject one half of either of the two above IM protocols deep in the gluteal muscles of each buttock.

## IV THERAPY: A METHOD FOR MAKING EXPENSIVE URINE?

Sometimes my patients tell me what their other physicians who practice drug medicine think of IV nutrient therapies. Many of them still proclaim that all IV therapies do is make expensive urine. It is a pathetic statement that reflects an appalling lack of understanding of how nutrients work. I discuss the *molecular* reasons for using IV therapies and the anticipated clinical benefits at length in the monograph *Intravenous Nutrient Protocols in Molecular Medicine.* I refer the professional reader to that monograph. Here, I include some brief comments for the general reader.

Actually, there is complete agreement among physicians about the clinical efficacy of intravenous nutrient protocols. Those who use these protocols are convinced of their enormous clinical value. Those who do not are equally convinced of their futility. It is easy to see why we in the first group are so enthusiastic about intravenous nutrient protocols. These protocols allow us to dramatically reduce the use of antibiotics and other types of drug therapies. They are extremely effective for resolving hard-to-define but unrelenting clinical symptoms such as fatigue, muscle aches, a sense of being "not healthy", stress and panic attacks, palpitations, mood and memory disorders, abdominal bloating, and symptoms of allergy and chemical sensitivity. Further, these protocols frequently allow us to successfully manage patients with chronic indolent degenerative and immune disorders who obtain little, if any, long-term relief from prevailing drug therapies. Finally, intravenous nutrient protocols are extremely valuable for some disorders for which there are no known effective drug regimens, i.e., incapacitating chronic fatigue.

It is not easy to see how the high priests of $N^2D^2$ medicine who never use intravenous nutrient therapies become convinced of their futility. How can anyone ever be really convinced of the futility of any therapy that he has never tried?

There are five essential molecular considerations in the formulation and administration of intravenous nutrient protocols.

## *First,*

is the issue of molecular medicine versus drug medicine — drug therapies are based on the patterns of tissue disease observed with microscopic study. The essential distinction here is this: The disease diagnosis based on structural injury to cells and organs tells us about tissue injury *after* the tissue has been injured. The study of molecular dynamics of health and disease, by contrast, gives us insights into the workings of the molecules, cells and tissues *before* the injury has occurred. This, indeed, calls for a major intellectual adaptation. Like all other adaptations, it can be expected to create considerable difficulties for physicians with intellectual subservience to $N^2D^2$ medicine. This is the *true* cause of the spurious controversy about the efficacy of oral and IV nutrient therapies.

## *Second,*

is the issue of growing oxidative stress on human biology, its impact on health and causation of disease, and what part nutrients play in providing a counterbalance. I discuss this issue at length in previous chapters of this volume.

## *Third,*

is the issue of correcting putative nutrient "deficiencies" with nutrient therapies versus the use of nutrients for their metabolic roles. The idea of using nutrients only for correcting narrowly defined nutritional deficiency is archaic and does not require any further comments. For example, the use of ascorbic acid only to treat scurvy is utterly irrelevant to the clinical problems we see every day. In my clinical practice, I use vitamin C liberally for its role in redox homeostasis — as a part of my global strategies to correct redox dysregulations that are always present in chronic fatigue states. I do not use vitamin C to prevent scurvy (of which I have never seen a case, nor do I expect to see one in my life).

## Fourth,

is the issue of holistic molecular relatedness in human biology. No molecule exists in biology alone, functionally or structurally. This is self-evident. And yet many physicians insist on diagnosing "a nutrient deficiency" to establish the presence of a "disease" that they can "cure" with "a nutrient therapy". The irony is that we continue to neglect all clearly established evidence against this simplistic and obsolete notion.

## Fifth,

is the issue of molecular benefits of nutrients versus the molecular burdens of drug therapy (drug detoxification). This critical point is rarely given any consideration. How do our molecular pathways deal with drugs? We talk about drug metabolism in abstract terms. We discuss hepatic breakdown of drugs and speak of renal clearance of drugs or their metabolites. This is where our discussions usually end. What is the true "molecular cost" of drugs? The fact is that molecule for molecule, drugs waste essential defense molecules of the body. Good examples of this phenomenon are the loss of vitally needed glutathione, glycine and taurine molecules. (The first two are used for conjugation of drugs and other xenobiotics, while taurine is a powerful quencher of hypochlorite radicals and serves as an important scavenger of free radicals.) These are the life-span molecules (see discussion below) that provide the necessary molecular counterbalance to the aging-oxidant molecules. From this molecular perspective, the essential difference between nutrient protocols and drug therapy becomes obvious. Drugs deplete life span molecules; nutrient protocols sustain them. Drugs add to the aging-oxidative burden of disease; nutrients drastically reduce such burdens. While drugs are essential for acute life-threatening disease, they are poor substitutes for nutrients to affect reversal of chronic molecular disorders.

## EFFICACY OF IV NUTRIENT PROTOCOL

In one of our studies, my colleagues and I assessed the efficacy of intravenous nutrient protocol in a series of 100 consecutive patients who suffered from chronic fatigue for more than six months. All these patients had received treatment according to the prevailing standards of therapy by their previous physicians without clinical benefits before they entered the study. Initially, all patients were managed with integrated holistic management protocols of nutritional and environmental medicine, self-regulation and were given training in slow and sustained physical exercise as outlined in the chapter On Reviving Injured Enzymes.

Initially, intravenous nutrient therapy was not deemed clinically necessary for 78 patients. Of these, 55 patients indeed showed satisfactory clinical improvement without intravenous nutrient therapy. The remaining 23 patients failed to show satisfactory clinical response as judged by improvement in general level of energy and symptom control in a follow -up visit after eight weeks of other nondrug therapies.

Some of these patients had been offered IV therapies earlier but declined it for a variety of reasons. We evaluated the clinical outcome with symptom scores. All but one patient of these patients showed significant clinical response within a period of six weeks. The average number of infusions administered to this group of patients was 6.5 (range: three to nine). Following are some data obtained with this study.

The following two tables show demographic and clinical outcome data comparing two groups of chronic fatigue sufferers: those who required IV therapies and those who didn't.

| CLINICAL DATA FOR IV OUTCOME STUDY: NUMBER OF PATIENTS: 100 | | |
|---|---|---|
| | **NON-IV GROUP** | **IV GROUP** |
| Sex M/F | 25/30 | 18/27 |
| Average Age | 40 | 48 |
| Range of Age | 6-70 | 26-81 |
| Duration of Symptoms (months) | 2.8 yrs | 6.1 yrs |
| Duration of Therapy (months) | 8 | 9.5 |

| EFFICACY OF IV NUTRIENT THERAPY: COMPARISON OF IV (45) AND NON-IV (55) GROUPS | | |
|---|---|---|
| **SYMPTOM** | **NON-IV GROUP** | **IV GROUP** |
| Fatigue | 2.41 | 2.78 |
| Allergy | 2.22 | 2.61 |
| Muscle aches* | 2.54 | 2.82 |
| Headache | 2.15 | 2.88 |
| Abdominal** | 2.2 | 2.5 |
| Depression | 2.1 | 2.25 |
| Anxiety | 2.5 | 2.39 |
| Sleep*** | 2.0 | 2.3 |
| Fever**** | 2.13 | 2.21 |
| Sore throat | 2.43 | 2.43 |
| **OVERALL** | 2.26 | 2.59 |

\*        Includes muscle aches, cramps and tender nodules
\*\*      Includes bloating, cramps and episodes of diarrhea
           and constipation
\*\*\*    Includes difficulty in onset and interruptions
\*\*\*\*  Includes low-grade fever and malaise

The following graphs specifically demonstrate the clinical benefits of IV therapy using fatigue protocol described in this chapter. The graph lines represent the initial symptom scores and clinical outcome scores for 23 patients who were managed with comprehensive nondrug therapies described in this volume initially and responded unsatisfactorily, and then were administered IV therapy. Thus, the difference between the pretreatment and post-treatment symptom scores for these patients truly represent the clinical benefits of IV fatigue protocol.

Of the 23 patients in the study, six received five or less infusions. Ten patients received 10 or less infusions. The remaining seven patients received more than 10 infusions, the highest number of infusions being 24 in one patient.

Clinical outcome was evaluated with symptom scores on a scale of 0 to -4 for intensity of symptoms and 0 to +4 for relief of symptoms. I recorded the presenting symptom scores at the time of initial consultation according to the symptom severity described by the patients. The clinical outcome data were collected by one of my research associates, Dr. Zarar Bajwa, based on patient interviews.

## SYMPTOM: CHRONIC FATIGUE

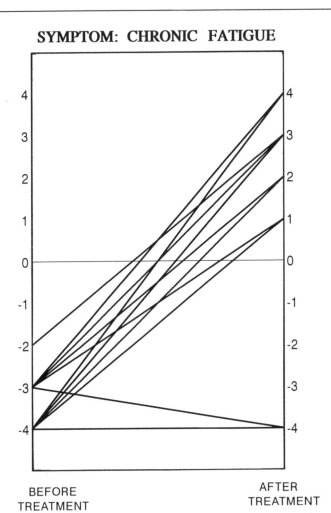

BEFORE
TREATMENT

AFTER
TREATMENT

Legend: Data point lines represent 23 patients. Four lines that show maximal clinical benefit (going from -4 or -3 to +4 or +3 scores) represent 12 patients. Two lines that show absence of clinical benefits represents one patient each (These two patients suffered from severe symptoms of chemical sensitivity, and were the only two individuals in this series of 100 consecutive patients who failed to show satisfactory clinical response with nondrug therapies.)

## SYMPTOMS: MUSCLE PAIN AND BOWEL SYMPTOMS

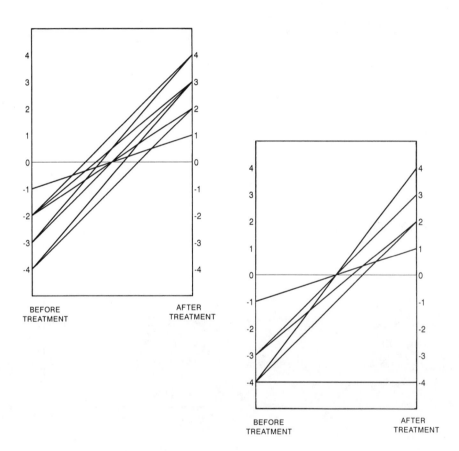

Legend: Data for relief of muscle symtpoms (upper left) and abdominal symptoms (lower left) are shown. Note that relief of bowel symptoms was observed in all patients given IV infusions.

## SYMPTOMS: ALLERGY AND HEADACHE

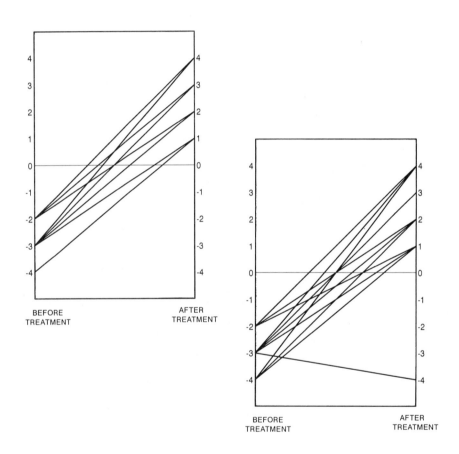

Legend: Data for relief of headache (upper left) and allergic symptoms (lower right) are shown. Clinical response for headache was satisfactory in every case in which it was a presenting symptom. Worsening of allergic symptoms in a single patient was considered to be caused by multiple seasonal exposures.

# SYMPTOMS: SORE THROAT AND SLEEP DIFFICULTIES

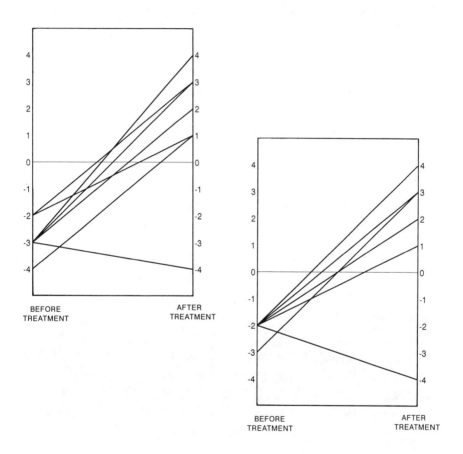

Legend: Data for symptoms of recurrent sore throat (upper left) and sleep difficulties (lower right) are shown.

---

## OXIDANT PROTOCOLS

Intravenous oxidant therapies —hydrogen peroxide infusions and hemo-ozone autotransfusion —are poorly understood but effective therapies. Many European physicians report good clinical outcomes with such therapies for a large number of immune, degenerative and infectious disorders.

In the United States, my colleague, Charles Farr, M.D., has pioneered in the use of intravenous hydrogen peroxide therapy, and has reported good clinical results for a host of clinical disorders including chronic fatigue states. At the November, 1993 conference of the American College for Advancement in Medicine, he told me that his data showed about 80% response rate in patients with chronic fatigue. My own experience with such therapy is too limited to draw any firm conclusions.

I include the following brief comments about oxidative therapy in this volume for one important reason. On the surface, the use of oxidative therapies to manage chronic fatigue states — that I believe are caused by accelerated oxidative injury — appears paradoxical, and may be considered strong evidence against my viewpoint.

How can oxidant therapies be effective for disorders that are caused by oxidative damage? Conceptually, my strong sense is that oxidant therapies work by modulating the redox regulation — they *shock* the normal restorative mechanisms by *exaggerating*the injury that caused the dysregulation in the first place. In a sense, it is the reverse of the Law of the Similars propounded by the ancients, among them, Hippocrates, the father of medicine. This law holds that whatever causes a disease can also reverse that disease process when used in suitable dilution. This is the core principle of homeopathy — and is validated by homeopathic physicians in their clinical work everyday.

To illustrate my viewpoint, I cite three examples in which proven effective therapies yield good clinical responses. The first example is that of the use of a cardiac defibrillator for life-threatening heart palpitations (ventricular fibrillation). It is a common observation that the sudden application of a powerful electric current to the fibrillating heart often restores the normal heart rhythm. Literally, the heart is shocked out of its senses; when it recovers in a few moments, it recalls its normal rhythm and begins to beat in a regular fashion. A second example of this phenomenon is that of electroconvulsive therapy for severe depression that does not respond to common antidepressant drugs. Here again, the deranged chemistry of serotonin and related neurotransmitters that causes depression is literally shocked to its senses by an electric shock that seems to break up the abnormal bioelectric circuits. The third example is that of provocation/neutralization technique for diagnosis and management of food sensitivities. Provocation of certain energetic-molecular events is followed by restoration of normal patterns with clinical relief. This proposed mechanism of the action of oxidant therapies, however, is pure speculation on my part at this time, and valid experimental evidence for it is not yet available.

Nitric acid and hydrogen peroxide are two molecules that

in my view, will prove to be of great clinical value in designing non-pharmacologic therapies for reversing chronic immune and degenerative disorders, and in the management of certain acute infectious processes. Nitric acid production and disposal are some of the fundamental events that occur at the peripheral level and regulate vascular tone — and so influence the perfusion of tissues. The effects of nitric acid on vascular tone are largely mediated by its effects on the muscle fibers. There is some clinical evidence that nitroglycerine may be of some clinical efficacy in the management of chronic fatigue.

Production and breakdown of hydrogen peroxide is one of the initial redox events that results from the activities of a host of enzymes such as oxidases, oxygenases (cyclo-oxygenases, lipo-oxygenases, peroxidases), myeloperoxidase, catalase and other related enzymes of redox homeostasis. Through these various reactions, hydrogen peroxide plays critical roles in the metabolic pathways involved in building up and breaking down various carbohydrates, lipids and proteins. Hydrogen peroxide production and degradation is also one of the initial responses of polymorphonuclear leukocytes to an assault by various microbial organisms.

## HYDROGEN PEROXIDE THERAPY

This protocol is intended for use along with other intravenous nutrient protocols in some patients who respond poorly to therapy. Before using this protocol, I strongly urge the reader to familiarize himself with several important issues relating to hydrogen peroxide therapy discussed at length in a monograph entitled *Workbook on Free Radical Chemistry and Hydrogen Peroxide Metabolism* prepared by Charles H. Farr, M.D. and published by IBOM Foundation (405-691-1112).

| HYDROGEN PEROXIDE PROTOCOL | |
|---|---|
| Hydrogen peroxide 3.75% | 0.35 ml |
| Sodium Bicarbonate | 2.5 ml |
| DMSO | 1 ml |
| Normal Saline | 250 ml |

**Administration Time:** Two to three hours

* Dextrose 5 percent may be used as the carrying solution.

### What is a weed?
An ecologically comfortable plant.

### What is a virus?
A strand of DNA that meshes irretrievably within the weave of the host DNA and yet retains its uniqueness.

### What is a bacterium?
A complete universe within a single cell.

### What is a yeast spore?
A bit of life smug in its envelope, ready to burst on the scene at the right signal.

### What is an intestinal parasite?
A wandering organism that becomes comfortable in a battered bowel ecosystem.


Weeds, viruses, bacteria, yeasts and parasites are living beings that have the same essential attributes of life as human cells. Ecologically, these life forms are as intricately involved with the human tissues as the human cells they are composed of. We cannot exclude these living beings from our environment any more than we can eliminate butterflies, ants and houseflies from our towns and cities. We cannot kill them without killing tiny parts of ourselves. We have to learn to *coexist* with them. This is the essential lesson of biology.

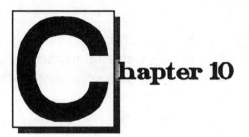

# Chapter 10

# Battered Bowel
# Ecology
## and
# Chronic Fatigue

The bowel ecosystem is *always* injured in chronic states, and its restoration is the *second* core thrust of my management philosophy for chronic fatiguers — the *first* core thrust being a global strategy for reducing oxidative stress.

## THE GUT IS A MISUNDERSTOOD ORGAN

In drug medicine, when the symptoms are directly related to the gut, the treatment strategy consists of symptom suppression with drugs. When the symptoms are not directly related to the gut, any suggestion of a possible role of a damaged bowel ecosystem in the cause of symptoms is unceremoniously dismissed.

In my view, the most remarkable phenomenon in the entire field of human biology is this: A vast number of clinical problems that are seemingly unrelated to the bowel spontaneously resolve when the focus of clinical management turns to *all* the issues in bowel ecology. How often do symptoms of persistent debilitating fatigue in young men and women clear up when an altered state of bowel ecology is restored to normal? How often do troublesome mood swings subside when therapies focus on the bowel? How often does arthralgia (pain and stiffness in joints with or without joint swelling) resolve when all the bowel issues are addressed? How often do we successfully prevent chronic headache; anxiety; palpitations; incapacitating PMS; recurrent attacks of vaginitis; asthma and skin lesions by correcting the abnormalities in the internal environment of the bowel? The answers to these questions will vary widely among physicians.

Physicians who regularly neglect the bowel (and those who never understood the issues of bowel ecology in the first place) will dismiss these questions with scorn. None of this has been proven with double-blind cross-over studies, they will strenuously protest. Other physicians who have learned to respect the bowel — as the ancients did — and care for their patients with a sharp focus on bowel issues will readily and unequivocally validate my personal (and fairly extensive) clinical experience.

## LIFE IN THE BOWEL ECOSYSTEM

The bowel ecosystem teems with life. Shrouded in metabolic mists, it is as rich in biologic diversity and as broad in biochemical interrelationships as any other ecosystem on this planet Earth. The ancients seemed to have an intuitive sense about it. Death begins in the bowel, they pronounced in more than one way. Leeuwenhoek studied fecal bacteria during his invention of the microscope in 1719, and, thus, was the first man to study life in the bowel ecosystem with modern scientific methods. Metchnikoff, the Russian biologist, who single-handedly developed the concept of the cellular arm of the immune system, became intensely interested in the aging process in his later years when he moved to Paris where he served as the head of the Pasteur Institute. He studied the longevity of Bulgarians and provided strong evidence that certain bowel microbes played important roles in preserving health and promoting longevity among them. He named the microbe he thought was most prominent in this field as *Lactobacillus bulgaricus*. Metchnikoff's work opened the floodgates of basic research on the bowel flora.

## WINDOWS ON THE WORLD

A cell looks at the world around it through its cell membrane. It is this membrane that separates the cell's internal order from external order. Although molecular host defense mechanisms of both immune and nonimmune types have progressed from simple single-cell forms to multicellular forms to highly developed complex organisms such as humans, the fundamental pattern of host defenses has remained the same: The cell membrane or its counterparts carry the primary responsibility for preserving the biologic integrity of the organisms. For the professional reader, I discuss at length the energy and biochemical events which occur at the cell membrane in health and disease in my monograph, *The Agony and the Death of a Cell,* published in the 1991 syllabus of the American Academy of Environmental Medicine.

*For humans, the gut mucosa is the true counterpart of the cell membrane of unicellular organisms.* From a phylogenetic perspective, the gut mucosa would be expected to be the primary host defense organ. This indeed is the case when one looks at health and disease from a *holistic* perspective.

In a biologic sense, man's gut lining is his window to the world around him. What do we ever get through our skin but a little vitamin D when we get a chance to bask in the sunshine? What do we get through our lungs? All our ancestors ever received through their lungs was oxygen. Now we receive —

unwillingly and under severe protest — a heavy load of environmental pollutants. Everything else that enters our biologic systems enters through the gut lining. It is important to recognize that the mucosal linings of the mouth, esophagus and stomach essentially are extensions of the gut lining. The states of health and absence of health are expressions of the dynamics of foods within the gut ecosystem — the effects on foods of the digestive-absorptive processes as well as the various life forms in the gut.

## HUMAN MOLECULAR DEFENSES EXIST AS PLANTS IN THE SOIL OF THE BOWEL CONTENTS

The ancients seemed to have known this intuitively. We seem to have taken a very circuitous route to grasp this most fundamental of all aspects of the immune system. I remember that the *hakim* (folk-doctor) in my village always prescribed laxatives for a headache. He prescribed remedies that seemed to work on the bowel for problems of the skin, joints, liver and other organs. Of course, I, then a medical school student, found it very amusing. It never occurred to me then why these folk-doctors would prescribe year after year remedies that couldn't work. More important, from my present perspective, I never wondered why people accepted those remedies year after year if they afforded no relief. I was into the science of medicine then. I wasn't into finding out what worked and what didn't. Nor did I ever doubt the science of my professors who doled out prescriptions for drugs by the dozens for sheer symptom suppression. That was then. And that was poor Pakistan. Now I question the science of an average American family practitioner when he prescribes drugs for chronic bowel symptoms. How scientific is his use of antacids for symptoms of burning or pain in the pit of the stomach? How scientific is his use of antispasmodic drugs for abdominal cramps? How scientific is his use of antidiarrheal drugs for diarrhea? How scientific is his use of steroids for inflammatory bowel disorders? Steroids suppress the immune system. How scientific is it to further suppress the immune system for problems caused by an errant immune system in the first place? How scientific is the use of anti-inflammatory agents, anxiolytic drugs, antidepressants, antispastic agents, antihistamines, and, of course, broad-spectrum antibiotics for treating various types of bowel disorders that we — by our own admission — do not understand the causes of?

## THE BOWEL PERPLEXES A PATHOLOGIST

How many different things can the bowel do? It cramps. It obstructs. It turns and twists. It ulcerates. It bleeds. How does the bowel know when to cramp and when to obstruct or bleed? And when to turn and twist?

For many years I have studied a host of clinical syndromes in which the symptom-complexes can be related to events occurring in the bowel. As a hospital pathologist, I have had the opportunity to examine more than 11,000 bowel biopsies during the last 25 years. Every time I peered at a bit of bowel through a microscope and saw inflammation — colitis in common jargon — I wondered where and how it might have started. We pathologists know quite a bit about how a damaged bowel looks, but we know little, if anything, about the initial energetic-molecular events that set the stage for tissue damage. What is the cause of ulcerative colitis? Pathologists will tell you it is not known. What is the cause of Crohn's colitis? The answer: unknown. What is the cause of irritable bowel syndrome and spastic colitis? Unknown. What is the cause of microscopic colitis and collagenous colitis? The answer is the same.

Why is it that we do not know the cause of any of these types of colitis? The reason is we search for answers in the damaged structure *after* the fact rather than in the events preceding the damage. None of these "diseases" can be understood except with ecologic thinking.

During the early 1980s, my research colleague, Dr. Madhava Ramanarayanan, and I introduced the micro-elisa assay for allergen-specific IgE antibodies. This research interest and several subsequent studies gave me important insights into immune and nonimmune events that inflict tissue injury. It also raised serious questions about many of the prevailing concepts regarding the role of food and mold allergy in the causation of numerous bowel disorders. As a clinician, I have cared for a fairly large number of patients with autoimmune and immunodeficiency syndromes. These microscopic, immune, molecular, and clinical observations — as disparate as they appeared in the usual clinical setting — began to take coherent and integrated forms before me. I began to recognize that events taking place in the bowel were clearly related to many clinical syndromes that seemed to have nothing to do with the bowel according to the prevailing concepts of pathogenesis of disease. The single most important insight into the workings of the human immune and nonimmune defense systems for me has been this: The integrity of human molecular defenses cannot be

---

preserved except through preservation of the gut ecology. My clinical work with chronic fatigue states allowed me to test and validate this fundamental concept with therapies founded on my view of injured bowel ecosystems.

---

## LAPs AND TAPs:
## THE GOOD AND BAD GUYS OF THE BOWEL

---

LAPs and TAPs are my abbreviations for lactic acid-producing and toxic agents-producing microbes in the bowel. LAPs preserve the normal bowel ecosystem, TAPs disrupt it.

In the chapters, What Is Chronic Fatigue? and Where Does It All Begin?, I discuss many elements that increase oxidative stress on energy and detoxification enzymes. It turns out that almost all these elements also suppress LAPs and — both directly by inhibiting LAPs and indirectly by other mechanisms — promote the growth of TAPs. This subject is of enormous significance in the normal aging process as well as in the accelerated aging process associated with chronic fatigue states.

LAPs confer many important host defenses upon the bowel discussed later in this section. TAPs are equally versatile in their functions and produce a very large number of noxious substances in the bowel. Among these are ammonia; phenols; tryptophan metabolites; vaso-constrictive amines such as histamine, tyramine, agmatine and cadaverine; certain steroid metabolites; and many toxins — most notably mycotoxins derived from fungi (yeasts). This area has received rather limited investigative attention, and it is almost certain that future research will uncover a host of as yet undetected bacterial and fungal toxins and metabolic villains. Finally, the bowel flora both produce and potentiate some carcinogenic substances.

Not unexpectedly, LAPs-TAPs dynamics are profoundly influenced by food choices. American and British individuals show overgrowth of some TAPs such as bacteroides and some types of clostridia as compared with Japanese, Indians and Ugandans (*Lancet* 1:95-100; 1971). It appears likely that these differences are due to an abundance of fats and beef in the former populations' diet.

## BACTERIA: THE MASTER CHEMISTS

Bacteria are living beings capable of executing an enormous number of biochemical reactions. Farmers used bacteria and fungi to turn compost into fertilizer long before biologists understood the metabolism of these single-celled bodies. A partial list of such reactions brought about by the normal bowel flora includes production of ammonia, conversion of amino acids into amines and phenols, inactivation of digestive enzymes such as trypsin and chymotrypsin and other enzymes located on the surface of cells lining the gut, deconjugation of hormones such as estrogen and bile acids, denaturation of bile steroids, breakdown of food flavonoids, hydrogenation of polyunsaturated fatty acids in food, utilization of certain amino acids such as $B_{12}$, conversion of some compounds into carcinogens, and many other enzymatic reactions.

I list below the three genera of LAPs and several genera of TAPs that most frequently populate the bowel ecosystem.

| LAPs | TAPs |
|------|------|
| Bifidobacterium | Proteus, Pseudomonas, Salmonella, Escherichia |
| Lactobacillus | Bacteroides, Clostridium, Peptococci, Peptostreptococcus |
| Streptococcus | Streptococcus, Staphylococcus |

About 30 species of LAP microbes have been identified. Some important members of these three groups (L, Lactobacillus; B, Bifidobacterium; S, Streptococcus) include the following:

L. acidophilus            B. bifidum
L. bulgaricus             B. adolescentis
L. lactis                 B. infantis
L. casei                  B. breve
L. helveticus             B. longus
                          S. faecium
                          S. thermophilous

Most byproducts of modern technology threaten LAP microbes. In addition, alcohol, nicotine, various pharmacologic agents, and highly processed and "preserved" foods have a negative impact on lactic-acid producers.

Normal fecal flora in man includes the following:

Bacteroidaceae (Bacteroides and Fusobacteria), Eubacteria, Lactobacilli, Bifidobacteria, Veillonellae, Acidaminococci, Megasphaerae, Peptococcaceae (Ruminococci, Peptococci and Peptostreptococci), Clostridia (C. perfrigens and other species), Enterobacteriaceae, aerobic Lactobacilli, Streptococci, Staphylococci, and yeast and fungi (often used interchangeably).

## LAPs: THE GUARDIAN ANGELS OF HUMAN CANARIES

The LAPs angels look after human canaries in many ways.

First and foremost, LAPs keep TAPs out. It appears that this essential role is played through different mechanisms that include simple physical crowding out of the potential pathogens as well as production of antimicrobial substances. L. acidophilus produces acidophilin, acidolin and bacterlocin; L. plantartium produces lactolin; L. bulgaricus produces bulgarican; and L. brevis secretes lactobacillin.

Second, they produce many life span molecules. Notable among them are members of the vitamin B complex, especially folic acid and biotin and vitamin K. Lactobacillic acid is an important fatty acid that is produced by some lactic-acid producers and is then converted into essential fatty acids. Another notable molecule in this context is tryptophan — this is likely to be one of the mechanisms by which yogurt has been reported to be beneficial in cases of chronic anxiety and other conditions.

Third, they play a pivotal role in digestion. Lactose intolerance is a very common clinical problem. It is often not fully appreciated that a major portion of lactose ingested in dairy products is actually broken down to simpler sugars by lactase enzymes produced by lactic acid producers. Lactic acid and lactase producers also play important roles in protein digestion. This is one of the primary reasons protein intolerance is so common among individuals with altered states of bowel ecology.

Fourth, LAPs actively break down some toxins produced during metabolism such as ammonia, free phenols and polypeptides.

Fifth, LAPs normalize bowel transit time and are effective in controlling infant and adult diarrhea.

Sixth, the antiviral and antifungal roles played by LAPs, having long been empirically suspected by nutritionists and holistic physicians, have recently been documented with research studies.

Seventh, the cholesterol-lowering effects of fermented milk have been attributed, among other mechanisms, to orotic acid, which facilitates fat metabolism in the liver.

Eighth, some LAP microbes suppress tumor cells in rats. This factor is not of direct relevance to human canaries — at least not yet, though in time accelerated oxidative damage is likely to increase the incidence of cancer in chronic fatigue states.

## ALTERED STATES OF GASTRIC ECOLOGY

Altered gastric ecology is one of the dominant chronic disorders of our time. Most — though not all — chronic fatiguers develop problems of indigestion and upper abdominal discomfort after variable periods of fatigue.

A fundamental difference in concept between the altered states of bowel ecology and gastric ecology in the past was that the former was predominantly a "bio-ecosystem" while the latter was essentially a "chemical ecosystem." This concept is rapidly changing; the most visible villain, of course, is the microbe Helicobacter pylori. I have a sense that we will encounter other microbes colonizing the gastric ecosystem in the future as the use of antacids, histamine receptor blockers, nonsteroidal drugs for joint disorders, steroids and other drugs becomes more pervasive.

Gastric acidity — secretion of hydrochloric acid by the stomach lining — is essential for the digestive efficiency of pepsin and for the absorption of minerals such as iron. It is one of the primary host defenses against viral and bacterial infections and against parasitic infestations. Pepsin digestion (and ongoing salivary amylase and other enzyme functions) within the stomach lumen is required for preparing food for digestive-absorptive functions in the small bowel. Normal gastric motility preserves the gastric reservoir function without which undigested foods would readily enter the bowel. A detailed discussion of the patho-physiology of the stomach and derangement of gastric function that lead to gastritis-peptic ulcer continuum as well as to the hypochlorhydria-malabsorption spectrum is outside the scope of this monograph. However, symptom-complexes induced by an altered gastric ecology have become pandemic. Further, bowel ecology disorders frequently cannot be reversed without carefully addressing gastric ecology.

Enzymes are proteins, and are easily injured by accelerated oxidative injury — the root of chronic fatigue. The enzymes of the stomach and intestines are no exception to this. I cite two examples of enzymes that are vulnerable to oxidative injury: $H^+,K^+$-ATPase and rodinase. One type of cell in the stomach lining (parietal cells) in the gastric mucosa secretes hydrochloric acid by a process involving oxidative phosphorylation. This is one of the most astounding phenomena in nature: These cells secrete hydrogen ions at a concentration of about 3 million times that found in blood. So intense is the process that one bicarbonate ion released into the blood as a reciprocal event for secretion of each hydrogen ion causes the *alkaline tide* in the blood Ph. A key enzyme involved in this proton pump mechanism is the specific enzyme, hydrogen-potassium adenosine triphosphatase ($H^+,K^+$-ATPase). Reciprocal bicarbonate release into the blood is mediated by parietal cell carbonic anhydrase.

Rhodanese is a sulfur-transfering enzyme in the surface of cells lining the intestinal surface. It takes cyanide from cyanogenic foods and combines it with thiosulfates to make thiocyanate —a molecule that is necessary for production of acid in the stomach. It is likely that many digestive symptoms in chronic fatigue—especially stomach fullness after small meals—are due to oxidative injury to rhodanese. Thiocyanates are also required for iodine storage as well as for optimal function of ATPase — another essential energy enzyme.

## HYPERCHLORHYDRIA AND HYPOCHLORHYDRIA

Hyperchlorhydria — too much acidity — is a gastric maladaptive response to the changes in gastric ecology in chronic fatiguers. Such persons are often given massive quantities of antacids for "regulating" abnormal patterns of gastric acidity — a sad reflection on our capacity for understanding the true nature of these problems. Antacids suppress gastric acidity when it is needed and promote it (through rebound phenomenon) when it is unnecessary. Antacids are a common source of aluminum overload and toxicity. The worst side-effect of antacids, in my judgment, is this: Antacids suppress the symptoms that draw our attention to the underlying abnormalities of the gastric structure and function.

Hypochlorhydria — not enough gastric acid — is much more common among human canaries. Gastric acidity normally declines as we age. Hypochlorhydria is almost a constant feature of atrophic gastritis in the elderly. It is seen with high frequency in patients with recurrent episodes of chronic gastritis. Studies on healthy college students have shown hypochlorhydria to occur following acute viral infections in one-third to one half of volunteers. Hypochlorhydria occurring as a consequence of acute viral infections in otherwise healthy subjects can be expected to resolve spontaneously within a period of a few weeks.

For suspected or documented gastric hypoacidity, my own clinical preference is to avoid the use of acid-containing products such as betaine hydrochloride. Such products often carry the risk of inducing excessive acidity. The use of herbal digestives (gastric protocol 4 [Floridex] described later in this chapter or similar products) is much more desirable. Patients must be prepared for a slow restorative approach, as is done for other patients managed with nondrug management protocols of molecular medicine. Digestive enzymes (gastric protocol 1) administered with or soon after meals significantly expedite restoration of gastric ecology.

## CLINICAL MANAGEMENT OF ALTERED BOWEL AND GASTRIC ECOLOGIES

The prevailing classification of various types of inflammatory disorders of the bowel is essential for the management of acute, life-threatening pathologic entities with drug regimens and/or surgical procedures. However, I do not address those issues in this volume. Several excellent texts exist to discuss the diagnosis and clinical management of such disorders. Here, my focus is on long-term, nondrug therapies that are designed and implemented to restore the normal bowel ecology and reverse the various disease processes that eventually lead to such bowel diseases as irritable bowel syndrome, spastic colon, inflammatory bowel disease and others. The optimal clinical management of altered states of bowel ecology, in my view, requires that the following issues be effectively addressed.

1. Bowel transit time
2. Bowel perfusion (blood supply)
3. Efficiency of digestive enzymes
4. Efficiency of absorptive mechanisms
5. Preservation and enhancement of normal bowel flora (LAPs)
6. Slow and sustained exclusion of pathologic microbes (TAPs)

Acute, life-threatening bowel disorders, I wrote earlier, require precise diagnosis and prompt use of drug therapies. This is not the focus of this monograph. Rather, it is my purpose to outline nondrug therapies that I have found to be effective for addressing the above elements and for restoring the bowel and gastric ecosystems to their normal states.

## BOWEL TRANSIT TIME

One of my criteria of health, I wrote in *The Butterfly and Life Span Nutrition,* is two to three effortless, odorless bowel movements each day.

This is one area in which I am very rigid in my clinical practice. I consider all treatment plans for diseases of the bowel utterly futile unless the problem of small, shrunken, infrequent stools is first resolved. The bowel transit time in health should range from 8 to 14 hours. This means healthy people should have two or three loose bowel movements a day. Indeed, in my own clinical experience, I find this approach equally important in the management of all chronic immune disorders. More often than not I see people who relate constipation to hard, dried-out stools. It does not seem important to them if they miss a bowel movement for a day or even for two or three days. *It is the bowel transit time that is of central importance to us when we think in terms of the bowel ecosystem.* The problem of hard, shrunken stools is but one aspect of this larger issue. I have had rather extensive experience with the use of nutrients and herbs for normalizing the bowel transit time. Vitamin C, nutrient protocols containing magnesium, bifidus and acidophilus microbes, and several herbs (described later in my bowel ecology protocols) are the best remedies for this purpose. Synthetic chemicals can and must be avoided.

Colonic therapy may be necessary in a very small number of patients with long-standing constipation and impaired colonic motility. Long-term use of colonic therapy for normalization of bowel transit time is not desirable. Some professionals add an oxidative component to their colonic therapies — by bubbling oxygen through their colonic enema fluid. Notwithstanding some temporary benefits such therapy might offer, I do not approve of it because of an enormous potential for oxidative damage to LAPs in the bowel ecosystem.

My specific recommendations for the use of vitamin C, nutrient protocols containing magnesium and bowel ecology protocols for normalizing the bowel transit time are discussed later in this chapter.

## HERBAL AND NUTRIENT PROTOCOLS

In my own clinical practice, I combine several herbs and nutrients to formulate my bowel ecology protocols (BEPs) for managing altered bowel ecology and some others to formulate gastric ecology protocols (GEPs) for managing disrupted gastric ecology.

Before prescribing specific doses of BEPs and GEPs, I prescribe for all my patients a broad basic coverage of vitamins, minerals and essential fatty acids, and some amino acids and herbs when necessary. For this purpose, I have organized a large number of important nutrients into the following nine basic protocols: anti-oxidant, anti-stress, mineral, vitamin C, circulation, omega-3, omega-6, TPM, allergy and amino acids. I use liberal doses of these protocols initially — often to the limit of bowel tolerance. I describe the compositions of these formulations and recommended daily dose schedules in *RDA: Rats, Drugs and Assumptions.*

Allergy and circulation protocols are used for patients with allergic and circulatory disorders. As the clinical picture improves, I gradually taper down the number and doses of protocols used. This is a point of great clinical significance. It is important to note that it is not my purpose to correct any "nutrient deficiencies" that might exist (these almost always exist). Rather, nutrients are the "drugs" I use to restore the various molecular pathways so often stressed in chronic indolent states of altered bowel ecology.

## SEED, FEED AND OCCASIONALLY WEED

A "seed, feed and occasionally weed" holistic approach to the problem of restoring a damaged bowel ecosystem is the centerpiece of my chronic fatigue management.

Seeding is the repopulation of the gut with microflora that have been destroyed by indiscriminate use of antibiotics or crowded out by the unrestrained proliferation of yeast and bacterial organisms such as the Proteus and Pseudomonas species. The "guardian angel bacteria" for bowel ecology belong to the Bifidobacterium and Lactobacillus species. Some other species also play protective roles. In health, these organisms provide the necessary counterbalance to the growth of yeast and pathogenic bacterial organisms. Beyond this, these organisms produce several molecules that play critical roles in our molecular defense systems.

Feeding is the use of some growth factors that the normal bowel flora require to flourish. These include biotin, pantetheine, Vitamin $B_{12}$ and others. We clinicians have used Vitamin $B_{12}$ for decades with good clinical results (to the great chagrin of those "academicians" who considered it quackery because they couldn't understand how this vitamin could ever help anybody except those with pernicious anemia). One of the principal mechanisms by which vitamin $B_{12}$ exerts its myriad beneficial effects is by serving as a "growth hormone" for health-preserving bowel flora. Of course, this vitamin has several other essential roles. It plays a role in the citric acid cycle (the main molecular pathway for energy generation where it facilitates the conversion of methylmalonyl-CoA to succinyl-CoA) and is essential for cell maturation. Further, Vitamin $B_{12}$ benefits many patients with neuropsychiatric disorders unassociated with anemia or macrocytosis (*N Eng J Med* 318:1720; 1988).

My friend, Choua, is fond of saying that the subject of the clinical uses of vitamins is a misunderstood subject, not because sound scientific information does not exist but because such information does not fit into the prevailing model of prescriptive $N^2D^2$ medicine.

Occasional weeding is the use of several natural substances that are known to suppress the overgrowth of pathogenic bacteria, viruses and yeasts. During initial treatment, I frequently use oral nystatin or fluoconazole (Diflucan) for short periods of two to three weeks, partly for diagnostic and partly for therapeutic reasons (how a person with one of the ABE states responds to these agents is useful in assessing the degree of damage to bowel ecology). Extensive clinical experience has convinced me that long-term clinical results are far superior when the use of drugs is kept to a minimum.

Simple-minded efforts to "get rid of the yeast" with nystatin and "yeast-free diets" usually yield poor long-term results. Cold hands are associated with "cold bowel." *Cold hands and cold bowel are the result of oxidatively-damaged thyroid enzymes (underactive thyroid gland), oxidatively-damaged autonomic nerve cells and fibers (dysautonomia) or an oxidatively-overdriven adrenalin gland (the relentless chatter of the cortical monkey).* None of these problems can be effectively managed with yeast-free diets and Nystatin. Of course, there are other essential issues of nutrition, environment, food and mold allergy, and fitness. In the management of battered bowel ecosystems, it is essential to consider the biologic individuality of the patient. It is necessary to adopt an integrated, long-term approach that addresses all relevant issues of bowel flora and parasites, bowel transit time, bowel ischemic patterns, IgE-mediated disorders related to candida and other yeast antigens, malabsorptive dysfunctions, and secondary systemic consequences.

## BOWEL AND GASTRIC ECOLOGY PROTOCOLS

Physicians who are not familiar with natural therapies for managing chronic bowel and gastric disorders are in for a pleasant surprise. A very large number of effective natural agents are available to them. Extensive clinical experience has convinced me that for nonlife-threatening, chronic disorders, natural therapies are far superior to the huge array of drugs that are foisted upon us.

Before giving the composition of several bowel ecology and gastric ecology protocols that I use in my clinical work, I want to make some essential points here:

### First,

all patients should be offered standard drug therapies for acute disorders when any question exists about impending clinical crises or risk of serious complications.

## *Second,*

all patients managed with natural agents should be prepared for *slow and sustained* recovery over weeks and months. It is my practice not to wean my patients off drugs prescribed by other physicians. Rather, my clinical strategy is to go for gentle restoration of bowel and gastric ecologies. The patients sense clinical improvement within several days or some weeks. It is at this time that they ask me if they should begin to reduce the dose of drugs they are taking, and I am only too happy to provide guidance on how to do so *gradually.*

## *Third,*

all patients are required to attend a full-day workshop in which I give detailed information about the devastating impact of internal and external environments on our biology. In addition, nutrition and exercise classes are given by the nursing staff at the institute.

## *Fourth,*

all patients must be managed with an overarching philosophy of *holistic molecular relatedness in human biology.* I repeat this essential point several times at the risk of offending the reader because it is the very *essence* of the new medicine that the problems of the 21st century call for.

## *Fifth,*

and this is of critical importance for the general reader, a self-help approach to health requires guidance from a knowledgeable professional. Safety first. This is the first principle of molecular medicine as it must be for all other types of medicine.

*Persons suffering from chronic fatigue must use the natural remedies I describe below under professional supervision.*

This caution I give above should not be dismissed as a mere disclaimer insisted upon by some attorney. It must be heeded. Disabling chronic fatigue is not a problem that can be resolved on a self-help basis.

| BOWEL ECOLOGY PROTOCOL 1 | |
|---|---|
| Bifidobacterium species<br>Lactobacillus species | Total count more than<br>one billion organisms |
| Biotin | 25   mcg |
| PABA | 2   mg |
| Pantetheine | 2   mg |
| L-Histidine | 5   mg |
| L-Arginine | 5   mg |
| Aloe vera | 2   mg |
| Spirulina | 10   mg |

| BOWEL ECOLOGY PROTOCOL 2 | |
|---|---|
| Alfalfa | 500 mg |
| Pau D'arco | 100 mg |
| Allicin | 100 mg |
| Licorice root (deglycerrizinated) | 200 mg |
| **BOWEL ECOLOGY PROTOCOL 3** | |
| Calcium caprylate | 50 mg |
| Magnesium caprylate | 50 mg |
| Grapefruit seed extract | 25 mg |
| Aloe vera | 1 mg |
| Spirulina | 10 mg |
| **BOWEL ECOLOGY PROTOCOL 4** | |
| Grapefruit seed extract | 50 mg |
| Allicin | 50 mg |
| Pau D'arco | 500 mg |

| BOWEL ECOLOGY PROTOCOL 5 ||
|---|---|
| Artemisia annui | 150 mg |
| Pau D'arco | 150 mg |
| Beet root fiber | 150 mg |
| Guar gum | 150 mg |
| **BOWEL ECOLOGY PROTOCOL 6** ||
| Echinacea | 200 mg |
| Golden seal | 150 mg |
| Astragalus | 150 mg |
| Burdock root | 150 mg |
| **BOWEL ECOLOGY PROTOCOL 7** ||
| Cascara sagrada | 250 mg |
| Alfalfa | 50 mg |
| Beet fiber | 50 mg |
| Goldenseal | 50 mg |
| **BOWEL ECOLOGY PROTOCOL 8** ||
| Defatted rice bran | 400 mg |
| Beet fiber | 100 mg |
| Guar gum | 100 mg |

| BOWEL ECOLOGY PROTOCOL 9 | |
|---|---|
| Tumeric | 200 mg |
| Milk thistle | 200 mg |
| Artichoke | 150 mg |
| Golden seal | 150 mg |

| GASTRIC ECOLOGY PROTOCOL 1 | |
|---|---|
| Papain* | 50 mg |
| Amylase | 50 mg |
| Lipase | 50 mg |
| Protease | 50 mg |
| Pancreatin | 100 mg |

| GASTRIC ECOLOGY PROTOCOL 2 | |
|---|---|
| Aloe vera gel | 2 mg |
| Deglycerrizinated licorice | 500 mg |
| Black currant seed | 75 mg |
| L-Arginine HCl | 25 mg |

*All enzymes in gastric ecology protocol 1 are derived from bovine tissue except for papain which is of plant origin.

| GASTRIC ECOLOGY PROTOCOL 3 | |
|---|---|
| Betaine hydrochloride | 75 mg |
| Ammonium chloride | 50 mg |
| Calcium chloride | 50 mg |
| **GASTRIC ECOLOGY PROTOCOL 4** | |
| Artichoke | 650 mg |
| Dandelion | 207 mg |
| Gentian root | 164 mg |
| Turmeric root | 118 mg |
| Milfoil (Yarrow) | 118 mg |
| Chamomile flowers | 74 mg |
| Fennel | 74 mg |
| Holy thistle seed | 30 mg |
| Buckbean leaves | 15 mg |
| Pear juice concentrate | 3.6 mg |

The above formulation is commercially available as *Floridex Bitters*. It acts as a herbal bitter and is recommended for patients with hypochlorhydria. It stimulates the secretion of acid and digestive enzymes in the stomach and intestine. Dose: two to four teaspoons 30 minutes before meals as an appetizer or after meals as a digestive supplement.

| BROMELAIN PROTOCOL | |
| --- | --- |
| Bromelain | 500 mg |
| Vitamin C | 50 mg |

## USE OF ANTIFUNGAL AGENTS

I write earlier that my basic philosophy for managing altered bowel ecology (ABE) states is my *Seed, Feed and Occasionally Weed* approach.

I generally begin my management of ABE with a short course of Nystatin, 500,000 units four times a day, usually for a period of two to three weeks, in tablet or powder form. Initially I reduce the dose to one-half tablet twice a day and then gradually build the dose to full dose of four tablets a day if there are any problems of tolerance. I have two objectives in this therapy. First, it reduces the bowel burden of yeasts and allows a rather quick clinical response and relief of many ABE-related symptoms. Second, it gives the patient and me a sense of the role played by yeast overgrowth in the bowel symptomatology. I do not think it is advisable — as I often see in patients consulting me after management by other physicians — to keep patients on Nystatin for periods of several months at a time. Not unexpectedly, prolonged Nystatin therapy eradicates the yeast strains that are sensitive to this antifungal agent causing other resistant strains to thrive. The result: a relatively simple problem is turned into a major one. This is one of the serious consequences of the simplistic notion that the "yeast can be cured." If considered necessary, short courses of Nystatin may be used after an interval of some weeks or months. Certainly, its use should be considered when the use of antibiotics cannot be judiciously avoided for persons with chronic ABE states.

In order to prevent initial symptoms of the so-called "yeast die-off," I often ask patients with severe ABE-related symptoms to begin with smaller doses (250,000 units of Nystatin twice a day), and then gradually increase the drug dose (250,000 units three times a day) to yet larger doses (250,000 units four times a day). As drug tolerance improves, the dose can be increased to the full dose.

Nystatin is given in doses of 500,000 units (capsules or powder form) four times a day. If tongue coating, foul odor or thrush is present, a Nystatin solution should be swished around in the mouth for 2-3 minutes before swallowing the solution.

Fluconazole (Diflucan) may be used in doses of 50 to 100 mg daily for a period of two to three weeks. This drug is prohibitively expensive, requires careful monitoring of liver function, and in my judgment does not offer significant advantages over the less expensive Nystatin. Still, it is a good alternative drug in uncommon cases where Nystatin intolerance exists. Nizoral carries a much larger risk of liver injury and requires careful follow-up with laboratory tests. I have not used this drug in several years so it is my sense that it is not difficult to avoid.

## GUIDELINES FOR THE USE OF BOWEL AND GASTRIC ECOLOGY PROTOCOLS

Following are some general guidelines for the use of various bowel ecology protocols (BEPs) based on considerable personal clinical experience as well as the experience of several colleagues. To reiterate, each patient requires an individualized management strategy. Also, the more natural and milder the agents used, the better the long-term clinical results. BEPs # 1 through 6 are given in doses of three to four tablets or capsules daily. Protocols 7 and 8 are used to optimize bowel motility and decrease bowel transit time. I usually recommend two to four tablets of these BEPs at night to assure two to three effortless, odorless bowel movements a day. The BEP 7 contains cascara and acts like a strong laxative. The usual dose is one to two tablets at bedtime. Protocol intolerance, if it occurs, is usually of short duration. It can be managed with gradual escalation of the dose (one tablet first day, two the second day and so forth). These protocols are given with the same dosage schedule for other variants of the ABE states. Diflucan is used in doses of 100 to 200 mg once daily. Sialic acid in doses of 500 mg four times a day may be added in some instances.

It is not unusual for some patients with battered bowel ecosystems to face some difficulty with initial tolerance of various BEPs (usually bowel cramps or diarrhea). I usually reduce by one half the dose prescribed BEPs. Sometimes, I also reduce by one half the dose of vitamin C and protocols that contain magnesium such as TPM. On rare occasions, I discontinue all protocols and begin slowly all over again.

## ACUTELY ALTERED STATES OF BOWEL ECOLOGY

It is essential to remember that acute, life-threatening bowel disorders require precise histopathologic diagnosis and prompt pharmacologic and/or surgical intervention. In such cases, I refer my patients to my colleagues in gastroenterology for standard drug therapies or surgical procedures. For the purpose of the management approach under discussion, acute altered bowel ecology (ABE) states are present when the symptoms are acutely distressing for the patient for a duration of less than three months, and yet there is no serious hazard in withholding standard drug therapies — for instance, standard drug therapies have repeatedly failed to bring clinical relief.

## INITIAL THERAPY FOR ACUTE ABE STATES

| | |
|---|---|
| Nystatin tablets* (500,000 units) | 3 or 4 tablets daily for 4 weeks |
| or Diflucan tablets** (100 mg) | One tablet daily for 4 weeks |

* In order to prevent or reduce initial problems of tolerance, I prescribe Nystatin in gradually increasing doses as follows:
> Days 1 and 2: one half with breakfast and one half with dinner
> Days 3 and 4: one half tablet with breakfast, lunch and dinner
> Days 5 and 6: One tablet with breakfast, lunch and dinner
> Days 7 to 28: One tablet with breakfast and lunch, and two tablets with dinner.

** Diflucan dose may also be divided in two halves with meals to reduce initial intolerance problems.

| INTERMEDIATE THERAPY FOR ACUTE ABE | |
| --- | --- |
| BEP 1: One tab four times a day<br>BEP 6: One tab twice a day | Alternate weeks |
| BEP 3: One tab four times a day<br>BEP 5: One tab twice a day | Alternate weekls |

I prescribe BEP protocols after the initial course of Nystatin (or Diflucan) is finished in order to reduce initial intolerance problems.

| FOLLOW-UP THERAPY FOR ACUTE ABE | |
| --- | --- |
| BEP 1 and BEP 6: one tab each<br>three times a day | Alternate weeks |
| BEP 2 and BEP 5: one tab each<br>three times a day | Alternate weeks |

BEP 3 or 4 may be substituted for BEP 6, and BEP 9 may be substituted for BEP 5.

---

## SUBACUTELY ALTERED STATES OF BOWEL ECOLOGY

I use this clinical term to refer to acute and persistent bowel symptoms of longer than six months duration. Not unexpectedly, there will be instances of overlap between this category and acute as well as chronic ABE states. I use this term more as a working definition for clinical work and do not imply specific histopathologic patterns of structural bowel injury.

| INITIAL THERAPY FOR SUBACUTE ABE | |
|---|---|
| Nystatin: one tablet four times a day with meals | Two weeks |
| or Diflucan: one tablet daily | Two weeks |
| INTERMEDIATE THERAPY FOR SUBACUTE ABE | |
| BEP 1: 1 tablet four times a day<br>BEP 3: 1 tablet four times a day | Alternate BEP 1 and BEP 3 on weekly basis |
| BEP 2: 1 tablet four times a day<br>BEP 5: 1 tablet four times a day | Alternate BEP 2 and BEP 4 on weekly basis |

Continue this weekly rotation for six weeks, then review results in follow-up visit. BEP 4 may be substituted for BEP 3, and BEP 9 may be substituted BEP 2 in case of limited initial intolerance.

| FOLLOW-UP THERAPY | |
|---|---|
| BEP 1: 1 tablet four times a day | Alternate weeks |
| BEP 2: 1 tablet three times a day | Alternate weeks |

Continue this weekly rotation for three months, then review progress in a follow-up visit.

## CHRONICALLY ALTERED STATES OF BOWEL ECOLOGY

It is important to prepare patients who have suffered from chronic, indolent bowel symptomatology for long periods of time for a slow and sustained recovery taking as long as several months. This category includes patients who have received prolonged broad-spectrum antibiotic therapy and those whose bowel ecosystems have been literally destroyed by long-term steroid and other immunosuppressive therapies and/or multiple surgical attempts to relieve chronic bowel symptoms. Not infrequently, patients in this group give a history of extensive antifungal therapy with Nystatin, Nizoral or Diflucan therapies. Both the patient and the professional in such cases fail to see the obvious: Prolonged antifungal therapies eradicate fungal strains that respond to the agent used and lead to overgrowth of resistant fungal strains, usually with disastrous results.

| INITIAL THERAPY FOR CHRONIC ABE ||
|---|---|
| BEP 1: one tab four times a day<br>BEP 6: one tab four times a day | Alternate weeks |
| BEP 2: one tab four times a day<br>BEP 5: one tab four times a day | Alternate weeks |

Continue this rotation for eight weeks and assess the outcome with a follow-up visit.

## FOLLOW-UP THERAPY FOR CHRONIC ABE

A holistic approach with a full focus on all the issues of nutrition, allergy and chemical sensitivity, stress, and fitness usually gives good results with the above therapy. If satisfactory results are not obtained within four to six weeks, I reevaluate the entire case and make appropriate changes.

I favor the use of natural substances over antifungal

drugs for patients  in this category. I indicated  earlier  that  in my
experience  long-term  results  are better  with this approach.  Of
course,  the  use  of  antifungal  drugs  sometimes  becomes
necessary  if acute  symptoms  develop,  for instance  with  the
onset  of a respiratory  or urinary  infection.

## MANAGEMENT  OF  ABE  STATES
## ASSOCIATED  WITH  PARASITIC  INFESTATIONS

Infestation  of  the  bowel  with  parasites  for  human
canaries  is simply  a matter  of time.  This for me is the  single
most important  issue  in parasitic  diseases  of the  bowel. Parasitic
infestation  should be assumed  — unless  specifically excluded with
appropriate  tests performed  with a rectal  mucus  swab  or other
suitable  methods  —  when  the  bowel  ecosystem  has  been
damaged.  For example,  giardiasis  is now endemic  in both  New
York City and the Rockies around  Denver,  and this parasite can
be detected  in many chronic fatiguers.

Intestinal  parasites  coexist  with us just  as other  living
beings do. Elimination  of bowel parasites  from our environment
is as simplistic  a notion  as banishing  ants and houseflies  from
our towns and cities. In health,  the high level of acidity in the
stomach  destroys  parasites  that enter  human  body with water
and  food.  Diminished  acidity  (hypochlorhydria)  is  now
pandemic,  and reduction  in acidity caused by pervasive abuse of
antacids  further  weakens  this essential  defense  system  of the
body against  parasites.

Blastocystis  hominis  in  many  regions  is  the  most

commonly encountered parasites. Other commonly found parasites are Dientamoeba, Giardia, and various amebas (Entamoeba histolytica, Entamoeba coli, Entamoeba hartmanni, Endolimax and Iodamoeba butschlii).

The treatment of acute parasitic infestation often requires specific drug therapies for specific parasites. For chronic parasitic infestation of the bowel, I describe below my comprehensive program of parasite eradication that employs several natural antiparasitic herbs, digestive enzymes, and small doses of hydrochloric acid. I might add here that I use bowel ecology protocol 5 containing Artemisia liberally whenever I suspect that parasitic infestation exists but cannot conclusively prove. This Chinese herb, of course, has other beneficial effects in restoring normal bowel ecology.

The issue of parasite pathogenicity — ability of the parasites to cause clinical disorders — is quite complex, and I discuss it at length in *Battered Bowel Ecology — Waving Away A Wandering Wolf*. The essential point in the context of chronic fatigue is this: Many parasites such as Blastocystis that are commonly regarded as nonpathogenic must be considered significant in the battered bowel ecosystems of chronic fatiguers.

## FOUR-WEEK UDARTE AND GOZARTE PROTOCOL

Udarte contains pringamoza, a component of South American herb Uda that is conjugated with Artemesia for enhancement of its antiparasitic activity. Gozarte contains gossypol that is conjugated with Artmesia to enhance its antiparasitic activity.

After the 8-week parasite is finished, I follow it with a 4-week Udarte-Gozarte protocol. I prescribe Udarte (one capsule three times day between meals) for one week and follow that with Gozarte (one capsule three times a day with meals) for one week. This two-week program is repeated to complete four-week program.

| EIGHT-WEEK SCHEDULE FOR PARASITIC INFESTATIONS | |
| --- | --- |
| Bowel ecology protocol 5 | 1 tablet four times a day with meals |
| Gastric ecology protocol 1 | 2 tablets one hour before breakfast<br>2 tablets one hour before lunch<br>2 tablets two hours before dinner |
| Gastric ecology protocol 3 | 2 tablets with breakfast<br>2 tablets with lunch<br>2 tablets with dinner |
| Bromelain | 2 tablets one hour before breakfast<br>2 tablets one hour before breakfast<br>2 tablets one hour before dinner |

\* Gastric ecology protocol contains betaine hydrochloric acid and should be used with caution in patients with history of gastric and duodenal ulcers.

This is a slight modification of a digestive enzymes and hydrochloric acid formulation that has been used successfully by many naturopathic physicians for decades. I have learned much from my colleagues in naturopathic medicine. I take this opportunity to express my gratitude to them.

The rectal mucus test for parasites should be repeated to assess the efficacy of the treatment.

Following is the patient instruction sheet my staff uses to facilitate the use of the eight-week protocol for intestinal parasitic infestations.

| PATIENT INSTRUCTION SHEET FOR EIGHT-WEEK SCHEDULE | |
| --- | --- |
| Breakfast | with breakfast: 2 tablets of GEP 3<br>one hour before breakfast:<br>2 tablets GEP 1<br>2 tablets bromelain protocol |
| Lunch | with lunch: 2 tablets GEP 3<br>one hour before lunch<br>2 tablets GEP 1<br>2 tablets bromelain protocol |
| Dinner | with dinner: 2 tablets GEP 3<br>Two hours before dinner:<br>2 tablets GEP 1<br>2 tablets bromelain protocol |

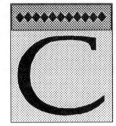

**C**hapter 11

# Limbic
# Exercise
# for Chronic
# Fatigue

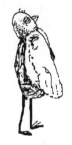

There are six important issues for chronic fatiguers in the area of physical fitness.

## First,

exercise is essential for the recovery process, although physical fitness through exercise understandably is the last concern of chronic fatiguers.

## Second,

exercise for chronic fatiguers must be slow and sustained, heeding signals from the tissues in the limbs.

## Third,

exercise with commonly recommended videos and hi-tech indoor training equipment should be avoided.

## Fourth,

exercise should never be done to test the limits of physical endurance in chronic fatigue states.

## Fifth,

exercise must be done in the morning to up-regulate energy enzymes — even if the energy changes may be imperceptible — and to free the musculoskeletal restrictions that always develop during sleeping hours.

## Sixth,

exercise should be combined with meditation and spiritual search. This may seem like strange advice to chronic fatiguers, but extensive clinical experience with persistent, severe fatigue has convinced me of its validity.

---

## BEATING UP ON INJURED TISSUES DOESN'T WORK

---

Commonly recommended exercise programs are unsuitable for chronic fatiguers. Many of my canaries were athletes, dancers and trainers participating in fitness programs before they developed chronic fatigue. Invariably they told of their attempts to simply pull themselves out of disabling fatigue with sheer willpower. Energy enzymes do not care for our mind-over-body notions of health and disease. All these patients succeeded in achieving were yet more sore muscles and bruised spirits. Tired tissues get more tired. Aching muscles ache further. Anxiety intensifies. Depression deepens.

---

## EXERCISE INCREASES OXIDANT STRESS

---

This should not come as a surprise after the discussion of spontaneity of oxidation and the redox reaction in the preceding chapters. Sudden and repetitive movements in exercise require sudden and repetitive bursts of energy; and energy, of course, can be obtained from oxidative activities in the body. Since chronic fatigue is fundamentally a state of oxygen dysregulation, oxidatively damaged energy enzymes can be expected to poorly tolerate further oxidative stress associated with physical exercise. This indeed does happen.

*"Dr. Ali, I exercised with a video last week. For the next three days, I couldn't move my legs. I couldn't even do the few simple things I could do before I did the darned thing with the video. Then my depression nearly killed me."*

A human canary

Blood circulation and metabolism in the brain has been studied in chronic fatiguers with SPECT and PET scans during demand-type exercise. The results of such studies, of course, have been entirely predictable. Blood flow in the brain in chronic fatigue actually decreases and metabolism slows down — both consequences of oxidative dysregulation.

Does that mean that chronic fatiguers should not exercise? Of course, not. As stated, exercise is essential for recovery from chronic fatigue. On the surface, this seems contradictory. On deeper reflection, it isn't.

In *The Ghoraa and Limbic Exercise,* I described two different types of exercise: cortical and limbic. These two types of exercise involve two different types of muscle fibers, employ different types of energy mechanisms, and create totally different types of energy and health effects.

## CORTICAL AND LIMBIC EXERCISES

Cortical exercises are intense, competitive, and goal-oriented. These exercises are of *the stop-and-go* type. In cortical exercises, Type II muscle fibers burn sugar to generate quick bursts of energy, much like a piece of dry paper burns to produce sudden heat with a flash but only for a few moments. These muscle fibers have fewer mitochondria and are poor in mitochondrial oxidative enzymes. Unable to use fatty acids for energy, they follow the path of least resistance and burn whatever sugars are available to them (the glycolytic or sugar-burning molecular pathways for energy generation).

Cortical exercises emphasize technique, style, duration and results. The best examples of cortical exercise are competition sports and athletics such as wrestling, bodybuilding, football, tennis, basketball and soccer. Sharply focused, highly intense and meticulously analyzed cortical exercises are evidently essential for such sports.

Limbic exercises are *continuous,* nonintense, nongoal-oriented, noncompetitive exercises. In such exercises, Type I muscle fibers burn fats to generate energy, much like a candle burns wax to generate light slowly but for a long time. These muscle fibers are rich in mitochondria — and the oxidative enzymes contained in them. They are designed to break down fats and utilize the fatty acids liberated from fats by their oxidative enzymes.

In limbic exercises, there is no hyperventilation nor perspiration. When done *limbically*, exercise ends with more energy than that with which it began. The essence of limbic exercise is the absence of focus. When we run limbically, we do just that — we simply run. There is no effort made to run well, to run at some predetermined speed, to run for some defined distance or to run to solve the problems of the day. When we walk, we simply walk. We make no attempt to solve our problems nor sit in judgment of how we walk. Limbic exercises are done with abandonment, with total disregard of all the demands of the thinking mind.

Cortical exercises are performed while taking commands from the thinking mind. Limbic exercises, by contrast, are exercises done while we take counsel from our tissues, counsel from muscles that contract to produce motion, counsel from tendons that carry the commands from the muscles to the bones, counsel from the ligaments that hold the bones together and counsel from bones that provide muscles their scaffolds. We take counsel from lungs that bring air into the body and from the heart that pumps the blood to spread nourishment to the body tissues. A period of listening to body tissues (and dismissing all demands from the thinking mind — the cortical monkey) is a necessary prelude to limbic exercise. It generally requires several minutes before we begin limbic exercises. With continued limbic exercise comes what I call "limbic openness."

Limbic openness is a period of inner reflection, meditation, prayer and deep visceral stillness. There is no rush of cortical thoughts. There is only a *limbic* flow of perceptions. I urge the reader to read the chapter Unto the Rising Sun in

*The Ghoraa and Limbic Exercise* for valuable insights into the state of limbic openness as well as practical suggestions for reaching this state.

---

## HIGH OXIDATIVE SPARKS, LOW OXIDATIVE FLAME

The critical issue in necessary exercise for chronic fatiguers is this: While high oxidative sparks of cortical goal-oriented, competitive exercise further feed the frenzy of the oxidative storms in chronic fatigue, the low oxidative flame of limbic exercise — with profound physiologic and energy advantages of the limbic state — do not pose such threat. The limbic state is a regenerative state — a healing state. This has been a gift of insight to me from my human canaries.

---

## CORTICAL AND LIMBIC PACING

Cortical pacing is the speed and intensity of exercise determined by professional trainers or by makers of exercise videos. It is a pace designed to keep tight schedules. Limbic pacing is a mode of exercise whereby a person allows himself to simply follow his inner "limbic voice." This voice may wish him to walk slowly or quickly, run with arms swinging from the shoulders or just hanging by the side; it may urge him to continue or stop.

## CORTICAL  GREED  AND  LIMBIC  GRATITUDE

Cortical greed is the irrepressible desire to "do exercise right." It is putting demands on injured tissues to perform according to some preconceived — and frivolous — notions of achievement. Cortical demands negate the very idea of allowing the limbs to lead. This is a point of enormous practical significance, and has been the most common initial obstacle encountered by my human canaries when attempting to learn limbic exercise.

Limbic gratitude is the sense with which we accept whatever responses we receive from our tissues when we do limbic exercise. It is gratitude in receiving, at a nonintellectual, limbic level.

Cortical greed breeds cortical clutter — the ceaseless chatter of the mind when we try to do limbic exercise. It consists of all the "What if", "Why couldn't it", "Why not", "Why me" and all of the other favorite lines we use for punishing our tissues. Unfortunately, canceling cortical clutter is easier said than done. There are other less threatening forms of cortical clutter, for example, planning your day during your walk, or examining somebody else running on the same track, or simply not wanting to exercise because it is Sunday or Saturday or the 4th of July.

Anger and hostility are the first casualties of self-regulation, I wrote in *The Cortical Monkey and Healing*. Limbic exercise in chronic fatigue states is one of the most rewarding ways of dissipating anger and hostility. I discuss this subject further in the chapter, On Hope, Spirituality and Chronic Fatigue.

## MORNING IS A DIFFICULT TIME FOR MANY CHRONIC FATIGUERS

Morning is a time for renewal — with the language of silence and a deep sense of gratitude for simply being alive. For chronic fatiguers who have not yet ventured into the world of silence and spirituality, these words might seem like a cruel joke.

Nights are often restless for chronic fatiguers. They often wake up just as tired as when they went to bed. Mornings bring yet more difficult days ahead. Morning is the best time for limbic exercise. I ask my human canaries to heed their mornings. The days, I know, will take care of themselves. I reproduce below some text from *The Ghoraa and Limbic Exercise* that is relevant to my comments about the morning for chronic fatiguers.

## FACING THE EASTERN SKY

In my view, whatever one does for exercise later in the

day, he must have a *daily* morning period of limbic exercise and silence facing the eastern sky, even if this time can be only a few minutes. Also, this time must include a few moments of initial neck, back and limb stretching, and some forehead and temple message. I have several sound reasons for this recommendation.

### First,

the morning sets the tone for the day. We usually wake up with the cortical monkey. This monkey, of course, loves to recycle the misery of our yesterdays. When that doesn't sustain him, he precycles the feared future misery of our tomorrows. All of us need to unclutter our minds in the morning. There is no better way of doing that than limbic exercise.

### Second,

the morning offers several physical and mechanical advantages over all other times for limbic exercise. The morning is the best time to relieve the strain on muscles, tendons, ligaments and other connective tissue that results from one's sleeping posture. Reverse isometric exercises for neck and low back muscles are essential preventive measures against chronic neck and backaches.

### Third,

the morning is the best time to obtain a state of slight overhydration for the rest of the day. Most of us stay in a state of dehydration when not making a conscious effort to drink fluids. I include a brief note about my own daily routine later in this section.

## Fourth,

most people can control their schedule best in the morning. All that is required is rising a little earlier (and going to sleep a little earlier, a small price to pay to start a new day right.

## Fifth,

the early morning hours are a time of high molecular turmoil. This time of day, I discuss earlier in this chapter, carries some well-recognized hazards for people with heart and vascular disorders. Limbic lengthening followed by slow, sustained exercise offers considerable protection from these risks.

## Sixth,

and most important from my personal perspective, morning is the best time for perceiving the energy of the native human condition. It is a time for limbic openness through limbic exercise. It is a time for silence. It is a time for achieving higher states of consciousness, a time for *being*. It is a time for seeking a link between the gentle guiding energy within us and the gentle guiding energy around us — the energy of that larger *presence* that surrounds each one of us at all times.

From personal observations I know that my general level

of energy and sense of well-being is profoundly affected by my
state of hydration. During the first one hour of the morning
before I leave for the hospital, I drink about 36 ounces of fluids
— half as plain water with my nutrient supplements and half
with a peptide and protein drink mixed with vegetable juice.
Five days a week, this carries me through to lunch time at about
1 P.M. Coffee or tea are not a part of my morning. Without this
much fluid, I sense a need for coffee the way I used to before
I changed from being a disease-doctor to a physician devoted to
health and preventive medicine.

## LIMBIC LENGTHENING

Limbic lengthening is a set of physical steps that allows
gentle, sustained lengthening of the muscles and connective
tissue — ligaments, tendons and other forms of tissues that hold
together muscles fibers and other tissues. The essential point in
limbic lengthening — by contrast to common methods of muscle
stretching — is this: We should *never* use a degree of force that
makes us uncomfortable. On the following pages are five steps
for specific lengthening exercises for the neck that are very
beneficial for people with chronic neck pain and stiffness.
Before you try these five steps, move your neck gently in a
circle and feel the presence or absence of any muscle stiffness
or pain. Now follow the five steps:

## *First Step*

Rub the neck and shoulder muscles between your two

palms to loosen them and warm them up for one or two minutes. Next do a temple message with a *gentle*, rolling motion of your palms placed on your temples as shown in the illustration below.

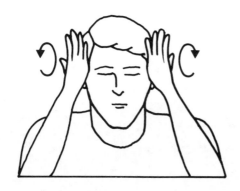

## Second and Third Steps

Turn your neck to the left as far as it will go without causing any discomfort. Put your right hand firmly on your left temple as shown in A. Push your neck firmly against the left hand. There should be no actual movement in the neck, the push of the neck should be balanced by the push of the hand. Count to 10 and let go. Repeat the same steps with the opposite side as shown in B.

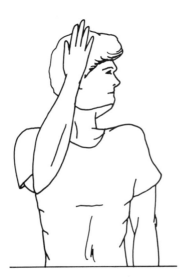 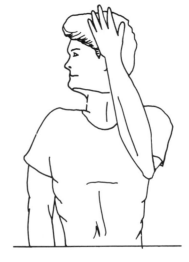

## *Fourth and Fifth Step*

Flex (bend forward) your neck as far as it will go without causing discomfort and put your two hands on the back of the head as shown in the diagram as shown in C. Push your head up against the two hands as much as you can without causing any discomfort. There should be no actual movement of the neck. Count to 10 and let go. Extend (bend backward) your neck and put your two hands on your forehead as shown in D. Follow the same instructions for bending your neck backward as for bending your neck forward.

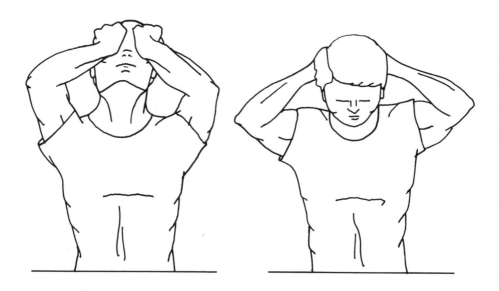

## Sixth Step

Move your neck in *gentle* circles, with the head rolling from right side to back to left and extension  as shown in the diagram given below and see how much freer your neck is now compared with the same movements before doing the preceding five steps.

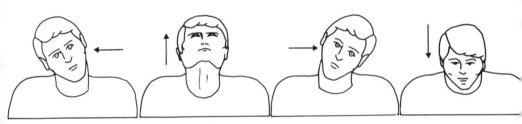

## LIMBIC LENGTHENING OF MUSCLES

Limbic lengthening for specific muscles of the shoulder, back, thighs and legs can be developed using the principle of reverse isometrics. If necessary, a professional may be consulted for learning lengthening exercises for different parts of the body.

Limbic lengthening that includes all major muscle groups should be done several times during the day even while working. The principle of limbic lengthening is the same regardless of what body tissues are in play: Muscles and ligaments are stretched in a gentle and sustained fashion.

Limbic lengthening of the connective tissue and muscle fibers is essential for success in exercise. The exercise illustrated below seeks gentle lengthening of ligaments, tendons and muscles of the back and the calf with gentle, sustained tension for two or three minutes. The arrows indicate the locations of gentle and progressive tension in the first step (A). In the second step, the direction of the gentle lengthening stresses on the back muscles changes as shown in (B).

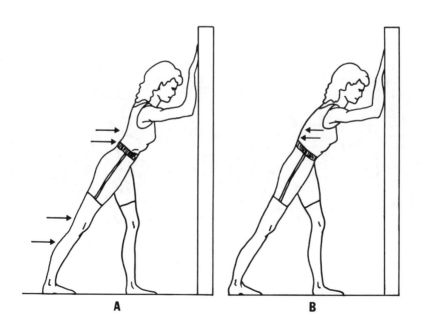

A        B

The diagram below illustrates gentle, sustained lengthening of a large number of muscles and ligaments in the thigh and leg, and the muscles of back when the individual leans forward to touch the wall.

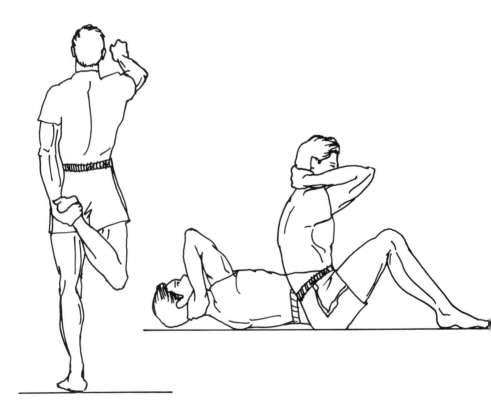

The diagrams given below illustrate gentle lengthening of the muscles of legs, thigh, abdominal, shoulder, neck and back muscles. These exercises are more demanding than those illustrated previously. Chronic fatigue sufferers should be very careful in putting undue stresses on their tissues. They may wish to do these exercises after finishing other exercises, when my muscles and ligaments have been warmed up and loosened with limbic exercise.

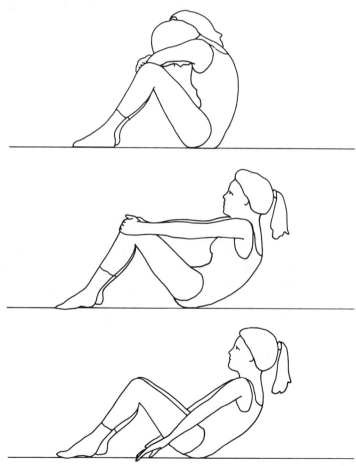

---

Some simple lengthening exercises that are suitable for work hours are shown below. It is a common mistake to think that exercise must produce immediate physical effects to be of any value. Such thinking is clearly not relevant to chronic fatigue sufferers.

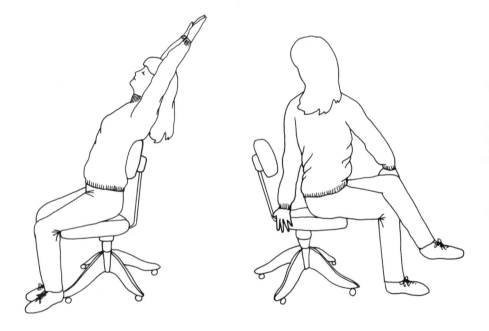

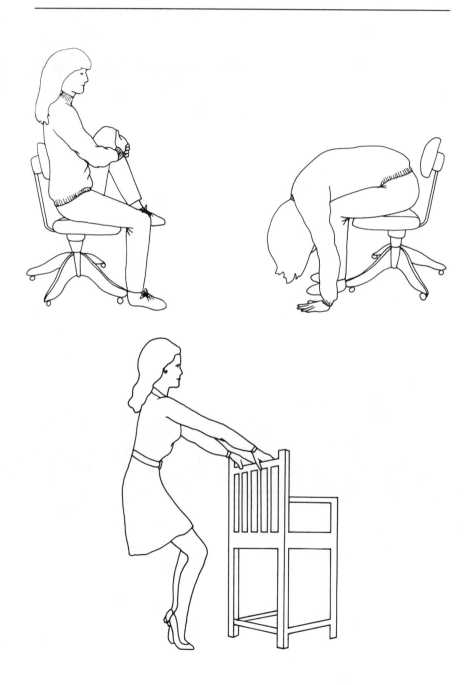

## LIMBIC WALK ON A TRAMPOLINE

"Limbic walk" on a trampoline is an expression I use for walking in place on a trampoline with limbic openness — without any affirmations, without any mind-over-body notions, without any demands on tissues and without any goals. Such walking on trampoline lengthens the connective tissue and invigorates the muscles more effectively than ordinary walking on flat a surface. Actual physical steps for limbic walking on a trampoline are illustrated in the two diagrams below. Note that the toes in the diagrams do not lose contact with the trampoline during the walk. This greatly reduces excessive stress on tired and aching muscles and weakened connective tissue in chronic fatiguers.

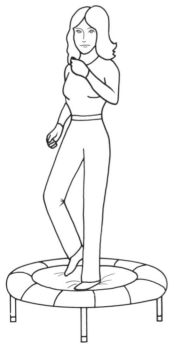 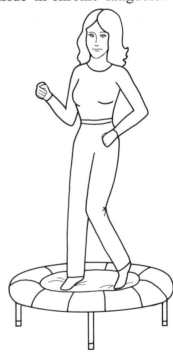

With some practice, chronic fatiguers can learn to walk with eyes half-closed or completely shut. Next, I recommend that the person begin to breathe slowly — with long, sustained breathe-out periods using the following counts: Breathe-in, two, three...hold, two three...breathe-out, two, three, four, five and so on. The breathing should be abdominal, with the abdominal wall moving out with each breathe-in phase and falling back in again with each breathe-out phase. The shoulder and chest muscles should be kept still. This, in essence, is the limbic breathing that I describe in detail in *The Cortical Monkey and Healing*.

Diagrams given below illustrate some other steps that are effective in freeing musculoskeletal restrictions in limb and torso muscles.

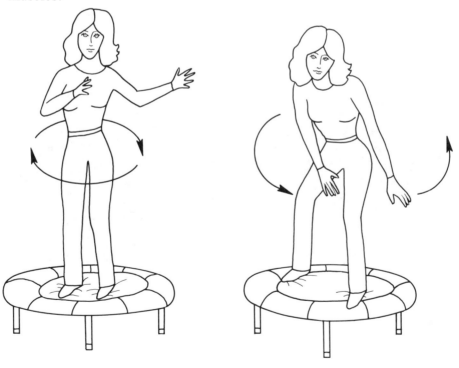

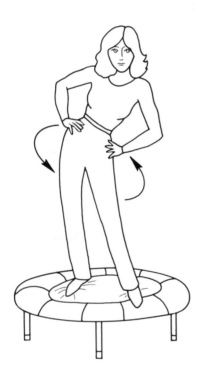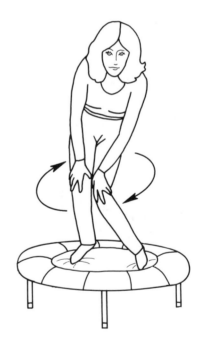

## LIMBIC EXERCISE CYCLING

For several reasons, I recommend that chronic fatiguers begin limbic exercise with an exercise cycle. The cycle used should be an inexpensive one without any electronic gimmicks. Flashing, ticking and beeping video screens on exercise equipment are cortical devices, pure and simple. They are completely and utterly irrelevant to our desire to achieve limbic openness through limbic exercise and the language of silence.

Three elements are essential for limbic exercise with an exercise cycle:

*First,*

we set no goals.

Goals are cortical devices. We do not need them in limbic exercise. In the context of limbic exercise, setting goals for exercise is nothing more than scheming to punish tissues. Consider, for example, the simplest of all goals: duration of exercise. How many of us think of doing exercise for 20 or 30 minutes, look at our watches, and decide that so much time simply cannot be dedicated to exercise that day? How many of us think of how hard we need to drive our muscles, hearts and lungs for the putative cardiovascular and respiratory benefits of exercise? How many of us invest money in expensive futuristic gadgets but seldom, if ever, use such equipment? How many of us see our impulses to exercise killed by a cortical censor?

## Second,

we let our eyes fall upon something and let them stay with it.

That something for the eyes may be a branch of a tree or a twig of a bush visible through a window, a patch of snow or grass, a cloud in the sky, or simply a picture of a flower if no suitable windows are available. With time, the eyes become heavy and want to close.

## Third,

we let our eyes close if they wish to do so.

As we learn to keep our cortical monkey out of the way of our eyes, our eyes begin to follow their own inner cues: Sometimes they want to stay closed, and at other times they wish to open. We must simply accept what they choose to do.

I repeat, any exercise is better than no exercise. Thus, exercises done with exercise videos, music or even with TV news all have some benefits. None of these exercises, however, leads us down the path of limbic listening. None of these exercises can banish the cortical monkey. None of these exercises can lead us the way the eastern sky lit by a rising sun does. Exercise with a treadmill clearly is not suitable if our purpose is to seek limbic openness. Treadmills define the pace for the individual and negate the very essence of the limbic state, which is defined as being free of any external programming, restraints or controls.

# LIMBIC BURSTS FOR CHRONIC FATIGUERS

All people doing limbic exercise sooner or later become aware of a physical phenomenon I believe to be universal. The speed of walking or running or cycling suddenly changes without any deliberate attempts on the part the exerciser.

My own usual limbic run in the morning is a slow, sustained running in place. I make no attempts to achieve any predetermined speed, pulse rate, or any specific breathing rate. Nor is it my purpose to reach any other goals. Yet I notice that at times my legs spontaneously break into a sprint and moments later I recognize this change. Initially, whenever this happened, I'd make deliberate attempts to break this burst and resume my regular pace. After some weeks or months I recognized that even this interference is a device of the cortical monkey in its desperate efforts to regain control over my body. Once I became aware of this interference, I let my limbs lead me. The limbs, I mentioned earlier, never mislead anyone. These bursts of speed interspersed with a slow, sustained pace became a natural order of things for me.

When the tissues of chronic fatiguers become strong enough, they also break into limbic bursts when the time is right. This is different from the goal-oriented, competitive exercises that are commonly recommended to chronic fatigue sufferers.

*"Doc, I know you are right. I shouldn't do exercise with any goals, set by myself or by others. Every time the staff at the rehab center push me to increase my exercise cycle time, I pay dearly for it. Once when they made me reach the target of 22 minutes, I could not get out of my bed for three days. I know it is dumb, but they are paying for my rehab program, and I cannot afford not to do what they want me to do."*

Just when I think I have heard about all the absurd notions of treating chronic fatigue, some one will tell me things I could never imagine. A rehab center pushes hard a chronic fatiguer to meet their predetermined goals for physical exercise even when such activity puts the patient into the bed for days! Who would have guessed that a rehab center would go to such lengths to justify their beliefs? Or could it be simply a strategy of *maximizing* revenues — protocols for "treatment" that many institutions set to meet their financial needs. How would a rehab center create billable services if all it could do was to teach chronic fatiguers how to let their tissues lead the way?

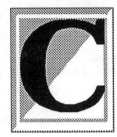

**C**hapter 12

Obsessive
Psychopathology,
Depression and
Chronic Fatigue:

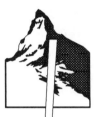

Immortals Strike
from
Mount Olympus

Choua came over one day, stood by my desk and started shuffling through my papers and journals piled up on the desktop. We all have our quirks. Certainly Choua has some of his own, and looking through my papers and journals is one of them. I really do not mind that and he knows it. I looked at him with amusement for a few moments and remembered the last tirade. He seemed absorbed in reading a newspaper clipping someone had sent me. I returned to my microscope.

"Did you see this?" Choua asked after a few moments, holding a newspaper clipping.
"Yes. Someone gave it to me at the last Academy meeting," I replied without looking up from my scope.
"Interesting stuff!" Choua murmured. "Listen to this:

*In our view, the origins most often involve obsessional psychopathology rather than environmental toxins."*

"Origins of what?" I asked.
"Origins of chronic fatigue and chemical sensitivity. That's what he is talking about."
"Who is he?"
"Some immunology professor." Choua replied.
"What paper is that?" I asked.
"*Minneapolis Star Tribune.*"
"Interesting! That's interesting. What made him make such a statement?"
"Some reporter asked him to comment on a story about a young woman with fatigue and chemical sensitivity that the

*Tribune* ran in its July 8, 1990, issue.
"To each his own." I responded.

Choua went back to the clipping and I to my biopsies.
Minutes passed. I looked up to pick up the requisition slip for
the next case. Choua was looking out the window, in deep
thought. I knew it had to be something about that professor and
his pronouncement that chronic fatigue and environmental
illness were nothing more than obsessive psychopathology.

"What do you think of obsessional psychopathology?" I
broke the silence.

Choua didn't answer. I looked out the window as well. It
was a clear day, the sky unusually dark blue, the tree leaves
bright green.

"What do you think, Choua?" I spoke again, "what do
you think of this diagnosis of obsessional psychopathology for
people with chronic fatigue and chemical sensitivities?" I asked.
"Obsessional psychopathology, my foot," Choua answered
with irritation, without looking at me.
"No, seriously, Choua, what do you really think of it?" I
ignored the irritation in his voice.
"Yes! Seriously, obsessional psychopathology, my foot!"
Choua snapped back.
"C'mon, Choua. What do you think of this diagnosis for
people who suffer from chronic fatigue?" I persisted. "Do you
think these patients are psychopathic?" I provoked him.
"What is psychopathic?" Choua turned, cocked his neck
and frowned.
"You know what I mean! Is environmental illness
psychopathic? Is the fatigue it causes psychopathic?"

"What is psychopathic?" Choua looked at me sternly.

"Psychopathic! You know what that is. The distortions of the troubled minds," I pushed Choua.

"That's funny coming from you." Choua's face softened.

"Surely, you don't believe problems of obessional psychopathic don't exist, do you?"

"What do I think of obsessional psychopathology?" Choua became serious again.

"Yes, what do you think of psychopathology?" I pressed.

"Obsessional psychopathology is the crutch for the ignorant and ...." Choua stopped in midsentence.

"And what?"

"And the days of psychiatry are numbered," Choua spoke flatly.

"What? What did you say?" I was taken aback.

"The days of psychiatry are numbered," Choua repeated without acknowledging my reaction to his glib words.

"C'mon Choua, you don't mean that, do you?"

Choua turned, looked out the window, and fell silent again. He often does that. He is good at sudden withdrawals from conversations, as if what we said wasn't said at all. He does that often when he has to answer a question that he would rather not answer. Some minutes passed. This time he broke the silence.

"There is no such nonsense as psychiatric illness," Choua turned his gaze at me.

"No?"

"No!"

"So when people suffer from mental illness what do they suffer from?"

"From contortions of brain chemistry."

"And phobias?" I followed.

"From dysfunctional neural synapses."

"And depression?"

"From dysfunctional neurotransmitters."

"And anxiety?"

"From molecular roller coasters! That's your expression, remember!" Choua taunted me.

"And bulimia?"

"Chemistry of sadness. Sparks of anguish brought back by memory of past abuses."

"And hyperactivity syndrome?"

"Food and mold and chemical sensitivity."

"In all cases?"

"And sugar roller coasters."

"And?"

"And God knows what else!" Choua showed signs of irritation. "You don't think you guys know everything there is to know about unfriendly molecules that surround you, do you?" Choua snapped.

"And neurosis? I mean what happens when a little meek girl becomes neurotic as she watches her bulky mom bully her timid father, year after year?"

"Neurones begin to misfire when they are so violated, year after year," Choua snapped back at me again.

"And codependency?" I goaded Choua.

"Oh yes, codepedency!" Choua chimed. "Codepedents are folks who never knew your stuff about energy and language of silence and spirituality." Choua said with a grimace. "They are in the hands of therapists who think they can *clever-think* their way out of every problem. These therapists are so sure of themselves. They think they can *cure* their hordes of codependents by teaching them how to clever-think their way out of all their troubles. Words! Words! Words! They think their words are their scalpels. They think they can lance the deep wounds of their codependents — let out all the purulent substance of dependency buried deep in the recesses of their psyche. They think they can excise fetid thoughts with their skillful use of words — just as surgeons excise cancer with scalpels — and the codependents will be codependents no more. Fascinating stuff! Isn't it?" Choua was heaving now.

"And obsessive thoughts? Are they also caused by neurones misfiring?" I chided Choua.

"What else can cause them?" Choua regained his calm.

"C'mon Choua, no one has ever shown any evidence for that," I tried to provoke him again.

"What do psychiatrists use Mellaril for?" Choua asked calmly.

"For what?"

"It's so odd how..." Choua didn't complete his sentence.

"What's so odd?"

"It's so odd how you can be so quick with your microscope and your oxidative stuff but so slow with ...." Choua stopped in mid-sentence again.

"Slow with what?" I said, flustered.

"Slow with common sense...I mean what is so obvious," Choua stammered a little as he recognized the insult his words carried..

"What are you rambling about, Choua?" I asked with annoyance.

"What do psychiatrists use Mellaril for?" Choua's voice softened.

"Mellaril? Why bring Mellaril into this discussion, Choua?"

"Yes, Mellaril! What do psychiatrists use Mellaril for?" Choua repeated his question.

"For controlling obsessive thoughts, I suppose." I

ventured a guess.

Choua grinned and turned to the window again. I looked
at the back of his head and wondered what was that all about.
And then I caught on to what Choua had been leading me to all
that time. If Mellaril, a chemical, can be used to prevent
obsessive thoughts, wasn't that the clearest evidence there can
be that obsessive thoughts were caused by some sort of
chemical imbalance. If some chemicals can prevent obsessive
thoughts, I realized, certainly some others can cause them.
Choua's approach may have been circuitous, but his logic was
unassailable. We were again silent for some minutes. This time
I broke the silence.

"And sadness after the death of a close family member,
Choua. What causes such sadness? Brain chemicals again?"
"In that case you would have to think of a deranged
brain chemistry if they didn't become sad."
"How about schizophrenia?"
"Go read Pfeiffer's book about schizophrenia, zinc and
vitamin $B_6$."
"Do you think psychiatry then has any place at all,
Choua?"
"Drugs help in acute crises."
"And you think that's all psychiatry is good for? Drugs?"
I challenged him.
"You know something I don't?" Choua cocked his head
again.
"You don't think analysis and counseling help?" I tried to
suppress my frustration.
"Compassion comforts. And it comforts regardless of
where it might come from, but you don't have to concoct all
those fancy and frivolous diagnostic labels if you want to

comfort the uncomfortable with compassion."

"I am talking about psychoanalytic theory and psychological counselling." I persisted. "What about Freud's theories?"

"Even *Times* magazine thinks psychoanalysis is dead. I mean that's what it said on the cover of its December 29, 1993, issue. Didn't it? And then it said that Clinton's folks were not going to include it in their Health Plan because there was no evidence it ever worked."

"So, you don't think psychotherapy ever works," I pressed him.

"It's okay if it brings some understanding of where the suffering might come from."

"What about homosexuality?" I changed the subject, and decided to give him some more ammunition.

"Oh yes, homosexuality!" Choua's face lit up. "Do you know for years your pundits at the American Psychiatric Association called homosexuality a psychiatric disorder. It was only in 1974 that those wizards came to their senses. Now we find out that alignments of some DNA sequence can set people up for such sexual orientation. But you have short memories. You forget how silly your theories were ...."

"So?" I interrupted Choua.

"So what?" Choua growled.

"So do you think psychiatry has any place?"

"Yes, unless ..." Choua stopped again.

"Unless what, Choua?"

"There is nothing wrong with talk therapy as long as these fellows with their wonderful diagnoses do not come in the way of people who are really trying — I mean those who are struggling to define the physical basis of suffering that psychiatrists glibly label as mental illness. I mean the people who are busting their behinds to figure out the physicochemical basis of such problems. And ...."

"Don't you think you're being dogmatic?" I interrupted him.

"There is no such nonsense as psychiatric illness. All illness has some basis. There is no suffering without a molecular-energetic basis—without some underlying physicochemical events. Twenty five years from now, psychiatrists will become molecular neurobiologists or they will have no patients." Choua winked.

"You don't really think that will happen. Do you?" I expressed my doubt.

"Once you know something you cannot unknow it. Those are your words," Choua spoke mockingly.

"I know! I know! But ...."

"But what? Those are your words. Remember! Malaria used to be caused by evil spirits. Now it is caused by a blood parasite. Alcoholism used to be a sin. Now it is a problem of aberrant brain receptor chemistry. And cocaine addiction used to be ..."

"I know what I wrote," I interrupted Choua in frustration. "We don't call alcoholism a sin because we know better."

"People are beginning to understand," Choua continued.

"Understand what? That there is no such thing as psychopathology?" I interrupted him.

"Where do you think mental diseases come from?" Choua ignored my question.

"I thought we were talking about psychopathology." Now I ignored his question.

"Where do you think psychiatric illnesses come from?" Choua pressed on.

"So we are going to have two conversations. You talk about what interests you and I will talk about what interests me," I said sarcastically.

"So, where do you think mental diseases come from?"
Choua persisted.

"I don't know, Choua. You tell me where do mental
diseases come from?" I sighed.

"From Mount Olympus."

"Mount Olympus?"

"Yes! From Mount Olympus. The Immortals did it."

"Did what?"

"Venus, Cupid and Psyche did it."

"Did what?" I asked with annoyance.

"Hid the source of mental diseases from you mortals."

"Choua,     I     thought     we     were     talking     about
psychopathology." I tried to return to the original subject.

"It isn't your destiny to know. Is it?" Choua frowned and
looked out the window again.

"You are schizoid today."

Choua turned, looked at me with piercing eyes, and then
returned to the window again. We were silent for some minutes.

"People are beginning to see," Choua suddenly spoke
without looking at me.

"See what?"

"People are beginning to see that diseases just do not
happen, even when the practitioners of drug medicine can't see
something that obvious."

"See what? Choua, is there an end to this? One minute
you talk about depression and the other about Mount Olympus
and Venus, Cupid and Psyche. I give up," I said in frustration.

"For every pain, there is a reason. For every suffering, a
basis," Choua ignored me again. "People are beginning to see
that diseases do not just happen. There are energetic-molecular

reasons for everything — for every form of suffering. Suffering that comes with bad thoughts is just as real as that which comes with low hormone levels or neurotransmitter dysfunctions. Once enough people find it out, you cannot put them back in your diagnostic boxes. Once people know, you cannot make them *unknow* it. How many people have you seen who suffer from natural light deprivation?"

"Some," I answered.

"What do psychiatrists now call it?"

"SAD! Seasonal affective disorder."

"How many thousands of people do you think spent how many hundreds of thousands of hours on the couches of their shrinks figuring out their childhood conflicts and repressed anger before they recognized light deprivation caused their mood and depression problems? How many hundreds of pounds of mind-altering drugs were poured into them to *cure* SAD before the *simple* truth about the ill-effects of light deprivation was recognized?" Choua pressed on.

"Choua, you know I am not a psychiatrist, and I don't keep such tallies," I responded curtly.

"How many patients with steroid psychosis have you seen?" Choua asked archly.

"It happens. I don't know, how often?"

"How many hours did these people spend on their shrinks' couches before they figured out cortisone was making them crazy?"

"I don't keep such tallies," I repeated my answer.

"How many folks were incarcerated in mental asylums for your psychiatric illnesses before that surgeon from Boston removed their parathyroid tumors so that they became sane again?"

"I know! I know!" I conceded.

Choua backed away from the window and walked out. He is usually not so disjointed in his conversations. Choua's logic is sometimes jarring. I thought about his ideas about psychiatry and wondered about how the old man, Freud, would have answered his questions had he been alive today. He was a smart fellow. He probably would have had some glib comebacks for Choua.

*************

Choua returned a few days later and read to me from a book called *The Ion Effect* by Fred Soya:

*Toward the end of 1965 I went back to the doctor again, and this time he recommended a psychiatrist on the grounds that if the problem wasn't physical it simply had to be psychosomatic. So for the next two years I spent four hours a week on an analyst's couch examining my life for hidden fears, conflicts, and guilt that had waited until my mid-thirties to emerge from the subconscious to haunt me. When I left New York to move to Geneva I was the kind of man who was impatient with people who turned to psychiatrists to solve problems that I felt they should deal with themselves. But having experienced firsthand the kind of suicidal despair that is beyond reason and self-help, I was forced to grow more tolerant. Even so,*

*after two years of analysis I felt no better.*
*Those diary entries in red ink still read: "Felt*
*terrible!" "Very ill, depressed, feel*
*discouraged" "Sleeplessnight — again!" "Get*
*out of Geneva!" "Felt like the dead, and*
*wish I were."I would still lie awake worrying*
*about little things — something idiotically*
*trivial at the office, or about the future. And*
*I worried about the fact that I was worrying.*

"So what happens  next?"  I asked  when  Choua  finished
reading  from  the  book

Choua  didn't  answer.  We  remained  silent  for  some
minutes.  I returned  to my paperwork.  Choua  broke the silence
after some moments,  pulling me away from my papers  a second
time.

"This fellow  has  a very  interesting  story  to tell," Choua
resumed,  "For about  ten  years,  he was healthy  when  in New
York and very  sick when  in Geneva.  Medical  specialists  he
consulted  couldn't  figure  out what  caused  his problems.  They
sent him to psychiatrists  whose  talk therapy  didn't help. Unlike
millions  of people  who  suffer  in silence,  he searched  and
searched and finally figured out what was causing the problems."
"And what was that?"  I asked.
"Changes  in  natural  electrical  charges  in  the  air.
Ionization!  Apparently  some  physicians  in Geneva  recognize this
health  hazard  in many  of their  patients.  It is like humans
blowing  their  fuses  when  patterns  of natural  and  man-made

ionization change abruptly."

"Interesting!"

"How many Fred Soyas are there in this world?" Choua asked. "Living out their miseries commiserating with their psychiatrists?"

I didn't answer Choua. His question carried my thoughts to clinical reports of electromagnetic sensitivity I had read in clinical ecology and other journals. Christian Bach, Director of Danish Air Ionization Institute, has written about his extensive experience with people who suffered from severe asthma and related respiratory disorders and whose health was restored with "passive" therapy comprised of eliminating sources of excessive ion generation from an overload of synthetic materials in their homes. Japanese customs require them to take off their shoes when they enter their homes — a practice that my wife, Talat, and I follow in our home, and that I recommend to my patients for two reasons: 1) It drastically reduces the pollutants we bring home with our shoes; and 2) It reduces the ion overload by literally "earthing" us. Such ideas are derided in the prevailing drug medicine because they do not lead to use of drugs. At a fundamental level, all living beings — and for that matter, all inanimate materials — are energy entities. That's an old saw since Einstein put together his concepts of substance, space, time and causality. But we physicians are still very uncomfortable about matters of energy in medicine, unless, of course, we can put tissues cooked by electromagnetic energy under our microscopes and invent specific "diagnoses" for them.

"You know what amuses me about psychiatry?" Choua's words brought me back from my thoughts.

"What?" I asked.

"Psychiatrists have forgotten all about the origin of the

name of their profession."

"How do you mean?" I asked.

"You remember the story of Psyche, the beautiful dame of Greek mythology."

"Sort of." I didn't know where Choua was going to take us this time.

"You know the story," Choua started, "Psyche was stunningly beautiful. The mortals who came under her spell began to ignore Venus, the goddess of beauty. Venus, smitten by jealousy, had Psyche's family told by the oracles of Delphi that Psyche was to be married to a monster who would destroy her. Immeasurably saddened and feeling utterly helpless, they took Psyche to the wilderness and left her there. The anger of Venus was not yet quenched. She dispatched her son, Cupid, to destroy Psyche, taking great caution not to lay eyes on her. But Cupid couldn't resist the temptation, saw Psyche, and was instantly overwhelmed by her transcendent charm. Cupid immediately decided to be Psyche's lover. Now Cupid couldn't openly defy his mother, the goddess Venus. So he took Psyche to a great palace filled with music of unseen musicians and the sounds of waterfalls coming from unseen streams. There he would visit her in the darkness of nights and whisper into her ears a thousand words of undying love for her. He told her he could never be seen by her, and that she must never to try to see him."

Choua stopped and looked out the window again. What does Psyche have to do with obsessive psychopathology of chronic fatiguers. I wondered? I didn't clearly recall the whole story. It went something like this: Psyche is tempted by her jealous sisters to disobey her lover and to shine a light at him at night to see what kind of a monster he really was. Poor

Psyche! She did that and lost her lover as well as her palace. Psyche once again rambled along in the wilderness, deeply sorrowful for the loss of her lover and her palace. After many hardships, Venus is finally persuaded by Cupid to relent and let him marry Psyche. The Olympian gods bless the marriage, and Psyche finally turns from a mortal to a goddess.

"So what does Psyche have to do with chronic fatigue and obsessional psychopathology?" I asked Choua after some moments.

"Those Greeks knew something about human nature, something about the human soul, something about spirituality."

"What did those Greeks know about chronic fatigue syndrome and psychopathology?" I asked sarcastically.

"The Greeks had a sense." Choua ignored my sarcasm. "They had a sense about the *unknowable*. That essence of the human soul — the spiritual. The story of Psyche has something to do with that unknowable — the spiritual."

"So what does Psyche have to do with chronic fatigue syndrome? Are you saying the causes of chronic fatigue are unknowable?"

Choua frowned, squinted his eyes, said nothing and turned to the window. Choua suffers from flight of ideas. It is not unusual for him to talk with disjointed sentences and shift from one irrelevant subject to another. Usually though he does return to the original point of discussion.

"So what does Psyche have to do with chronic fatigue and obsessional psychopathology?" I asked again after a few moments.

"The Greeks had a sense about things unknowable, our psychiatrists do not."

"Speak plainly, Choua. I don't know what you're talking about," I said with some irritation.

"When the Greeks talked about psyche, they talked about something *unseeable* — something that had to do with the essential spirituality of humankind. Psyche to them represented the hidden, the mystic aspects of the human experience — that unknowable *presence* that surrounds each of us, and yet cannot be known with our bodily senses or the reach of our intellect. Psyche to the Greeks was that *presence* that extends beyond the ordinary human experience. Psyche for the Greek was not about the diseases that arise from deranged brain chemistry. Psyche's story was about the mysticism and spirituality, and not about the disorders of brain receptors and neurotransmitters. Your psychiatrists should know that. They should know something about the Greek deity that gave them the name of their profession. They should have a sense what Psyche's story was all about. Yet, to this day they adamantly hang on to their fixation that diseases come from somewhere else — somewhere, elsewhere, anywhere. They are smug about their couches and their classifications of psychiatric *diseases* — forever spinning tales of obsessive psychopathology for people made sick by chemical sensitivities, allergy and nutritional disorders, merrily incarcerating the sick into their models of mental diseases. "

"You don't have any great love for psychiatry, do you?" I prodded him along.

"You have had generations of psychiatrists who believe that the causes of psychiatric disorders cannot be physical, and hence will always be beyond scientific scrutiny. They don't see the absurdity of this notion. They think psychiatric disorders will always be the domains of their couches and they will forever sit by their prostrate subjects dispensing their superior wisdom into the inner workings of the mind, forever doling out prescriptions for psychoactive drugs."

"Choua, I think you are hopelessly opinionated. Just as dogmatic as the psychiatrists you ramble about. No! You are worse. You are delusional." I provoked him.

"Opinionated and dogmatic! Yes, that I am. Delusional? That I'm not! You watch! Your anxiety states and phobias and schizophrenia will be found to have energetic-molecular basis just as you are beginning to see the energetic-molecular basis of depression and addictions. Your professors who pronounce chronic fatigue is obsessive psychopathology may not be around by then, but it will happen. You watch, if the bomb does not put us back into caves, there will be no such nonsense as psychiatry in fifty years."

"So it was 25 years just a few minutes ago and now it is 50 years," I teased Choua.

Choua stepped back from the window, swung on his heels and was gone.

## BRAINLESS PSYCHIATRY AND MINDLESS NEUROLOGY

Choua returned after some days. My thoughts drifted to the mythic story of Psyche, Cupid and Venus, and then to depression in chronic fatiguers.

"Tell me, Choua, what do you think of depression in chronic fatigue?" I asked him.

"Folks get depressed when they are tired and when their muscles ache all day long." Choua shrugged his shoulders.

"I know that, Choua, but that's not what I meant."

"What did you mean?" Choua looked at me, puzzled.

"You know what I mean. Don't you?"

"No! I don't know what you mean."

"Get serious Choua!" I protested. "The whole medical world is perplexed about the relationship between chronic fatigue and depression. Psychiatrists cannot figure our how much fatigue comes from chronic fatigue syndrome and neurologist cannot evaluate how much depression comes from depression. And all you can say is that folks get depressed when they are tired all the time."

"Brainless psychiatry and mindless neurology!" Choua spoke with a twinkle in his eyes.

"C'mon Choua, you are impossible today. What does brainless psychiatry and mindless neurology have to do with what we are talking about, Choua?" I asked with annoyance.

"Neurologist define chronic fatigue syndrome by the presence of two of the three major criteria and six of the eleven minor CDC criteria. Psychiatrists do the same. They define major depressive syndrome by the presence of either depressed mood or anhedonia and at least four associated features included in their DSM III-R classification. Both group make their diagnoses by processes of exclusion, and that, by definition, means they do not know what they are dealing with. You don't diagnose breast cancer by a process of exclusion, do you? Nor do you make any other pathologic diagnosis by a process of exclusion, do you? Neither neurologists nor psychiatrists truly search for the root causes of these problems of fatigue and depression." Choua shrugged his shoulders and started to walk to the window.

"Don't do that!" I nearly screamed at him in exasperation. "Don't just turn away in the middle of the argument and disappear into the clouds."

Startled by my words, Choua froze in his feet. I felt sorry for having raised my voice. We were quiet for some moments.

"Why are you so caught up in this debate of depression and fatigue?" Choua asked softly as he recovered.

"Choua, I didn't mean to scream at you, but it is really an important issue for me. I have to write something about it. I mean I think my fatigue book should say something about this subject, shouldn't it?" I tried to be conciliatory.

"Oh! your book." Choua grinned a little. "That's what is troubling you. Why don't you *simply* write about what your patients tell you about fatigue and depression. Why do you have to get embroiled in this debate of brainless psychiatry and mindless neurology?" Choua now spoke condescendingly.

"Some people give history of depression before they came down with chronic fatigue and some do not. Those who have previous history of depression require antidepressants more often." I summarized my clinical sense about the problem in two senteneces.

"That's it! That's it!" Choua perked up. "You just said the right thing. Don't say anything else."

"That's all what you want me to write about depression?" I asked with disbelief.

"You *really* do not need to write anything more." Choua counseled firmly.

"Choua, get serious! I just can't..."

"Okay! Okay! I know your problem." Choua interrupted. "I tell you what! Write about Carol. That should do it."

## CAROL AND A YOUNG PHYSICIAN

A young physician who is interested in my work was

visiting me when Carol first consulted me for chronic fatigue. She was very distraught and spoke with disjointed sentences, sometimes struggling to put sentences together, at other times speaking breathlessly and repeating endlessly her words. At times, she was clearly disoriented, bordering on acute psychosis. She spoke with bitter irritation about her fatigue, bloating, unending headaches, mental confusion, brain fog, depression and the death of her dog and brother-in-law. She broke down frequently in her long monologue.

Such patients often speak frantically as if afraid that their time will be up before they can say everything that their doctor must hear, and as a result become incoherent and repetitive. They are aware of their incoherence and repetitiveness, and that further feeds the fury of their anguish. Carol seemed to sense all this as her husband, my physician-visitor and I tried patiently to listen to her. Sometime during the visit, she suddenly pulled a picture out of her wallet, thrust it up close to my nose, broke down and sobbed uncontrollably:

> *Look, Dr. Ali, look what has become of me. I was a model. Look at the way I used to look. And look at what has become of me. My skin is all broken out. I am obese, grotesque. I can't do anything. I am depressed. I am tired. I can't think straight. What will become of me. I am young. I don't have any children yet. Look what has become of me.*

During the rest of the initial interview, she passed from

periods of complete lucidity to incoherent muttering. We finished the interview and then proceeded with the physical examination. As I came out of the examination room, the young physician-visitor looked at me and said,

"This is acute psychosis. She obviously suffers from severe psychiatric illness. You don't think you are going to succeed with your nondrug methods with her, do you?"
"We'll see." I replied.

The young doctor looked at me as if I was losing my mind. Then he recovered, and spoke,
"Dr. Ali, if she can get better with your methods, anyone can get better with your methods."
"We'll see." I repeated.

Next, the images from my first visit with Carol were replaced by those from a recent visit, about 14 months after the first visit. This time around Carol literally was waltzing around showing her waist line to other patients she knew in our IV therapy room. She had lost about 40 pounds. Most of the blemishes on her face were gone. She was full of energy, and excitedly talked about the distance she had yet to go. She had started playing tennis. Then she recalled how hopeless things had seemed to her. Her husband shook his head as Carol talked. He had been so completely supportive of his wife. I wondered how much he had to do with her continuing recovery. Then I recalled how my young, visiting physician had challenged me. Some months into our treatment, I had told Carol about what that physician-visitor had thought about her problems. "I'm glad you think differently," Carol had answered with a smile. Carol that day reminded me of his words.
"I know some of my enzymes are back to life now.

Maybe you should call that young doctor and ask him to return and see how I am doing," she exulted.

I saw Carol recently, about three years after I first saw her. She looked tired and sullen. "She does so well when she stays with her treatment, but then she becomes careless and gets tired again," her husband remarked.

"Carol has a message for your chronic fatiguers who get very depressed." Choua's words brought me back from my thought. "That message is simple: Depression and psychosis of chronic fatigue do lift when the aching muscles do not hurt anymore." Choua spoke softly but firmly.

"And when clinically depressed people come down with chronic fatigue?" I prodded him.

"Then it is much tougher. Then they need more of your stuff of the language of silence."

"And antidepressant?"

"Yes, that too! Chronic fatiguers do get depressed. And yes, sometimes they slide into psychotic periods. But their depression, their psychosis and their *mental illness* are caused by your oxidative fires. And yes, their psychosis is *reversible* when those oxidative fires can be put out. That's your stuff, isn't it? You shouldn't have any problems with that." Choua stopped and stretched his back.

"So what do you think of depression and chronic fatigue?" I returned to my original question.

"You don't get it, do you?" Choua stiffened and his eyes narrowed. "Amazing!" he exclaimed after some moments. "You cannot figure out something *that* simple. Amazing!" He shook his head and left.

*An ancient legend has it that the gods hid spirituality deep within men's hearts for they knew that was the last place they would look for it.*

*Or could it be that God put spirituality deep within men's hearts so they could never be far away from Him?*

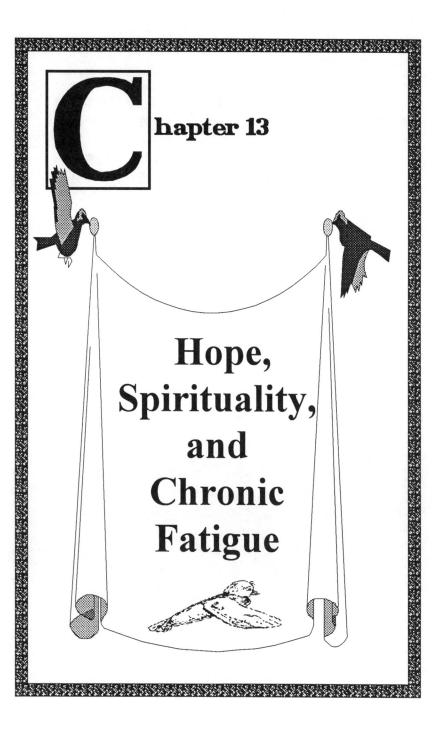

# Chapter 13

## Hope, Spirituality, and Chronic Fatigue

I began this book by predicting four major changes in the medicine of the 21st century. First, chronic fatigue will be the dominant chronic health disorder. Second, chronic fatigue will reorient the disease doctors of drug medicine to a new medicine that will focus on health rather than disease. Third, chronic fatigue will usher in participatory medicine — the patient will actively guide the physician, informing him how his body is responding to therapy. Fourth, hope and spirituality will become integral parts of medical jargon. This last chapter of this book is devoted to the last of these four changes.

Hope *is* healing. Hope is life. Indeed, the human life span is incompatible with true absence of hope.

Absence of hope is *the* most difficult problem I face when seeing patients who have suffered from severe, paralyzing fatigue. They have usually undergone extensive diagnostic testing and received multiple drug therapies before I see them. Hopes were dashed as each new set of drug therapies left them weaker and sicker. Thus, my first task is to create hope, and the second to sustain it. I prepare my patients for recovery by explaining that the therapy may take several weeks, sometimes several months.

When is hope false? When is it true? When is holding out hope for someone inappropriate? When is it pure deception?

*"Dr. Ali, Billy was such a stunningly beautiful baby no one could look at him only once. Then he grew into a strong six-feet-two young man. His grades in high school were so good. When we drove him to MIT, my husband and I thought we were the luckiest people in the world. And now this! I see him struggle, going from one room to another. He used to weigh 168. When he came down with this thing — whatever it is — he went down to 148. God knows we saw enough specialists. And they did enough tests and prescribed enough antibiotics and antidepressants. For a while, his weight stayed at 148. Now he is down to 140. No one knows what is eating him from within. He is just melting away, right before his mother's eyes and there is nothing she can do." Bill's mother broke down.*

I sat motionless, looking at a Monet reprint hung on the office wall, not wanting to look into Bill's nor his mother's eyes. I had no ready answers for either of them. Did I see absence of hope for Bill? No! Did I think I could tell them about it flatly? No. Can hope be dispensed from a prescription pad for every chronic fatiguer? Is every patient ready for the firm assertions that I make in this book about chronic fatigue? There are times when all a physician can do for a patient is to grieve with him.

After a while I looked at them. Bill and his mom were studying my face with intense eyes. "You will get better." I forced a smile and started asking some questions.

## HOPE MYOPIA

Hope is *never* false in medicine provided that we have the courage to dismiss the narrow-focused proclamations of drug medicine when its tools fail. Hope is never false if we accept the enduring truth that every form of suffering carries with it a possibility for some spiritual search and rewards — an opportunity for enlightenment. Enlightenment, Jean-Paul Sartre wrote, begins on the other side of despair.

Hope myopia — paucity of hope based on a lack of understanding of the true nature of the healing process — is a pervasive problem among the disease doctors of drug medicine. Physicians are trained to look for quick responses from their drugs and scalpels. Such strategies work well when problems we confront are acute and life-threatening but fail utterly when we have to deal with slow, insidious, degenerative and immune disorders. The disease doctors of drug medicine are incarcerated in mental boxes of their own making. The fact is that serious environmental, nutritional, degenerative and immune disorders can be managed — and their recurrences prevented — only through focus on nutrition, environment, self-regulation and spiritual search. Chronic viral syndromes also fall in the same general category. Unfortunately, such an approach has come to be regarded as quackery by the mainstream medicine in the United States.

---

## SIMPLE TRUTHS
## AND COMPLICATED LIES

*The chronic fatigue syndrome reflects a complex interaction between cerebral dysfunction, trigger factors, and social attitudes, and is complicated by secondary symptoms. There will be no simple explanation.*

*British Medical Journal* 306:1558; 1993

The *Journal* does not see any hope for understanding the fatigue problem. I do.

The public will believe a simple lie in preference to a complicated truth, de Tocqueville wrote in his commentary on early Americans. If de Tocqueville were to return and visit our chronic fatigue centers today, he would find the opposite: Our fatigue experts prefer complicated lies to simple truths.

The story of chronic fatigue syndrome has become a web of complicated lies, and our fatigue experts continue to weave new yarns everyday. On a positive note, chronic fatiguers are beginning to see the simple truth. Here is how a patient put it to me recently,

*"Dr. Ali, it took me a long time to finally understand what you have been trying to explain to me. I know now that only I can pull myself out of this problem. You can only guide me. Of course, IV drips and immunotherapy shots and auto-reg do their part."*

Chronic fatigue states are reversible. We need simply to suspend our disbelief of the enormous restorative potential of nutritional, environmental and self-regulatory methods and simply try them.

## HOPE
## AND DISEASE DOCTORS OF DRUG MEDICINE

How can a rheumatologist ever dare to create hope for a cure for a patient with rheumatoid arthritis? After all, he knows that his steroids only further suppress an injured immune system, and gold injections, as useful as they may be in reducing symptoms, never cure rheumatoid arthritis.

How can a gastroenterologist create hope for a cure for a patient with ulcerative colitis? He knows his steroids suppress the immune system and his azulfadine never cures ulcerative colitis.

How can a dermatologist ever create hope for a cure for a patient with eczema? He knows his steroids suppress the immune system and his skin creams only hide the underlying problem.

How can a pulmonologist create hope for a cure for a patient with asthma? He knows his steroids suppress the immune system and his bronchodilator drugs cannot normalize the underlying molecular derangements.

How can a cardiologist create hope for a cure for his patient with coronary heart disease? He is absolutely convinced the heart disease of his patient is completely irreversible.

There are yet other reasons why hope myopia continues to flourish among the practitioners of $N^2D^2$ medicine. There are lawyers who advise physicians against hope — it is the fabric that lawsuits are made of, they assert. There are insurance companies that advise against hope — promise nothing so you may be sued for nothing, they say in words that cannot be heard, only understood. The editors of our medical journals do their part — what's not double-blinded and crossed-over is not to be trusted, they admonish. Hope, of course, can neither be blinded nor crossed-over. There is even a new genre of quality assurance personnel in our hospitals — brainwashed by the gurus of *total quality management* (TQM) at the Joint Commission on Accreditation of Healthcare Organizations — who believe that what cannot be *quantified* cannot be *real*. Thus, hope being unquantifiable, is of no interest to them. Hope myopia is forever growing in $N^2D^2$ medicine.

Is it hard, then, to understand why disease doctors of drug medicine do not like the subject of hope in medicine? Why would they?

Can every chronic fatiguer wholly regain his full energy level? If not full recovery, what percentage can he recover? How shall we compute the percentage points by which we must reduce hope for him? How do we measure the "quantity" of hope? Who should decide that? An editor of some prestigious journal? Someone sitting on some state licensing board? A medical ethicist? Or should it be some lawyer? Or perhaps a judge?

Some years ago, I heard a physician vehemently petition a group of physicians to have the hospital seek a court order allowing him to operate on his patient. The woman in question — a bag lady hospitalized for a large abscess around her rectum that caused a blockage — had steadfastly fought all attempts by her surgeons to persuade her to sign a surgical consent. The principal argument of the physician was that the patient was most assuredly going to die if this operation was delayed for too long, and that she clearly was not intelligent enough to understand the risks she faced. Some days later, I ran into the physician, and asked him about the woman with the rectal abscess. "Her abscess burst into her rectum, she passed out all the junk in her stool and signed out against medical advice." He shrugged his shoulders and walked away.

## I DON'T THINK I WILL MAKE IT TO 45

"I have to move every hour in bed, however I sleep. No matter what part of my body is under pressure, it begins to hurt after an hour," Ronald, a 31-year-old contractor, told me in response to my inquiry about the quality of his sleep.

Here are some of his other words:

"There were things in my childhood that made coping with life difficult.

"Sometimes I have to ask people their names three times. Sometimes I write things down, then I forget where I put the paper that I wrote the stuff on.

"Sometimes I get nightmares. Most of the time, I can't breathe. I suffocate. I struggle hard to breathe. I want to move away. When I lived at home, I used to have them often. When I moved out, I almost stopped having them.

"The more I sleep the more tired I get. You would think more sleep would help. Well, it doesn't!

"Sometimes I ate ice cream before I slept. I would wake up after an hour and try to reach for a glass of water on the end table. My hands would tremble. I quit eating ice cream after I saw what was happening to me.

"Sometimes when I get behind a truck, I begin to feel lightheaded and eventually dizzy. So I have to get away from that truck.

"I can only use one brand of cleaners. Every other brand bothers me.

"When I suffer a lot of stress, the left side of my face

goes numb.

"I have to eat every half an hour or so. If I don't, I slow down to a crawl — and then I get a headache or an adrenaline problem.

"When I tell my gastroenterologist about foods that bother me, he doesn't listen. No doctor ever advised me to have allergy tests.

"I was extremely energetic as a teenager — I used to ski and lift weights. I used to camp, ride motorbikes and everything. Now I can do none of that. And I am only 31. Last time I played softball, I just collapsed. That was about it. I never tried after that.

"I am good at work. If I wasn't, I don't know what would have happened. That's what keeps me going.

"I was born when my folks were forty. Now that has got to have caused some weakness. Isn't that right?

"My Lyme disease doctor gave me stiff doses of antibiotics for almost a year."
"Was the Lyme antibody test positive?" I inquired.
"No."
"No?" I asked, surprised.
"No. But my Lyme disease doctor said I probably had had Lyme disease for at least five years. I had a lot of antibiotics even before that. I was given tetracycline for a year for acne."
"You said there were things in your childhood..."
"I was abused as a child," Ronald interrupted me. "I don't

know if I was sexually abused. I know my sisters were. My mom knew about that. But what could she do? She was beaten up badly so often. I remember the commotion in the house and screaming and crying. I was a little boy but I knew exactly what happened. I was once going to kill my father. He was about to kill my brother and that was all I could do. I almost strangled him."

"Why are you smiling as you tell me about one horror after another?" I asked.

"Perhaps because I am still alive," he smiled with a wink. "I'm 31 but I don't think I will make it to 45."

How does one tell Ronalds of this world they can heal?

---

## YOU SEE THINGS YOUR WAY, YOU SHOULD LOOK AT THEM OUR WAY

---

During the early years of my focus on chronic fatigue, there were many times I became very disillusioned about the clinical outcome of my therapies. In some cases, weeks turned into months, but still I saw no improvement. Diagnostic tests and therapies for chronic fatigue are expensive, and many insurance companies go to all lengths not to support chronic fatiguers. I wondered if it was right for me to continue to spend their scarce resources on treatment methods of doubtful validity. At times, I wanted to discontinue my therapies. My patients would ask me what I would do in their predicament. I'd tell them I would continue, and so they would. Still, it was hard for me to keep seeing them. Sometimes, I simply did not want to see them anymore.

Then a woman — a practicing registered nurse before she became disabled — taught me an essential lesson. During a follow-up visit, she sensed my deep disappointment and desire to terminate my therapies.

"Dr. Ali, if you lose hope, where will I go?" she asked. "I tried the medical school. I tried the chronic fatigue centers. I tried the private doctors. All they did was to tell me they didn't know what it was, and then they gave me antibiotics and antidepressants and anxiety drugs. At least, you have a game plan to repair the damaged energy systems. That's all I can hope for under the circumstances. Dr. Ali, you see things your way. You should look at them our way."

A companion in grief! A companion in hope! That's how I learned that a physician must be prepared to play this role when his therapies fail utterly and for long periods of time. I found out how wrong I had been. Even in my failure, I had been of some value to them — I *was* hope for them. How do I know this? They told me so.

## WHAT IS THE SPIRITUAL?

*The spiritual reflects the essence of life — not what we sense or think. It is unknowable* except through the changes it brings in our visible lives.

The spiritual is that *core* quality of life that exists beyond all needs to differentiate, beyond all needs to unify, beyond all judgment, beyond all concepts of right or wrong. The spiritual is *oneness* with that larger presence that surrounds each of us at all times and yet cannot be perceived with our senses nor imagined with our minds. Indeed, everything we can sense with our bodily senses or know by our mental faculties, by definition, would have to be considered matters of the body or of the mind — and not the spiritual.

The spiritual is the change that we can see but not know where it came from.

## DR. ALI, YOUR SWORD STORY DID IT

Andrew had been disabled with chronic fatigue for about a year when he first consulted me.

I sensed something different about Andrew within moments of his entering my office. I finished scanning the chronic fatigue questionnaire I use in my practice and looked up to ask him some questions about his health. He stared at me with sad eyes. As I asked questions regarding his medical problems, he kept interrupting his answers to talk about his two daughters who apparently suffered from many of the symptoms he described. Finally, I said,

"Your daughters are not here. You are. Once you get better, we can take care of your daughters."
"No, you won't," Andrew blurted.
"Okay, then we won't." His answer took me by surprise but I recovered quickly. "Let's talk about you."
"You can't help my daughters, Doc," Andrew spoke softly

this time.

"Fine! Fine! Tell me when did you..."

"You can't help my daughters because my wife won't let you," he interrupted me.

"Let's just talk about you, Andrew," I said with some frustration.

"Doc, I wish you could help my daughters, but you can't because my wife thinks your work is hocus-pocus." Andrew became sad and then sat up quickly. "My wife is a successful businesswoman. And she is a very strong woman. I have been disabled with this thing and can't do anything for my daughters. They are sick every month and I see their pediatrician prescribe antibiotics every month, just the way my pediatrician did for me. I'm very afraid for them."

I saw Andrew 10 weeks later for a follow-up visit. There was no sign of any improvement. I saw my notation, "concerned about two daughters," in his clinical chart and wondered how the situation at home might be. I decided not to ask him any questions about that.

Andrew continued to receive immunotherapy from our office but did not keep his appointment for a follow-up visit with me until several months later. Then he came in one day, his face lit up with joy. I wondered if the situation with his daughters had changed but said nothing. Next, I started to make entries in the chronic fatigue outcome sheet that I use in my practice for research studies.

"Tell me Andrew, how is your energy level these days?" I asked.

"Excellent!" he beamed.

"Excellent?" I asked in disbelief.

"Excellent. I am running a marathon," he crowed.

"Running a marathon?" I was stunned.

"Yup! I am running a marathon." Andrew became serious.

Chronic fatigue patients do not run marathons — not those who have been disabled for months. I was not prepared for this. Without being too obvious, I thumbed through the chart to see if I had the right chart, to ensure he was the patient I thought he was, the father of two daughters. "Concerned about two daughters," I saw my notation in the chart and knew that there was no mistake there.

"I'm not sure that's a good idea, Andrew," I began. "Marathons shouldn't be run by people who are just coming out of chronic fatigue," I counseled.

"I knew that's what you would say, Doc. But I am not coming out of chronic fatigue now. I have been out of chronic fatigue. I waited for three months before I decided to come and tell you about it. Your story did it. Yup, your story did it for me." Andrew grinned broadly.

I tell a lot of stories to my patients to help them understand the nature of this beast of chronic fatigue, and to help them cope with their unique brand of suffering. What story was Andrew talking about? I wondered. I looked up. Andrew was studying my face with his intense, blue eyes.

"Dr, Ali, your sword story did it. You remember your sword story, Doc. Don't you?" Andrew flashed a smile.

I often tell my patients the sword story to make some points about spiritual search and rewards. It goes something like this:

There was a ferocious captain in Genghis Khan's army during the invasion of India. He killed people with his sword at the least provocation and often without any provocation at all. His reputation preceded him whereever he went. On this occasion, after he entered a town, he thunderously demanded from his lieutenants to know if there was anyone left alive.

"No one, sir! No one except for this spiritual man," a lieutenant answered.

"Aha! A spiritual fool!" he thundered. "Take me to the fool," he ordered.

His lieutenant led him to an ancient small temple with a broken wooden door. The captain ordered the door smashed down. Within moments, his lieutenants smashed it. The captain entered the tiny courtyard. A thin man in a loincloth and wooden sandals stood still in the middle of the courtyard. The captain contemptuously looked at the spiritual man and roared,

"Do you know who I am?"

"No, I don't," the spiritual man answered meekly.

"You don't know who I am?" the captain asked, shaking with rage.

"No, I don't," the spiritual man repeated his words timidly.

The captain pulled his sword from its sheath and flashed it with his full might. "I can slice through your body and not blink an eye," he thundered again.

Everyone standing behind the captain froze, their eyes

fixed on the spiritual man. Time seemed to stop. The spiritual man stood silently, looking back at the captain with vacant eyes. Then he asked in a whisper, "Do you know who I am, sir?"

"Who are you?" the captain roared again, thrusting his sword forward until it nearly touched the spiritual man's abdomen.

"I could have your sword slice through me and not blink an eye," the spiritual man answered.

The captain trembled in his feet and walked out without saying a word.

********

"How did the sword story help you?" I asked Andrew in good humor.

"Your sword story did it, Doc. I'm serious," Andrew began with a grin. "A few months after I saw you last, my wife took a lover and threw me out. Suddenly, there I was. I had no wife. No home. No job. And I couldn't see my daughters. What would I tell my daughters anyway? I had nothing left. There was no reason for me to go on. No reason to fight back at all. No reason to live. There was nothing there. Just darkness. Then into that darkness came the sword and the man in the loincloth and wooden sandals. Then I don't quite know what happened — except that I wasn't afraid anymore. Nothing mattered anymore. I wasn't afraid. I think that did it! I wasn't afraid anymore. I guess I was just like that spiritual man. I thought I could have anyone slice through me and I wouldn't blink an eye — just like the man in the loincloth and wooden sandal. I began to move around and then I found the energy to start walking and then running. Before I knew it, I was preparing for the marathon. This is how it all happened. I was free at last — free of fear and free of anger. I wasn't a victim anymore. I knew there was something out there. I didn't know what, but *it* was out there, and it didn't seem to matter that I couldn't know *it* any better. I wasn't tired anymore. Honest Doc, that's what happened." Andrew shook his head warmly. There was nothing for me to say.

The story came back to me some weeks after I saw Andrew. In a flash, I saw him the way he looked during the first visit — distraught, deeply hurt, interrupting his answers about his health to talk about his daughters. Then I saw clearly what I had failed to see then: He was going through a profound change then — a spiritual change, through his suffering for his daughters. He didn't see it then, nor did I. Now I know it was not the sword story that did it. It was his love for his daughters that did it. He suffered for his daughters, and, through that suffering, he came to the truth — that there is something, *someone,* beyond our bodily senses and beyond all reach of the intellect that can sustain us when nothing else does. He went to that third dimension — the spiritual — that none of us is destined to know, and returned with a change, a transformation that neither he nor I could have known with our bodily senses nor with our clever-thinking. The spiritual man in the loincloth and wooden sandals in the sword story was just a little spark that he saw during his journey.

## THE EARLY MAN AND THE SPIRITUAL

Body, yes! We have bodily senses. Mind, yes! We think, imagine and dream. Spirit, why? What is it that we can know except with our bodily senses and faculties of the mind?

At the time I began work on this book, I knew I would have to tackle with this problem of the spiritual. No one can work with seriously ill patients for long months without observing a spiritual dimension to their suffering, and the profound changes that are reflected in their visible lives. Writing about such changes, however, is a different thing altogether.

It was difficult finding the correct approach to this subject. I suppose the spiritual has fascinated humankind for as long as it has looked with wonderment at the world around it. I have had the privilege of listening to many scholars define what the spiritual is, in spoken as well as written word. Almost always, these scholars define the spiritual by what it isn't rather than what it is. But here was Andrew — and many other Andrews like him — who were undergoing changes in their visible lives as they worked with what I call the language of silence. This language has no mind-over-body notions, no grand designs for clever thinking, not even affirmations with beautiful words. It does not protest illness nor demand health in prayers. A patient once put it thusly:

*"Dr. Ali, the silence is now coming to me. I am returning to myself. I'm discovering things I didn't know existed. Can it be real? I mean, do you think I am hallucinating? Could it be a part of the psychiatric problems in chronic fatigue everyone talks about?"*

I told her I didn't think it was a psychiatric problem, though I really didn't know what the psychiatric problems in chronic fatigue might be. (She smiled knowingly.)

The problem of writing about this essential part of my work with chronic fatiguers persisted. One morning during my ghoraa run — meditative running in place that I describe in *The Ghoraa and Limbic Exercise* — an image arose before me: It was a primitive man wearing an animal skin and facing the rising sun with closed eyes, just as I was. Then there were periods of mere openness, fields of energy and yet more images — the types of experiences or absence of them that come during my ghoraa runs.

Later that day at the hospital, the image of the primitive man in animal skin returned to me. Why was he facing the sun with his eyes closed? Why wasn't he looking at the rising sun with open eyes? What was it that he hoped to see with closed eyes that he couldn't see with open eyes?

The image of the man, and the thoughts provoked by it, led me to wonder how the early Man knew the spiritual existed? How did he know something existed beyond what he could know with his bodily senses or with the reach of his mind? I had never before reflected on this question.

I asked some of my friends if they could recall any experience in their lives that was outside their bodily senses or beyond the reach of their minds. Most of them simply acknowledged the question with repressed smiles and said nothing. Some thought for a few moments and then answered in the negative. The question loomed larger for me. The earliest records of humankind indicate a clear fascination with the spiritual. Man could have related his total being to what his bodily senses could experience or what his mind could comprehend. Why was he led instead to invoke the spiritual?

My thoughts turned to the early Man who first sensed the need — or the existence — of the spiritual, something beyond his bodily senses and beyond the reach of his mind, something different, unknowable, the *spirits.* How did he come to know of the spirits, and the spiritual. There is no indication that he struggled to put spirituality into some physical or intellectual context, as we, his progeny and disciples of Freud, continue to relentlessly do.

So we continue to write about spirituality in terms of what it isn't rather than what it is. Sometimes we see spirituality in the context of ethics or morality, and sometimes in those of the ritual or the religious.

## WHAT IS NOT SPIRITUAL

Ever since early Man came to "know" the spiritual, humankind has tried to define the spiritual by what it isn't rather than by what it might be. So we assert:

The spiritual is not what we might see with our eyes closed, listening to some familiar drumming or rattling sounds, as some tribal traditions hold. During a training session in my autoregulation laboratory, I once asked a patient if she saw anything with her closed eyes. "Yes! I saw a big load of stinking laundry," she replied in a matter-of-fact way.

The spiritual is not the psychic. What we call psychic in common language is, in reality, the ability to perceive that which may seem out of the reach of ordinary bodily senses and mental faculties. The psychic may see farther than others, and hence may proclaim superior faculties, a personal power. The spiritual does not recognize personal powers.

The spiritual is not the ritual, though we often mistake one for the other. The ritual is periodic reaffirmation of what the mind holds as "sacred." The sacred, of course, changes with time and place and culture, and so does the ritual. Today we consider most tribal rituals of the past barbaric and abominable. (How much of what we do today will be considered barbaric and abominable in the future? I wonder.) The spiritual is unchangeable, timeless.

The spiritual is not ethical. The ethical pertains to the standards of conduct of a given profession established primarily to maintain internal control. (For decades, American medicine considered it unethical for physicians to advertise — a clear design of those in power to keep newcomers out of their territories — until the courts struck down this absurdity.) The spiritual is silent on such human preoccupations.

The spiritual is not moral. The moral is the distinction between right and wrong and focuses on what is deemed righteous and virtuous at any given time, in any given place, in any given culture. Though often ascribed to the spiritual, the moral, in reality, reflects concepts of common good, social consensus, a basis for judgment about right and wrong. Like the ritual and ethical, the moral also changes. The spiritual transcends time, place and culture, and is unchangeable.

The spiritual is not the religious. The religious dogma differentiates, and so denies and excludes. How ironic? The religious seeks the spiritual as one of, if not the ultimate, path to salvation. Yet, it is a set of beliefs that so often turns into a dogma, a path that promises to lead to the realm of spirituality. Regrettably, as we all know, religious dogmas violate other people's beliefs, often violently. The spiritual never violates anyone's belief. The spiritual is nondifferentiative, nonseparative and nonexclusive.

Some gurus of spirituality write about states of spirituality. Now we cannot write about states of anything if we only know what isn't, can we?

The spiritual to early Man was *unknowable*. So we sort through our intellectual assertions and return to where we started from: The spiritual is being outside the capacity of our bodily senses and the reach of the mind. Spirituality lies outside the bounds of the human senses and sensibilities — beyond the needs of the body or the demands of the mind. Good teachers of spirituality may take us to the limits of our bodily and mental experience — to the gates of spirituality — but they cannot lead us into it. *No one can show anyone what is the spiritual, no one can make anyone else spiritual.* This is what early Man must have known — through some spiritual journey — when he conceived the body-mind-spirit dimensions.

*There is, however, something about the spiritual that everyone can see and know — the visible reflection of the spiritual in the lives of those who go in and return, not seeing anything, not hearing anything, not imagining anything, not knowing anything.*

I write about spirituality briefly in a book devoted to problems of energy and fatigue for pragmatic reasons. I have seen relentless, paralyzing fatigue destroy many lives. I know of some people who still live destroyed lives. I also see many such lives become "undestroyed" with persistent efforts to repair injured enzymes with nondrug therapies outlined in this book.

I often wonder what separates the Andrews from the Johns of the world of chronic fatigue. Some differences are easy to see: The Johns of chronic fatigue were given drugs for years — and their energy enzymes systems badly damaged — before they had any chance of undergoing restorative work with a knowledgeable professional. Some other differences are not so easy to discern.

I write about spirituality with regard to persistent, disabling chronic fatigue for pragmatic reasons. I have seen it work where all madical therapies failed. I have seen it work where all clever-thinking schemes failed. I have seen it work where the popular mind-over-body gospel simply proved to be extra salt on the wounds, nothing more than a cruel joke, .

Being in an *unknowable* state is the surest way to escape the tyranny of the knowable. It is as true of patients with disabling chronic fatigue as it is for those with cancer.

---

## THE FIRST GIFT OF SPIRITUALITY: FREEDOM FROM THE NEED FOR CONTROL

---

Once I was asked to give a nutrition lecture to an association of psychologists. I entered the hall a few minutes before I was due to speak and took a seat in the back. The speaker finished his lecture, and the conference moderator opened the floor for questions and answers. Within moments, the hall was resonating with excitement. And within minutes it became obvious to me what the core point of that excitement was: the need for control. Everyone who asked a question, gave an answer or otherwise commented, asserted the need of their clients for control in their lives. I realized how far this world of psychology was from my own world of silence and spirituality.

Absence of control, I was being vehemently told, is the root of the dominant problems of the mind. But that is not what my patients teach me every day. I see people with lives destroyed by severe fatigue and unrelenting chemical sensitivities recover not when they achieve control over their destroyed lives, but when they free themselves from the *need* for control. Control is a cortical device and its absence, a gift of spirituality forever to be treasured.

## THE SECOND GIFT OF SPIRITUALITY: FREEDOM FROM THE NEED FOR BEING A VICTIM

None of us are victims. All of us are victims.

There is a canary within each of us, only the cages look different. Each of us can fly out.

This sums up my view of the natural order of things. A predator cannot exist without a prey. New life can spring forth only through the death of old life. Biology has its own sense of order and disorder, of purpose and randomness. Why me? is a question without redeeming value. And yet who can resist it?

The cortical monkey loves to recycle misery. When that is not enough, it thrives on precycling the feared future misery. We can forever revisit the places of our past hurts — reinflict the wounds of the memory. The search for a villain never fails to produce one. Some victimizer is always around, materializing from the distance of decades at the command of the cortical monkey.

The cortical monkey thrives on the "victimhood," forever inventing and reinventing new ways of defining victimhood, forever wearing the badge of victimhood on its sleeve.

Who among us has not been harmed by another? Who has never been a victim? Who can plan not to be a victim?

Intellectually, it's so easy to understand — a random bullet, a reckless teenage driver, an infected drop of blood in the laboratory, an oxyradical hitting a DNA molecule at the wrong time and siring a cancer. That's all there can be to life.

Spiritually, none of us is a victim. To be a victim, one needs to be aware. How can one become victim in a state that has no awareness? How ironical! We waste long years yearning for awareness, not knowing the bliss of *unawareness*.

## THE THIRD GIFT OF SPIRITUALITY: FREEDOM FROM ANGER

Angry people do not heal.

Anger separates the world of psychology from that of silence and spirituality.

Psychology and psychiatry recognize anger as the root of many disorders of the mind, but their basic restorative approach to anger is quite different: Empowerment through unleashing their rage, they exhort their angry clients, is the right answer to the problem of the anger.

A nurse once told me how her marriage fell apart after a prolonged struggle with mutilating breast cancer surgery, radiotherapy and chemotherapy. Her anger was palpable during her first visit with me. Some weeks later, she waved her arm resolutely as she told me about her leaving her husband after reading "an eye-opening book" about female empowerment. I had no illusions about how she would have regarded my pleas for some spiritual search at that time, so I kept to myself my reservations about the role of empowerment in healing. She wanted to talk about her yeast and food allergy problems, and I let her do that. Then she left. I saw her several months later. She was now back with her husband, and together they regularly carried their disputes to a marriage counselor. She still brimmed with anger — unrelenting anger and suffering this time, I thought, had softened her somewhat. I wondered if she was now ready for my language of silence.

"What if some spiritual search could free you of the need to be proven right?" I gently broached the subject.

"Autoreg?" She became serious.

"Yes! Autoreg, language of silence, spiritual search, whatever you want to call it." I became hopeful.

"I'll take anything that would work." She smiled laconically.

"What if the spiritual could free you from the need for control?" I continued. "What if it could free you from the need for empowerment? What if it didn't matter at all what your husband did or didn't think about you? What if the yesterdays simply weren't there? What if there were only tomorrows? What if you could see all the evil men in the world just as people — different, difficult to like, hard to know — but simply people, including your evil husband?"

She winced a little at *evil husband*. There is a spark of spirituality there, I thought. There was hope. I talked some more about the difference between her previous approach of empowerment through power games with clever thinking and the alternative spiritual approach — the reach for the spiritual through the language of silence. In the spiritual, I told her, there are no scores to be evened, no need for empowerment, no strife for control, and no room for unleashing anger. In the spiritual, I added, there is only silence, energy, peace and love.

"I'm ready for your stuff now." She allowed herself another smile.

---

## THE FOURTH GIFT OF SPIRITUALITY: FREEDOM FROM REGRETS

Regret is a thief — it steals life. And living with regret is a life that gets stolen before it arrives.

I know people who know much about Sartre and his existence before essence. They know much about the inner workings of human mind — the deep, dark recesses of the subconscious. They know so much , and yet cannot see how regrets of the past come in the way of the living in the present. I know someone who once *knew* "something special" as a teenager, and who has spent a life time since struggling with his therapist to decipher what that something special might have been.

How often is "working out" the childhood problems a euphemism for unrelenting self-inflicted punishment? I know of persons who have successfully *worked out* the problems of their past — a thousand times, just like smokers who successfully quit smoking a thousand times or obese persons who successfully lose weight a thousand times. I do not belittle anyone's anguish. I write these few lines only to suggest that perhaps there is a chance of "unworking" out the problems of the past with the language of silence. Perhaps there is a chance of freedom from destructive probing —that so often passes for enlightenment —if we seek spirituality the way early Man did — without the use of his bodily senses and without any clever-thinking schemes.

## FREEDOM FROM FEAR:
## THE ULTIMATE GIFT OF SPIRITUALITY

Fear poisons hope. Fear paralyzes intuition.

Fear flows from uncertainty of the unknown. And the unknown, of course, carries fear of loss.

The spiritual is the unknown without any uncertainty. Fear cannot exist without a sense of loss, and there cannot be any sense of loss in the spiritual where there is no awareness. In the spiritual, we do not plead for freedom from fear of suffering, but for the heart to reach a stillness that is *beyond* any concept of freedom from fear.

We search for faith, seldom seeing the obvious: fear is a sworn enemy of faith. We yearn for freedom, rarely realizing that freedom is incompatible with fear. We look for friendship, not recognizing that we lose our friends through fear of loss. We plan for security, not knowing that fear is what creates insecurity.

*A stone I died and rose again a plant;*
*A plant I died and rose again an animal;*
*An animal I died and was born a man;*
*Why should I fear? What have I lost by*
*death?*

Rumi

## THE LANGUAGE OF SILENCE

How do we learn to become spiritual? We don't. How do we become spiritual? We just do. That's what early Man knew. That's what we need to know. Early Man chose the language of silence to break through the barriers of the bodily senses and the schemes of the mind. And that's what we need to do.

Bill now weighs 147 pounds, the inexorable beating of chronic fatigue is beginning to let up. Silence was painful for him during his early training in autoregulation. (And so it was for his mom who once wrote me a sarcastic note asking me what this "auto-wreck" class was that I wanted Bill to attend. We have since become friends.) Andrew sees his daughters only once a week but as he put it with a twinkle in his eyes, "They are with me all the time." I saw Ronald the other day. He is taking his nutrients and immunotherapy injections. He said he couldn't come for autoregulation because he has been too busy with his work. Some day perhaps he will discover that the language of silence never diminishes anyone's efficiency.

## SPIRITUALITY SPRINGS FROM SUFFERING

Is suffering from chronic fatigue really too high a price for a lifetime of enlightenment? I do not ask this question in jest.

Someone once told me how wonderful it would be if he could only know then what he would 15 years later about the right thing to do on that day. I thought the answer was quite simple: All he had to do that day was exactly what he wanted to do that day. That way, 15 years from then he could look back and say, "I did then what I really wanted to do." How can anyone really regret a time when he actually did what he most wanted? The trick, though, is to know what one really wants to do at a given time. The language of silence is hard to come by.

Someone said he should have been allowed to live his life backwards — from old age back to infancy. Then he could live his youthful years with the knowledge and wisdom of the old age. An impossible dream! Not really.

*He who finds the way in the morning*
*gladly dies in the evening.*

A proverb

Every severe chronic illness carries with it the promise of realizing this impossible dream of living backward — living each moment fully knowing that it is the *last* moment of *that time*. These are hard lessons to come by when life is "good." Suffering tears down safe assumptions of life — and intense suffering intensely dissipates the barriers and distinctions with which we surround ourselves. The language of silence melts away long-held beliefs of separateness and individualism. The oneness of spirituality prevails. Oneness with that larger *presence* that surrounds each of us at all times permeates a person's entire being.

**\*\*\*\*\*\*\*\*\*\***

*Dear friend,*

*Please know as you pass me by*
*As you are now, so once was I*
*As I am now, so you will be*
*Prepare yourself to follow me*

Inscription at the feet of a statute
of a princess of Babylon

MAJID ALI, M.D.
95 East Main Street
Denville, New Jersey 07834
(201) 586-4111

Name _____ Jane Smith _____ Age _____

Address _____ Date 1-3-94

Rx

Lord,
Today may I simply be in your presence for a
few moments.
Today I protest nothing.
Today I demand nothing
Today may I simply be in your presence for a
few moments.

☐ Substitution
Permissable _____
☐ Do Not Substitute _____
☐ Refill _____ Times          _____ M.D.
☐ Label                                   DEA #AA4904404

I offer the above prayer on a prescription sheet
(imprinted with a stamp) to many of my patients. They accept
this prayer prescription with good grace and often mention its
value in follow-up visits.

# APPENDIX

## *Hypothesis: Chronic Fatigue is a State of Accelerated Oxidative Molecular Injury*

Journal of Advancement in Medicine
Volume 6, Number 2, Summer 1993

# Hypothesis: Chronic Fatigue is a State of Accelerated Oxidative Molecular Injury

## Majid Ali, MD

*ABSTRACT:* A hypothesis is proposed that chronic fatigue is a state of accelerated oxidative molecular injury. Evidence supporting the hypothesis includes the following: 1. Spontaneity of oxidation in nature is the basic cause of the aging process for organisms capable of aerobic respiration. Redox dysregulations represent the initial events that lead to clinical disease processes. 2. Incidence of chronic fatigue is increasing, as is the oxidant stress in the Earth's atmosphere. 3. Evidence for oxidative cell membrane injury in chronic fatigue is furnished by changes in intracellular and extracellular ions. 4. Immunologic abnormalities that occur in chronic fatigue are consistent with initial oxidative injury. 5. Commonality of association of antigens of HLA-DR3 region with chronic fatigue syndrome and with other immune disorders such as rheumatoid arthritis, pemphigus vulgaris, systemic lupus erythematosus, and IgA and gold nephropathies. 6. Direct morphologic evidence of increased oxidative stress on the cell membrane is shown by the fact that we have found membrane deformities in up to 80% of erythrocytes in blood from chronic fatigue syndrome patients. These deformities are quickly reversed by administering ascorbic acid intravenously. 7. Changes in electromyopotentials observed in chronic fatigue patients are consistent with intracellular ionic and membrane changes. 8. Clinical entities commonly associated with chronic fatigue are known to increase oxidative molecular stress. 9. Clinical evidence obtained with relief of fatigue and related muscle symptoms with the use of oral and intravenous anti-oxidant nutrient therapy. From a clinical standpoint, this model for the molecular basis of chronic fatigue is useful for making therapeutic decisions for successful management of chronic fatigue without drug regimens.

### Introduction

Undue fatigue is a well known phenomenon as a problem for the physician. It is often traced to George Beard's 1869 description of undue

---

Majid Ali, M.D., is Associate Professor of Pathology at College of Physicians and Surgeons of Columbia University, New York, and Director, Department of Pathology, Immunology and Laboratories, Holy Name Hospital, Teaneck, New Jersey.

Address correspondence to 95 East Main Street, Denville, NJ 07834.

fatigue which he termed neurasthenia(1). Since then, undue fatigue has often been viewed as nervous weakness. The terms "Shirker's syndrome" and "Yuppie plague" represent attempts to cloak this bias in contemporary vernacular. Since Beard's description, the search for the cause of chronic fatigue has often focused on infection with a host of organisms, including Brucella, Epstein-Barr virus and, more recently, retroviruses.

In 1985, a group of investigators at the Centers for Disease Control (CDC) formulated a set of criteria for the diagnosis of what they called chronic fatigue syndrome (CFS)(2). These criteria have done little to elucidate the true cause of the syndrome, but have served as a diagnostic label to test the efficacy of therapeutic regimens using one or more pharmacologic agents.

It seems likely that chronic fatigue will be the dominant chronic health disorder of the next century. Twenty one percent of 500 patients visiting a primary care clinic in Boston(3) and 24% of 1159 patients at two adult care clinics in Texas(4) complained of chronic fatigue. The CDC estimates that there may be 100,000 patients in the United States who suffer from CFS(5). This is clearly a gross underestimation.

The state of chronic fatigue cannot be understood through the current simplistic, singe-agent single-disease model. What is required is a holistic "systems study" of man and his environment, including nutritional and fitness status, the impact of microorganisms on human biology, and the stress of modern life. What is needed is an integrated program of fundamental research into human energy dependent mechanisms, and how they are adversely affected by incremental molecular oxidant stress. Recognition and elimination of specific causes of increased oxidant stress, whenever possible, and nutritional and self-regulatory antioxidant techniques remain the primary approach to clinical management of chronic fatigue.

## Diagnostic Criteria

In 1985, the CDC proposed the major and minor criteria for the diagnosis of chronic fatigue syndrome(2). Rigid criteria of this nature are not usable in our model of accelerated oxidative molecular injury, in which there are 2 important issues:

1. How much fatigue interferes with the patient's life?
2. What is the molecular basis of the fatigue?

The CDC criteria indicate that chronic fatigue syndrome may not be diagnosed when secondary to an existing organic or psychiatric disorder, basically a reductio ad absurdum. It is the essential molecular duality of oxygen, and its impact upon human biology, which is being proposed here as the real culprit(6,7).

## Oxidant Stress, Redox Dysregulation and Chronic Fatigue

The life span of an organism is governed by the essential balance between metabolic oxidant stress and antioxidant defense. This is supported by considerable experimental evidence(8-13), indicating the role of oxidant stress and free radicals in pathogenesis of degenerative and immunologic disorders.

Knowledge of basic redox dynamics and free radical pathology is essential for understanding both the aging process and the initiation and progression of disease processes. The redox reaction, as well as determining life span, also determines the rate of metabolism and tissue auto-oxidation. Degenerative and immunologic disorders represent premature and accelerated molecular and tissue aging. Molecular injury and molecular repair are energy dependent. Cellular injury, expressed in morphologic terms, is a late event. Thus, clinical disease in its initial stages might be seen as redox dysregulation. Evidence exists(14) for evolution of mitochondria and other cellular organelles from oxygen using pro-karyote which migrated into proto-eukaryotic cells, thus protecting them from oxygen toxicity.

## Molecular Defense Pathways

Our concept of chronic illness is facilitated by understanding the balance that must be maintained between oxidant and anti-oxidant molecules(6,7); oxidants, which accelerate the wear and tear caused by environmental stress, are counter-balanced by anti-oxidants.

### Molecular Defenses

Oxidative metabolism is the first line of defense against environmental attack. Clinical symptoms associated with initial molecular and energy events are vague, hard to define, attributable to multiple organ systems, and often include chronic fatigue. Not unexpectedly, physical examination in patients with chronic fatigue often yields no clues to the cause of chronic fatigue.

Oxygen, though essential to life, is toxic. Cells need it, but they are aged by it. Of this, we generally have little understanding in the clinical practice of medicine. Oxidation is a spontaneous process. Reduction requires expenditure of energy. This molecular duality of oxygen represents the economy of nature at its best.

The primary molecular defenses against oxidant tissue damage are mediated by superoxide dismutase, catalase and glutathione peroxidase intracellularly, by plasma proteins and ascorbate extracellularly, and by the lipid soluble anti-oxidants tocopherol and carotene predominantly in the hydrophobic cell membrane compartment(15, 16). An inverse relationship between plasma levels of certain dietary antioxidants and incidence of cancer has been documented(17). There is some indirect evidence showing inadequate protection of cells by normal levels of plasma anti-oxidants against DNA damage caused by oxidant overload(18). Increased redox stresses play central roles in the pathogenesis of chronic immune, degenerative, allergic, and chemical sensitivity disorders.

The integrity of plasma membrane and mitochondrial oxidative enzyme systems is essential for initial electron transfer events that preserve molecular defenses and cellular health. Diseases begin when these initial electron transfer defenses fail as a consequence of oxidant injury. The occurrence of disease in specific organs is determined by the impact of environmental factors upon the genetic make-up of the individual. The oxidative stresses of interest in this context include enzyme induction and inactivation involving dysregulation of acetylation, methylation, conjugation, glucuronidation, carbon and sulfur oxidation, plasma membrane receptors, membrane peroxidation, oxidative protein cross-linking and molecular permutations of oligo- and polysaccharides caused by oxidative injury.

For example, cysteine oxygenase plays a role in the formation of sulfoxides from S-carboxy-L-methylcysteine, a reaction which varies widely among individuals(19). Impaired sulfur oxidation has been documented in many autoimmune disorders including primary biliary cirrhosis(20), rheumatoid arthritis(21,22), and systemic lupus erythematosus(23). An inadequate supply of inorganic sulfate limits the rate of formation of non-toxic conjugated sulfates, so this is clinically significant.

Evidently these lines of molecular defenses are ineffective against dioxins, chlordane and other related molecules which have a long half life. Enzymes frequently activated by xenobiotics include cytochrome P-450 systems and enzymes frequently inactivated by them include choline esterases, sulfite oxidases and phenol sulfotransferases.

In chronic fatigue, evidence for enzyme induction as well as inactivation can be developed by the study of their by-products and metabolites of xenobiotics. For example, increased urinary levels of D-glucaric acid indicate induction of hepatic enzyme induction by xenobiotics and some viruses (Pangborn J. Personal Communication). Similarly, mercapturic acid serves as an indicator of the detoxification process that involves oxidant glutathione complex (Pangborn J. Personal Communication). An increased urinary clearance of mercapturic acid has been reported in patients with chronic fatigue. The enzymatic efficiency of sulfite oxidases and enzyme systems involved with trans-sulfuration steps are of special importance to individuals with chronic fatigue associated with IgE-mediated disorders such as asthma, autoimmune diseases, and chemical sensitivity and toxicity. These functions can be assessed by measurements of urinary sulfites and sulfates.

Evidence is accumulating that the pathogenetic mechanisms of environmental disorders involve complex inter-relationships between exogenous toxins, genes, enzymatic inductions, and structural and functional impairments of immune cells(24,25). Toxins can directly bend or disfigure DNA molecules so that they become vulnerable to deletion or transcription by a host of proteins. In health, DNA is usually packed tightly within the nucleus and is hard to reach. When disfigured it becomes more accessible to proteins in its vicinity. Thus injured, DNA may encode specific enzyme systems. The enzyme activation so caused may persist for long periods of time and eventually lead to clinical disorders. This is illustrated by the example of DNA injury caused by dioxins(24,25).

Finally, the classical immunologic mechanisms of Gell and Coombs must be considered. While this classification has been of enormous value in delineating essential mechanisms underlying clinical and morphologic patterns of disease, it sheds little light on molecular events that initiate immunologic injury and lead to chronic fatigue. An exception to this is the case of IgE mediated disorders—clinical states in which the incriminated triggers can be effectively managed with proper diagnostic and therapeutic approaches, in general with excellent clinical responses.

Subcellular and cellular structural changes observed with morphologic studies are late events. Such changes are not relevant to our discussion of the causes of chronic fatigue. In any case, such morphologic changes have not been described in chronic fatigue.

## Experimental and Clinical Evidence in Support of the Hypothesis

### 1. Spontaneity of Oxidation in Nature and Aging

Bjorksten(26) and Harmon et al(8,13,27) advanced their theories of protein cross-linking and free radical injury respectively as the basic mechanisms of aging in man. These phenomena are the result of oxidative molecular injury which may be regarded as the *true* nature of the aging process(6,7). Tissue capacity for anti-oxidant generation provides the counterbalance to spontaneous oxidation. There is a large body of clinical and experimental data to support this(8-13).

### 2. Increasing Oxidizing Capacity of Earth

It is predicted that tropospheric ozone will decrease by up to 1% per year over the next 50 years(28). Man today faces accelerated oxidative molecular damage much like protoeukaryotes did millions of years ago. It would seem to be a defensible assumption that these rapid increases in oxidant stress of human biology have some pathogenetic relationship to the rising incidence of chronic fatigue unassociated with specific clinico-pathologic entities. Reports of vague, poorly defined states of ill health in many veterans of the recent Persian gulf war appear to fit into a category of illness related to high oxidant stress. Whatever criteria is used for the diagnosis of chronic fatigue(2-5), it is evident that the incidence of chronic fatigue in the closing decades of the 20th century far exceeds that reported in the opening decades.

### 3. Cell Membrane Ionic Channel Gating Proteins, Oxidative Injury and Chronic Fatigue

A cell propagates and integrates electrical signals by means of its membrane channels. Transfer of ions across the channels is regulated by gating proteins with multiple subunits containing voltage sensors. The function of gating proteins is finely orchestrated to attain a high order of subunit cooperation(29,30). Oxidative damage to ion channel proteins in the cell membrane can be expected to increase membrane permeability, leading to efflux of the intracellular ions, magnesium and potassium, and influx into the cell of the extracellular ion, calcium. Strong evidence for this is furnished by clinical studies showing efficacy of calcium channel blockers for a growing number of clinical entities linked to oxyradicals(31). It is also supported by the efficacy of intravenously administered magnesium and potassium for chronic fatigue and many other pathologic states associated with increased oxidative stress(32).

Lowered levels of intracellular ions have been documented in chemically-induced cell membrane injury, chemical sensitivity, food allergy and viral infections. Strong clinical evidence for severe gating derangements at the cell membrane in patients with chronic fatigue is furnished, as we shall see later in this article, by studies with intravenous magnesium and potassium infusions in almost all cases (33).

Human gene encoding specific enzymes can be induced by oxidative injury(34). Evidence that a deletion polymorphism in the gene encoding angiotensin-converting enzyme is a risk factor for myocardial infarction has been recently reported(35,36). Comparative study of epidemiologic data for coronary artery disease at the beginning and the end of this century strongly support the possibility of this being caused by oxidant stress. It seems probable from these considerations that deletion polymorphism in the gene encoding oxidative and detoxification enzymes will be found in time in patients with chronic fatigue.

### 4. Immunologic Abnormalities in Chronic Fatigue

A very large number of immunologic abnormalities have been described in chronic fatigue states. These include depression of cell-mediated immunity, phenotypic and functional deficiencies of natural killer cells, and diminished ability of mitogenically stimulated mononuclear cells, thought to represent cellular exhaustion(37,88). Variable changes in CD4 and CD8 lymphocytes have been reported, including depletion of CD4 and CD45RA cells, and alterations in humoral responses such as mild IgA deficiency and elevated levels of immune complexes. Other reported abnormalities include the presence of autoantibodies such as rheumatoid factor, antinuclear antibodies and cold agglutinins, and increased B cells(39-44). Evidence of T-cell activation is furnished by studies showing elevated blood levels of IL-2 and T8 receptors and increased numbers of CD3, CD20 and CD 56 cells(44). Blood levels of both 2'5' A synthetase and RNAase are elevated, indicating activation of lymphocytes by viruses or exposure to interferon(40). These changes appear to represent polyclonal B-cell activation. These observations have led some investigators to consider CFS as an acquired immunodeficiency state caused by one or more viruses belonging to the Herpes or enterovirus families. Indeed, in a very small subset of patients, strong circumstantial evidence suggests an important initial role of viral infections. In the hypothesis proposed here, these immunologic aberrations are regarded as consequences of accelerated oxidative molecular injury rather than primary cause of chronic fatigue.

### 5. Association of HLA-DR3 Antigens with CFS and with Some Autoimmune Disorders

The association of several autoimmune disorders with HLA-DR4 region antigens is well established(44). It has been reported that 46% of a group of patients with chronic fatigue were positive for antigens of HLA-DR3 region(45). This suggests a genetic predisposition for individuals with these HLA antigens for autoimmune injury and development of autoimmune syndromes. Can chronic fatigue be considered as a part of the spectrum of autoimmune response? Patients with chronic fatigue show clear evidence of autoimmune injury(37-42). It has already been pointed out that abnormal autoimmune responses are associated with, and most likely triggered by, induction or inactivation of certain enzyme systems by oxidative injury(19-23, Pangborn J. Personal Communication). These lines of evidence lend support to the proposed hypothesis, and further suggest that oxidative injury to certain enzyme systems may be the molecular pathogenetic mechanism involved in immunologic derangements observed in chronic fatigue.

### 6. Morphologic Evidence for Accelerated Oxidant Stress on Cell Membrane

Morphologic abnormalities of cell membranes have been observed with high-resolution, phase contrast microscopy, in 50-80% of erythrocytes in patients with persistent chronic fatigue(46). Abnormalities included crenation, sharp angulation, spike formation and rigidity, most accentuated during acute exacerbations of fatigue during acute and subacute allergic reactions. Studies repeated 15 minutes after infusion of 15 grams of ascorbic acid showed reversal of the membrane abnormalities in over 80% of the previously affected cells.

### 7. Galvanic Skin Responses and Electromyopotentials in Chronic Fatigue

A consistent pattern of markedly diminished galvanic skin responses and increased electromyopotentials is observed in patients with chronic fatigue as compared with healthy subjects and patients with essential hypertension (Ali M. Unpublished observations). Diminished perfusion and decreased glucose utilization in certain parts of the limbic system have been reported in patients with chronic fatigue(47). This is consistent with the consequences of oxidative injury to neurons. During training sessions in effective self-regulatory methods, many patients with chronic fatigue show moderate to marked reductions in electromyopotentials for short periods of time. With long-term training in slow, sustained breathing patterns with prolonged unforced expiration, reduction in muscle potentials is achieved by most of them.

## 8. Viral and Other Infections Associated with CFS

The cause of chronic fatigue has been considered to be chronic Epstein-Barr infection(48-51). Recent laboratory evidence has pointed to retroviral sequences(52). Occurrence of viral infections does not necessarily indicate that they are causative. They have been shown to increase oxidative stress, and mortality from acute influenza infection in mice can be drastically reduced with the use of superoxide dismutase(53). Viral infections do not lead to chronic persistent fatigue when they are managed with aggressive oral and intravenous antioxidant therapies and other necessary supportive measures (Ali M. Unpublished observations). Apparently, viral infections lead to chronic fatigue only in states of suppressed molecular defenses caused by food and mold allergy, extensive use of antibiotics, stress, anxiety and depressed states. They appear to be the proverbial straw to break the camel's back of molecular defenses.

Recently, several cases of chronic fatigue syndrome have been shown to meet the diagnostic criteria of idiopathic CD-4 T-lymphocytopenia (ICL), commonly known as AIDS-like illness in HIV negative individuals(54). Serologic evidence of past Epstein-Barr virus infection was seen in about two thirds of a group of patients and about one third had very high titers of IgG antibodies, presumably reflecting ongoing viral replication. One patient with long standing chronic fatigue showed serologic evidence of HTLV-III infection. She responded well to nutrient therapy and obtained near-complete relief within 8 weeks (Ali M. Unpublished observations).

## 9. IgE-Mediated Allergy in Chronic Fatigue

We investigated the prevalence of IgE antibodies with specificity for 8 molds, 12 pollens, 6 foods, and cat and dog epithelial antigens in one hundred consecutive patients with the clinical picture of CFS of more than six months duration. Micro-elisa assays for allergen-specific IgE antibodies were performed with a previously described method(55). Ninety-eight gave a history of past or present allergy symptoms. IgE antibodies with specificity for three or more molds were detected in all cases. Prevalence of IgE antibodies with specificity for pollen of grasses, trees and weeds ranged from 62% to 78%, and those for foods from 84% to 83%.

Although allergy is a well recognized cause of short-term fatigue, prevalence of specific IgE-mediated antibodies suggest that an underlying IgE-mediated allergy may play an important and perhaps a pivotal role in pathogenesis of chronic persistent fatigue.

## 10. Chemical Sensitivity and Toxicity

Chemical toxicity is largely a dose-dependent phenomenon, and chronic fatigue associated with exposure to industrial toxins is well established(56). Chemical sensitivity, by contrast, is dose-independent. Chronic fatigue associated with it is clinically well recognized, though the pathogenesis has not been fully elucidated. Both chemical toxicity and sensitivity clearly result from oxidizing potential of these agents, as already discussed.

## 11. Metabolic Derangements

Metabolic immunodepression resulting in impairment of cell-mediated immunity and a phagocytic dysfunction of macrophages has been proposed as a major contributory cause of the chronic fatigue syndrome(57). Factors that lead to immunosuppression include disturbances of carbohydrate and lipid metabolism, proposed by Dilman. These include glucose intolerance, post-prandial hyperinsulinemia, raised serum levels of free fatty acids and LDL cholesterol and accumulation of oxidized lipids in the plasma membranes of T-lymphocytes and monocytes. Many clinicians recognize chronic fatigue as an important aspect of the clinical syndrome of rapid hyperglycemic-hypoglycemic shift that are followed by similar peaks of insulin and adrenaline. Catecholamines are powerful oxidizing agents(58). Glucose autoxidation causes oxidative protein damage in the experimental glycation model of diabetes mellitus and aging(59). Both factors support the proposed hypothesis.

## 12. Anemia, Mercury Toxicity and Chronic Fatigue

Fatigue is a well recognized symptom of anemia, and is considered as a consequence of lowered oxygen carrying capacity of blood. However, anemia as a major or as a contributory cause of fatigue was not observed in a single case of 100 consecutive cases of chronic fatigue cited above. Diminished blood levels of oxyhemoglobin were observed in a majority of patients with mercury toxicity and chronic fatigue, and a lack of oxygen was proposed as a possible molecular basis of chronic fatigue(60). This observation is consistent with the proposed hypothesis. Mercury and other heavy metals are known to bind with the reducing potential and/or with the reducing function such as the sulfhydryl group of enzymes and other proteins, thereby inactivating them(56). As a consequence of this, the natural reducing mechanisms are impaired and oxidative mechanisms potentiated. Indeed, this mechanism is likely to play a role in the etiology of chronic fatigue in patients with heavy metal overload in the study cited above.

## 13. Clinical Evidence: Efficacy of Intravenous Anti-Oxidant Nutrient Therapy

Strong clinical evidence of the hypothesis is furnished by studies demonstrating the efficacy of oral and intravenous anti-oxidant nutrient therapies(33). Of 100 consecutive patients with the chief complaint of chronic fatigue who were treated at the Chronic Fatigue Clinic at the Institute, 46 met the CDC criteria for chronic fatigue syndrome. IgE antibodies with specificity for at least three mold antigens were present in all 100 patients. Eighty eight patients gave a history of extensive antibiotic therapy and symptoms indicative of altered states of bowel ecology. Elevated blood levels of one or more heavy metals (Pb, Hg, Al, Cd and As) were found in 37 patients. Serologic evidence for active viral replication was not detected in the majority of patients. Major stress (as assessed by the patient) preceded the onset of chronic fatigue in less than 10% of patients. All patients were managed with integrated treatment protocols of oral and intravenous nutrient therapies, antigen immunotherapy for IgE-mediated allergy, training in effective methods for self-regulation and a program for slow, sustained exercise. The intravenous nutrient protocol was formulated to provide a strong nutrient anti-oxidant support, and not to correct any putative nutritional deficiencies. The outcome data for these 100 patients with chronic fatigue were as follows: Excellent response (symptom relief > 80%), 68%; good response (symptom relief between 60% and 80%), 12%; modest response (symptom relief between 40% and 60%); and poor response (symptom relief between 0 and 40%), 12%.

## Conclusion

Chronic fatigue is emerging as the most dominant health disorder of our time. It is proposed that the state of chronic fatigue is the result of accelerated oxidative molecular injury caused by the impact upon our genetic make-up of environmental, nutritional, microbiological and stress-related factors. This model of molecular-energetic basis of fatigue is useful for designing successful, nondrug therapies to reduce oxidative molecular stress and relieve chronic fatigue.

## References

1. Beard G. Neurasthenia or nervous exhaustion. Boston Medical and Surgical Journal 1869; 3:217-220.
2. Holmes GP, Kaplan JE, Gantz NM, et al. Chronic fatigue syndrome: a working case definition. Ann Int Med 1988; 108:387-89.
3. Buchwald D, Sullivan JL, Karmaroff A. Frequency of chronic active Epstein-Barr virus infection in a general medical practice. JAMA 1987; 257:2303-2307.
4. Kroenke K, Wood DO, Mangelsdroff AD, et al. Chronic fatigue in primary care: Prevalence, patient characteristics, and outcome. JAMA 1988; 260:929-934.
5. Research News. On the track of an elusive disease. Science 1991; 254:1726-1728.
6. Ali M. Molecular basis of environmental illness. 1990. Syllabus of 1990 Instruction Course, American Academy of Environmental Illness. Denver, Colorado.
7. Ali M. Intravenous Nutrient protocols in Nutritional Medicine. 1991. Institute of Preventive. Denville, New Jersey.
8. Harman D, Eddy, DE. Free radical theory of aging: effects of adding antioxidants to maternal mouse diet on the lifespan of their offspring, second experiment. Age 1978; 1:162-168.
9. Tolmasoff J, Ono T, Cutler R. Superoxidase dismutase: Correlation with lifespan and specific metabolic rate in primate species. Proc Nat Acad Sci 1980; 77: 2777-2781.
10. Miquel J, Fleming J, Economos AC. Antioxidants, metabolic rate and aging in Drosophila, Arch Geriatral. Geriatr. 1982; 1, 159-163.
11. Cutler RG. Peroxide-producing of tissues: Inverse correlation with longevity of mammalian species. Proc Nat Acad Sci 1985; 82:4798-4810.
12. Halliwell B, Gutteridge JMC. Free Radicals In Biology And Medicine. Clarendon, Oxford, 1985.
13. Harman D. The aging process. 1981; Proc Nat Acad Sci USA; 78:124-128.
14. Marguilis L, McMenamin M. Marriage of convenience: The motility of modern cell may reflect an ancient symbiotic union. The Sciences. Sept/Oct. 1990 Pages 31-36.
15. Frie B, England L, Ames B. Ascorbate is an outstanding antioxidant in human blood plasma. Proc Nat Acad Sci USA 1989; 86:6377-6381.
16. Pauling L. Evolution and need for ascorbic acid. Proc Nat Acad Sci. 1970; 67: 1643-1646.
17. Ames BN, Saul RL, Schwiers E, et al. Oxidative DNA damage as related to cancer and aging: the assay of thymine glycol, thymidine glycol, and hydroxymethyluracil in human and rat urine. In: Sohal RS, Birnbaum LS, Cutler RG, eds. Molecular Biology of Aging: Gene Stability and Gene Expression. New York. Raven Press; 1985:137-144.

18. Cutler RG, ed. Molecular Biology of Aging: Gene stability and gene expression. New York: Raven Press 1985: 137-44.
19. Mitchell SC, Waring RH. S-oxygenase 111:human pharmacogenetics, In: Damani LA ed. Sulphur containing drugs and related organic compounds. Vol 11A Chichester; Ellis Harwood, 1989; 101-119.
20. Olumu P, Vickers C, Waring RH, et al, High incidence of poor sulphoxidation in patients with primary biliary cirrhosis. N Eng J Med 1988; 318:1089-1094.
21. Bradley H, Emery P, et al. Reduced thiol methyl transferase activity in red blood cell membrane from patients with rheumatoid arthritis. J Rheumatol 1991; 18(12):1787-1789.
22. Emery P, Panayi G, Huston G, et al, D-penicillamine induced toxicity in rheumatoid arthritis: the role of sulphoxidation status and HLA-DR 3. J Rheumatology. 1984; 11:626-631.
23. Gordon C, Bradley H, Waring RH, et al, Abnormal sulphur oxidation in systemic lupus erythematosis. Lancet 1992; 339:25-27.
24. Poland A, Knutson JC. 2,3,7,8-tetrachlorodibenzo-p-dioxin and related halogenated aromatic compounds: examination of the mechanisms of toxicity. Ann Rev Pharmacol Toxicol 1982; 22:517-554.
25. McKinney JD. Multifunctional receptor model for dioxin and related compounds toxic action: Possible thyroid hormone-responsive effector-linked site. Environmental health perspectives. 1989; 82:323-36.
26. Bjorksten J. Cross-linkage in protein chemistry. Advances in Protein Chemistry. 1951; 6:343-381.
27. Cross CE, Halliwell B, Borish ET, Harman D, et al. Oxygen radicals and human disease. Ann Intern Med 1987; 107:526-545.
28. Thompsen AM. The oxidizing capacity of the earth's atmosphere: probable past and future changes. Science 1992; 256:1157-1165.
29. Tytgat J, Hess P. Evidence for cooperative interactions in potassium channel gating. Nature 1992; 359:420-423.
30. Ism LL, De Jongh KS, Patton DE, et al. Primary structure and functional expression of the $B_1$ subunit of the rat brain sodium channel. Science 1992; 256:839-842.
31. Katz A. Molecular basis of calcium channel blockade. Am J Cardiol 1992;69: 17E-22E.
32. Ali M. Oxidative plasma membrane injury and magnesium. Environmental Physician. Summer 1992. American Academy of Environmental Medicine, Denver, Colorado.
33. Ali M. Experience with intravenous nutrient therapy for allergic patients with chronic fatigue. American Academy of Otolaryngic Allergy Abstract Summer 1992;p 23.
34. Keyse SM, Emslie EA. Oxidative stress and heat shock induce a human gene encoding a protein-tyrosine phosphatase. Nature 1992; 359:644-647.
35. Cambien F, Poirier O, Lecert L, et al. Deletion polymorphism in the gene for angiotensin-converting enzyme is a potent risk factor for myocardial infarction. Nature 1992; 359:641-644.
36. Miller C. Ion channel structure and function. Science 1992; 258:240-241.
37. Caliguiri M, Murray C, Buchwald D, et al. Phenotypic and functional deficiency of natural killer cells in patients with CFID. J Immunol 1987; 139:3306-3313.
38. Klimas NG, Salvato FR, Morgan R, et al. Immunologic abnormalities in chronic fatigue syndrome. J Clin Microbiol 1990; 28:1403-1410.
39. Targan S, Stebbing N. In vitro interactions of purified cloned human interferons on NK cells: enhanced activation. J Immunol 1982; 129:934-935.
40. Suhadolanik RJ, Reichenbach NL, Sobol RW, et al. Biochemical defects in 2-5A synthetase/RNAase pathway associated with chronic fatigue syndrome with encephalopathy, In: The Clinical and Scientific Basis of Myalgic Enceplalomyeltitis/

Chronic fatigue syndrome. Byron Hyde, ed. Ottawa, Canada. The Nightingale Research Foundation. [Chapter 67] 1992; 613-7.

41. Buchwald D, Cheney PR, Peterson DL, et al. A chronic illness characterized by fatigue, neurologic and immunologic disorders, and active human herpesvirus-6. Ann Int Medicine 1992; 116:103-131.

42. Linde A, Anderson B, Svenson SB, et al. Serum levels of lymphokines and soluble cellular receptors in primary Epstein-Barr virus infection and in patients with chronic fatigue syndrome. The J Inf Dis. 1992; 165:994-1000.

43. Gupta S, Vayuvegula B. A comprehensive immunological analysis in chronic fatigue syndrome. Scan. J. Immunol 1991; 33:319-327.

44. Tiwar JL, Terasaki PI. HLA and disease associations. New York, Springer Verlag. 1985.

45. Teresaki P. In: Chronic fatigue Syndrome. Goldstein J, ed. Chronic fatigue Syndrome Institute, Beverely Hills, CA, 1990.

46. Ali M. Ascorbic acid reverses abnormal erythrocyte morphology in chronic fatigue syndrome Am J Clin Pathol 1990; 94:515 (Abstract).

47. Mena I. Study of cerebral perfusion by neurospect in patients with chronic fatigue syndrome. Symposium on myalgic encephalomyelitis, page 21, Cambridge, England, April 1990. SPECT SCANS.

48. Salvato F, Fletcher M, Ashman M, et al. Immune dysfunction among chronic fatigue syndrome (CFS) patients with clear evidence of Epstein-Barr (EBV) reactivation. J Exp. Clin Cancer Res. 1988; (suppl) 7: 89-91

49. Okano M, Matsumoto S, Osato T, et al. Severe chronic active Epstein-Barr virus infection syndrome. Clin Microbiol Rev. 1991; 4:129-135.

50. Dubois RE, Seeley JK, Brus I, et al. Chronic mononucleosis syndrome. South Med J. 1984. 77:1376-1382.

51. Jones JF, Ray CG, Minnich LL, et al, Evidence of active Epstein-Barr virus infection in patients with persistent, unexplained illnesses: elevated anti-early antigen antibodies. Ann Int Med 1985; 102:1-7.

52. DeFreites E, Hilliard B, Cheney P, et al, Retroviral sequences related to human T-lymphocyte virus type II in patients with chronic fatigue immune dysfunction syndrome. Proc Nat Acad Sci USA 1991; 88:2922-2926.

53. Oda T, Akaike T, Hamamoto T, et al, Oxygen radicals in influenza-induced pathogenesis and treatment with pyran polymer-conjugated SOD. Science 1989; 244: 974-977.

54. Cases of AIDS-like illness (ICL) may double if chronic fatigue patients add. AIDS Weekly 1992; September

55. Ali M, Ramanarayanan M. A computerised micro-elisa assay for allergen-specific IgE antibodies. Am J Clin Pathol 1984; 81: 591-601.

56. Handbook of Toxicology Vol 1. Spector WS. ed. W.B. Saunders, Philadelphia, 1956 Pages 184-5. 1956.

57. Yutsis P. Metabolic immunodepression and chronic fatigue. Presented at the Spring Conference of the American College for Advancement in Medicine, Colorado Springs, Co. May 1992.

58. Singh A. Chemical and biochemical aspects of superoxide radicals and related species of activated oxygen. In Active oxygen and medicine (a symposium). Can J Physiol. Petkau A, Dhalla NS. Eds. 1982; 1330-1345.

59. Hunt JV, Dean RT, Wolff SP. Hydroxyl radical production and autooxidative glycosylation. Biochem J 1988; 256:205-212.

60. Denton SA. Fatigue—A lack of oxygen? Terf Momentum. Published by The Toxic Element Research Foundation, Colorado springs, 1992.

# Index

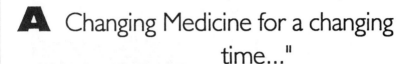
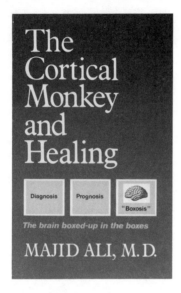

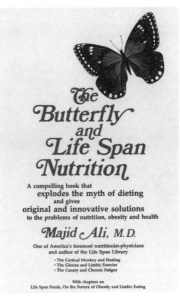

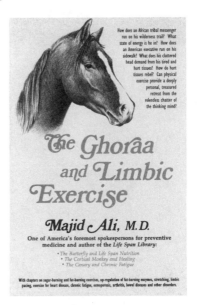